Forensic Medicine in Western Society

D1571381

The first book of its kind, *Forensic Medicine in Western Society: A history* draws on the most recent developments in the historiography, to provide an overview of the history of forensic medicine in the West from the medieval period to the present day. Taking an international, comparative perspective on the changing nature of the relationship between medicine, law and society, it examines the growth of medico-legal ideas, institutions and practices in Britain, Europe (principally France, Italy and Germany) and the United States.

Following a thematic structure within a broad chronological framework, the book focuses on practitioners, the development of notions of 'expertise' and the rise of the expert, the main areas of the criminal law to which forensic medicine contributed, medical attitudes towards the victims and perpetrators of crime, and the wider influences such attitudes had. It thus develops an understanding of how medicine has played an active part in shaping legal, political and social change.

Including case studies which provide a narrative context to tie forensic medicine to the societies in which it was practiced, and a further reading section at the end of each chapter, Katherine D. Watson creates a vivid portrait of a topic of relevance to social historians and students of the history of medicine, law and crime.

Katherine D. Watson is a senior lecturer in the history of medicine at Oxford Brookes University. She is the author of *Poisoned Lives: English Poisoners and their Victims* (2004), *Crime Archive: Dr Crippen* (2007) and editor of *Assaulting the Past: Violence and Civilization in Historical Context* (2007).

Forensic Medicine in Western Society

A history

Katherine D. Watson

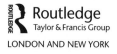

Routledge
Taylor & Francis Group

LONDON AND NEW YORK

First published 2011
by Routledge
2 Park Square, Milton Park, Abingdon, Oxon OX14 4RN

Simultaneously published in the USA and Canada by Routledge
270 Madison Avenue, New York, NY 100016

Routledge is an imprint of the Taylor & Francis Group, an informa business

Typeset in Times New Roman by Taylor & Francis Books
Printed and bound in Great Britain by CPI Antony Rowe,
Chippenham, Wiltshire

British Library Cataloguing in Publication Data
A catalogue record for this book is available from the British Library

Library of Congress Catalog-in-Publication Data
Watson, Katherine (Katherine Denise)
Forensic medicine in Western society : a history / Katherine D. Watson.
p. cm.
"Simultaneously published in the USA and Canada"--T.p verso.
Includes bibliographical references and index.
1. Medical jurisprudence--Western countries--History. 2. Forensic
sciences--Western countries--History. I. Title.
RA1022.W47W38 2010
614′.1--dc22
2010017797

ISBN 13: 978-0-415-44771-3 (hbk)
ISBN 13: 978-0-415-44772-0 (pbk)
ISBN 13: 978-0-203-84029-0 (ebk)

Contents

Acknowledgements

In writing this book I have benefited from the scholarship of many historians whose work has been both inspiring and thought-provoking, and from the support of friends (much more than mere colleagues!) at Oxford Brookes – thank you all. Special thanks are owed to Cathy McClive for reading and commenting on various chapters, to Yves Mausen for providing many helpful (and hard-to-find) references, and especially to Eve Setch at Routledge, who has been integral to bringing this project to fruition. Thanks also to Fortunata Oates for her generous translations from the Italian. I am grateful for the financial support of the Wellcome Trust, which enabled me to travel, to read more widely than I had ever done before, and to consolidate key portions of the manuscript. This book is the product of my long interest in the history of forensic medicine, and in writing it I have learned a great deal about medical practice, law and crime in the West over a period of many centuries. But there is clearly so much more to be discovered, and I hope that others will be encouraged to explore this stimulating and rewarding area of history, in the archives and in the classroom. I therefore dedicate this book to all historians of forensic medicine, past, present and future.

Introduction

Every politically organized society is regulated by laws which its government must enforce, and it is in this context that forensic medicine is to be understood, as the application of medical knowledge and practice to the clarification of uncertain issues that come before the law courts. The importance of forensic medicine thus rests on its ability to contribute to the fact-finding processes typical of both the pursuit of legal solutions to disputes between individuals, and of the state's duty to promote public security by preventing crime. The relationship between medicine and law is therefore one of shared responsibility in the areas of legal enquiry in which they meet, including criminal trials for a variety of forms of interpersonal violence and civil examinations into personal characteristics such as sanity and sexual potency. However, the relationship has not been equally developed at all times or in all places, for reasons largely to do with the organization of Western legal systems; although the history of forensic medicine is centuries old and its sphere of activity wide, its practice has been inconsistent. Medical practitioners have been asked to provide specialist opinions to help the courts reach just decisions, but the degree to which they could truly be considered expert has changed over time, as have their interests, methods and techniques. This book is concerned with the practice of forensic medicine in the West, with the main areas of the law to which it contributed, the development of notions of expertise, and medical attitudes towards the victims and perpetrators of crime and the wider influences such attitudes had. By the end of the book the reader will understand how medicine has played an active part in shaping legal, political and social change.

The origins of Western forensic medicine lie on the European continent; although the forensic activities and writings of the Chinese pre-date European developments, there is no evidence of their direct influence in the West.[1] European terminology has a particular history that it is essential to understand in order to define and explain what we mean by forensic medicine now. Most of the descriptive titles in the field have specific national origins, and the earliest texts in the Western world were Italian, of which the two most influential works had general titles which 'emphasized the *interrelationship* of the subject to both medicine and the law'. In 1598 Fortunatus Fidelis (1551–1630) of Palermo published a fairly comprehensive volume on forensic medicine entitled *De relationibus medicorum* (*On the Relations of Doctors*), but this was quickly superseded by the text of Paolo Zacchia (1584–1659), who was the medical consultant to the Rota Romana, the Papal Court of Appeals under canon (church) law. Published in 1621 and expanded in subsequent editions, his *Questiones Medico-Legales* (*Medico-legal Problems*) compiled information on a vast range of medical and legal subjects, and outlined actual cases brought before the Rota. This was the first text to use the hyphenated adjective 'medico-legal' to describe the field, but the term today is so common that many writers delete the hyphen.[2]

One of the most durable terms, 'forensic medicine', arose in the German states in the middle of the seventeenth century. The first formal lectures under this title were given in 1650 by Johann Michaelis (1607–67), a professor of medicine at the University of Leipzig, but the course was primarily medical in content, not legal, and it was designed for the training of physicians employed by municipal authorities in caring for the poor, dealing with contagious diseases, and investigating deaths.[3]

The adjective 'forensic' comes from the Latin *forensis*, 'of the forum', referring to the common meeting place of the Roman state, where civic affairs were conducted and legal controversies settled. In English the word has come to be associated with legal or court affairs, and forensic medicine is thus taken to mean that part of the medical field concerned with the presentation of medical information in courts of law or other judicial venues. In the nineteenth century the Germans dropped this term in favour of one that means 'legal medicine' (*gerichtliche medizin*), but which modern translations often render as 'forensic medicine'; the term *Rechtsmedizin* is also used.[4]

We gained the term legal medicine, *médecine légale*, from the French in the late eighteenth and early nineteenth centuries. Practitioners also used the term *médecine judiciaire*, judicial medicine, defined as 'l'art de mettre les connaissances médicales au service de l'administration de la justice'. The French also gave the world the term 'expert', which was originally limited to technical consultants to the French courts. In addition to the issues of interest to criminal and civil courts, legal medicine also included other medical areas of legal significance, such as the diagnosis, treatment and rehabilitation of criminals and the criminally insane.[5]

The Anglo-American contribution to the terminology of our subject was introduced in Scotland in 1791, when the Edinburgh professor Andrew Duncan (1744–1828) used the term 'medical jurisprudence' for his lectures, the first in the British Isles on the medico-legal field. The expression was not his, but one he borrowed from the academic Latin of earlier textbooks published in Europe. He used it to mean a mostly medical field of study, but the word 'jurisprudence' was essentially a synonym for 'law' and thus correctly interpreted his term meant 'medical law'. However, it was imported into the United States by Edinburgh graduates and freely used by American and British authors throughout the nineteenth century to refer to medico-legal matters. In modern times the word jurisprudence is used to mean the philosophy of law, and what used to be known as medical jurisprudence is now termed either legal or forensic medicine.[6] But this was not the end of the terminological story.

During the eighteenth century there was a parallel development, largely in the German states and France, and via France to Scotland, whereby new scholarship in public health established itself as a separate discipline from forensic medicine, with which it had initially been associated. The term most often used to describe this branch of medical service to the state was 'medical police', a broad field that later came to be known as 'state medicine' both in Europe and in Britain and America. It covered three areas: public health regulation; public welfare medicine for the poor and chronically ill; and forensic medicine. The link between medical police and forensic medicine survived into the early decades of the twentieth century, particularly in Scotland and the United States, but these three broad fields have now long since gone their separate ways.[7]

Today in any Western country one can generally say 'legal medicine' or 'forensic medicine' and be understood to mean largely one thing – forensic pathology and death investigation. Numerous related fields now have their own specialist titles and areas of coverage, but in this book we will follow the definition laid out by Michael Clark and Catherine Crawford in their introduction to *Legal Medicine in History* (1994): forensic medicine (a term that we shall consider as interchangeable with legal medicine) will be taken to be 'the application of medical knowledge in the broadest sense to help solve legal problems or satisfy legal requirements';[8] the adjective 'medico-legal' encompasses these activities. This definition is intended to include two key areas of practice. First and the one that readers will be most familiar with, is post-mortem investigation carried out by medical practitioners on the instructions of some agent or institution of the law. Second, all kinds of medical evidence presented to investigating magistrates, coroners' courts, and criminal and religious courts, in either written reports or oral testimony. The book does not cover what Clark and Crawford describe as 'medical matters which were merely the subject of legal proceedings', such as disputes over fees, medical ethics or medical malpractice, nor does it include the provision of medical certificates and testimonials for legal or quasi-judicial purposes such as prison administration or insurance policies. Purely civil disputes, concerning feigned illness and malingering, insurance claims, tests of mental capacity, inheritance, and divorce (in which one party or the other might allege that they had been given a sexually transmitted disease by their spouse, or that the spouse was of unsound mind), will not be addressed for practical reasons: the historical literature is simply too small to permit effective international comparison.[9]

The forensic practice that occurred in the principal legal arenas of the Western world could involve either the living or the dead. Ecclesiastical courts were concerned by impotence and persons of unclear gender. Criminal courts were concerned with crimes against the person, such as rape and other sexual offences, homosexual encounters (then illegal), murder, manslaughter, suicide, bodily injury, poisoning and infanticide; in many of these cases the issue of the insanity of the defendant might be raised, allowing for yet another area of medical study to enter the courtroom. A 'crime' was simply an act that was penalized under the criminal law, and which could thus vary between nations and periods. The history of forensic medicine cannot be understood simply as a branch of medicine, therefore, but must be considered in its relation to the law: it was the law that drove medico-legal practice and thus much of the intellectual content of what, in the nineteenth century, became the academic discipline of forensic medicine. Throughout we will see how political factors and social change also fed into and affected the scope of medico-legal practice.

There is now a considerable distinction between forensic medicine and forensic science, and this book focuses mainly on the former in the period up to the beginning of the twentieth century, before the division between the two became as clear-cut as it is at present. One of the things that will become apparent, however, is the essentially interdisciplinary character of our subject, so it is certainly not the case that we can always stay on one side of a medicine/science divide. However very different disciplines have emerged in the modern era, so that we now have forensic medicine, essentially pathology, and forensic science, of which many different sub-specialities exist, as well as criminology, which had its origins in forensic psychiatry in the late nineteenth century.

Anyone who follows the media's preoccupation with the world of forensic investigation will have a good idea of what forensic science is. Today it encompasses a large range of laboratory-based techniques for identifying criminals and their victims, including DNA analysis of blood and biological fluids and, with the advent of the computer, facial and voice recognition software. There is also toxicology, the study of poisons, which tends today to be concerned mainly with illegal drugs, but toxicologists are involved in death investigations (suicides, accidents and murders) when poison is suspected. Forensic chemistry deals mainly with materials that can be analyzed and identified by their chemical composition, like paints, flammable liquids used in cases of arson, and illegal drugs (when they have not been ingested, in which case toxicology is more relevant). Modern forensic chemistry is to a large extent concerned with the analysis of blood and urine samples in cases of suspected drink driving. The examination of firearms, known as ballistics, is an important aspect of forensic science, perhaps more so in the United States than in Europe, and probably less well known is the scientific analysis of disputed documents, often associated with cases of fraud.

These subjects fall clearly within the realm of forensic science, based for the most part in chemistry, biology and physics. How then is this different from forensic medicine? The key point to bear in mind here is that forensic medicine is concerned with the body, and with the effects on the body of acts of violence. The field of medicine that is today associated with forensic practice is pathology, from the Greek words *pathos* (suffering) and *logia* (the study of). Medicine's claims to being scientific are anchored in pathology as the study of disease, as a system of knowledge used to draw conclusions about illness and death. There is a difference between forensic pathology and pathology, because the latter is highly diagnostic in intention and its findings are used to help determine treatments for other people suffering from the same disease, or to supply evidence that the treatment undertaken was indeed the best course of action. It does this by using the post-mortem (after death) examination.[10] Forensic pathology also relies on the post-mortem, but its purposes are rather narrow: it is largely concerned with cases of sudden or unexplained death; in identifying cause and manner of death; and, where any doubt exists, establishing the identity of the deceased person, who can in forensic cases be described as the victim. The terms post-mortem and autopsy have long had the same meaning in all countries, though Americans tend to use the latter in preference to the former. The more correct term is necropsy (examination of the dead), but it is not commonly used. Pathology is a recognized field of modern medicine, but its formal professional history is relatively short, dating from the mid nineteenth century, although post-mortem examinations were for centuries carried out as and when necessary by surgeons who were not necessarily skilled in autopsy techniques.

The greatest changes in medical knowledge and practice have undoubtedly occurred over the past century, but for our purposes as historians of forensic medicine, histories of drugs and disease, health and healing are far less relevant than the working presence of medical personnel in society, the roles that they carried out, the status that they held and the institutions that employed them. There are four key types of medical practitioner relevant to our study: physicians, surgeons, apothecaries and midwives. They could be employed by the state, the military, a town or district, a hospital, or an individual, but the vast majority were in private practice and competed for business with a range of unorthodox practitioners such as herbalists and homeopaths. By the middle of the fourteenth century most European jurisdictions required some form of licence, obtained through examination by a guild, a public authority, or a university. Training occurred either in universities (physicians) or by a system of apprenticeship (everyone else until the nineteenth century). Most were men, with the exception of midwives, and as male professionals began to attend the births of the wealthy in the seventeenth and eighteenth centuries they came increasingly to dominate that area of medical practice too.[11] Some towns paid midwives to act in an official capacity in cases concerning female illness and infant care, and they also tested for virginity or sterility, and certified infant deaths. But the history of medical professionalization is the history of a shift from pluralistic health care to a monopoly of a powerful, and largely male, orthodoxy,[12] and this was reflected in forensic practice.

After the scientific revolution of the seventeenth century – a term which reflects the widespread transformation of thought about nature, from a basis in Greek and Islamic writings and medieval reflections on the ancients, to one founded on experimental observation and focused on theoretical explanations for actual events – European doctors began to frame illness in scientific terms.

Medicine lost its religious overtones and doctors' independent power began to grow. 'Charters of autonomy were granted to physicians and guilds of barber-surgeons, first by cities, then by nations. Being a professional medical practitioner was defined by membership in a body of practitioners who held the privilege of examining, licensing, and disciplining' their members.[13]

In the United States as early as 1760, irregular medical practice became recognized as a problem, and New York passed the first law requiring the examination and licensing of all who wished to practice medicine. A few other states followed suit, but the widespread official recognition of an acceptable course of medical training came only after the Revolution, when medical schools were empowered to grant licenses to their graduates. As the new nation expanded, so did the number of medical schools, leading to a rise in the number of badly trained doctors. State boards of examination were first set up in 1835, but the competition between orthodox and irregular practitioners meant that they were largely ineffective in regulating what was still seen very much as an art. As a more scientific form of medicine grew in influence, this situation changed, so that state boards of medical examiners were again set up in the 1870s and continue today to license all medical doctors in the United States.[14]

Surgery and medicine are mutually dependent, but have not always been considered part of the same discipline. The word 'surgery' is derived from the Greek *cheirourgikē*, via the Latin *chirurgiae*, meaning 'hand work', and prior to the modern era Western culture tended to rank hand work below that done by the mind. Surgeons were thus traditionally seen as inferior to physicians, and were on a par with barbers who earned a living by shaving, cutting hair and pulling teeth; 'minor operations were incidental'. Barber-surgeons learned their trade by apprenticeship, unlike the physicians who studied for a degree at university 'and rarely saw patients until after they had graduated'.[15] In general, physicians had authority over internal medical problems and surgeons over external ones such as wounds and fractures. Apothecaries formed a third branch of the medical profession: they sold drugs, filled prescriptions and frequently acted as the poor man's doctor.

The distinctions between medicine and surgery became important in the Middle Ages when the two separated. University-trained physicians were part of the three traditional professions of theology, law and medicine and, as elites, treated the rich; although since antiquity towns employed them to treat the poor also.[16] Separation led to professional rivalry until the eighteenth century, when a movement began, originating in continental military medical schools, to draw medicine and surgery closer together; greater cooperation between the three 'official' groups became evident. From 1794 French medical schools deliberately attempted to unify medicine and surgery by instituting a common education for physicians and surgeons, supplemented by specialized postgraduate training.[17] The growth of medical schools and increase in the number of hospitals – institutions that provided places for doctors to practice and learn – across Europe and North America during the eighteenth and especially nineteenth century, led to the establishment of organized national training programmes for all types of medical professionals, stressing clinical instruction, research, and professional boundaries delineated by examination and licensing.[18]

As is in some respects still the case today, the medical profession across Britain, Europe and the United States in the past was extremely hierarchical, with physicians at the top and everyone else below them. Since the hierarchy was largely based on education and practical focus – surgeons, apothecaries and midwives were trained by apprenticeship and in the broadest sense were involved with manipulating the bodies of patients, while physicians performed the more intellectually demanding tasks of diagnosing illness and prescribing medications – it should be fairly evident how this hierarchy may have been translated into forensic practice. Prescriptions were filled and sold both by apothecaries (forerunners of modern pharmacists) and apothecary surgeons (forerunners of modern general practitioners), and this gave them a familiarity with drugs and poisons that could involve them in forensic work. Midwives were useful when it came to issues involving women's bodies. The surgeon's knowledge of bodies was possibly the most relevant in the numerous cases of violent deaths and wounding that came before the courts. Finally, physicians' familiarity with the internal workings of the body made them the most likely to be consulted on matters to do with the mind and brain or, in other words, issues to do with sanity or the lack thereof.

In comparison to the other areas of history to which it is closely related – history of medicine and science, legal history, criminal justice history – the history of forensic medicine has not been the object of such extensive research. Few studies approach the subject through an international comparative structure, and the best example of this genre is now sixteen years old.[19] Many of those book-length national or comparative overviews which do exist are not accessible to audiences who can read only English,[20] while those that are tend to consider only Britain or the United States.[21] Furthermore, relevant secondary literature in the form of articles and chapters is widely dispersed in a bewildering range of publications, many written in languages other than English. No single work of synthesis unites these varying strands in the academic study of the history of forensic medicine, but the interested reader will surely agree that this history touches upon multiple subjects, actors and activities which had important consequences in Western society, and which might therefore most effectively be studied in cross-national comparison. This book consequently offers a first attempt to provide a broad overview of the history of forensic medicine in the West, focusing for the most part on Britain, France, Germany, Italy and the United States. It tries, within the limits posed by the existing primary and secondary literature, and the author's language skills, to give each topic a comparative element, so that the emphasis never lies too much on one country, theme or period.

Chapter 1 reviews the legal inheritance, contrasting common law and the jury's importance in Anglo-American practice with the trial procedures that evolved in continental Europe following the medieval hybridization of Roman and canon law, which excluded juries and allowed the torture of suspects. Under both systems, rules of evidence shaped the need for and reception of medical testimony in legal proceedings – oral testimony under the accusatory common law, the written record under inquisitorial Roman law. Chapter 2 surveys medico-legal practice from the medieval through the early modern period, presenting an overview of the types of cases that medical practitioners handled, the evidence that they gave and the growing importance of their presence in the legal setting. In cases of injury and death investigation doctors and midwives were clearly held to have privileged knowledge.

Chapter 3 is on experts and expertise, including the institutionalization of the discipline of forensic medicine and how that process helped to foster legal acceptance of the opinions of individuals who became recognized as a distinct class of witness. The nineteenth-century association of 'expert witnesses' with cases of poisoning, highly complex and difficult for the lay person to penetrate unaided, will be explored as a case study. But the capacity for medico-legal controversy was nowhere so evident, long-lived or widespread as in relation to the insanity defence; Chapter 4 considers criminal responsibility and by extension the criminally insane within Western legal systems. The emergence of a group of individuals with specific knowledge of the insane led to the new medical discipline of psychiatry and further scope for the creation of a cadre of medico-legal experts. The identification of insanity with mania, or total delirium, had long existed in Western medicine, but the 1820s' introduction by French psychiatrists of the concept of homicidal monomania opened the door for an increasing use of expert psychiatric testimony in trials where the insanity of the accused was by no means apparent.

Chapter 5 addresses the medicalization of deviant behaviour: the years around 1760 marked the beginning of important changes in attitudes to insanity that furthered the acceptance of medical explanations for criminal behaviour. In the case of infanticide, early modern viciousness to unmarried mothers who killed their newborns slackened in the eighteenth century and was in the nineteenth century replaced by relative leniency: new laws allowed women who killed their infants to be tried under different terms than other murderers. Other areas to be considered include suicide, deviant sexual practices and impotence. Finally, Chapter 6 takes the history of forensic medicine into the twentieth century by investigating some of the areas of medico-legal practice that became characteristic of the modern era, including the 'discovery' of child abuse and the rise of forensic science and its con-stituent branches. Although the practical features of contemporary forensic practice are significantly different from those of earlier centuries, its core aims and ideals remain unchanged.

1 The legal inheritance

Why is it, asked Catherine Crawford 16 years ago, that medico-legal publications were rare in early modern England but comparatively abundant in Italy, France and especially Germany?[1] Although there may have been a certain lack of enthusiasm for this type of work, given its association with unsavoury crimes and public trials, recent studies have shown that medical professionals, primarily surgeons and apothecaries,[2] were present as witnesses in English law courts during the seventeenth and especially eighteenth centuries, but in a much less systematic manner than in continental Europe.[3] The problem seems, in effect, to have been one of failure to record the experience for the benefit of others, rather than an absence of forensic practice. In what has proved to be the definitive solution to the mystery, Crawford identified one fundamental factor: differences between legal systems and specifically between standards of proof and evidence.

This chapter considers the Western legal inheritance, that is, the system of laws and official practices which emerged in medieval Europe, to explain the evolution of and differences between the two major legal systems that have shaped the development of forensic medicine. These were the Continental system, based on Roman and canon (church) law, and the Anglo-American system, based on English common law. Every nation in the modern Western world can trace the history of its civil and criminal laws to these two traditions, but it was their differing methods of proof that were to be the driving factors in stimulating the need for and reception of medical testimony in legal proceedings. Despite common historical foundations and shared trends in the systems of rational proof that emerged during the twelfth and thirteenth centuries,[4] the rules of evidence created on either side of the English Channel worked in opposing ways with regard to witness testimony in criminal trials. In England, juries became the finders of fact and based their decisions on oral eyewitness testimony; there was no formal mechanism for obtaining evidence from anyone who had not been a direct observer of the events in question. On the Continent, by contrast, judges investigated crime and determined guilt or innocence on the strength of the evidence that they gathered and compiled in written dossiers; their need to establish the facts of a case required them to seek out relevant information from anyone who could provide it. It was this feature of Continental practice that was to provide medical practitioners with a key point of entry to the legal system.

Early medieval justice

To understand how European legal systems evolved, we must turn briefly to the later history of one of the most important political entities of the ancient world, the Roman Empire, which spanned the continent. Partitioned in the year 395 into east (with its capital at Constantinople, later Byzantium; modern Istanbul) and west (Rome), the western empire was subject to a series of fourth and fifth century in-migrations by Germanic tribes seeking new lands. Predictably, the Romans objected to this breach of their borders and fought a series of wars against the invaders.[5] Where they could, however, they reached agreements with them, resulting in the integration of the peoples whom they called 'barbarians', because they could not speak Latin, into Roman society, notably the military. This was a risky strategy, however, and in 476 Odoacer, a barbarian who had risen to high rank in the army, deposed the reigning emperor and declared himself king of Italy, thus ending the empire in the west. It continued in the east, but the tribes that had settled in western Europe during the fifth century created their own kingdoms and, in theory, retained their own customary laws, though these had probably been influenced by Roman law.[6] There was thus not one law but several legal systems in force across Europe after the fall of the Western Empire.[7]

When historians refer to 'Roman law' of the period they generally mean the written text known as the *Corpus Juris Civilis*, the 'body of civil law' which brought together and codified the entire law of the citizens of Rome; the use of the word civil in this context is to be distinguished from its use in a modern sense. Issued between 529 and 534 by the eastern, or Byzantine emperor Justinian (483–562), the central attribute of the *Corpus* was the reliance it placed on oral and written testimony, which required rules of evidence and proof much as modern legal systems do. Moreover, the Roman system gave significant investigative or 'inquisitorial' powers to the judge, while the burden of proof usually lay on the accuser, so that it was their responsibility to find credible witnesses to support their allegations.

But this written law co-existed with customary law, a fact that Justinian noted and accepted,[8] and it is in the links between the written and unwritten Roman civil law that we can see clear points of similarity with the key features of so-called barbarian law, which gave a central role to tribal custom. Today notable for its very different legal principles, barbarian law was personal, that is, it was considered to reside in the individual, not the territory where he lived. It relied on monetary payments called *wergeld* to right illegal or wrong actions; and used unique ways to prove the guilt or innocence of an accused person – the so-called irrational proofs, which included ordeals, oath swearing and trial by battle.[9] The Romans had also accepted the notion of compensation for injury, however, custom sanctioning it as a payment to cover medical treatment and loss of income, while there is evidence that they used oaths, long held to be Germanic in origin, as a way to counter the flaws inherent in the use of torture, the most widely used Roman method of securing proof.[10] What seems to have been entirely lacking in Roman law, however, was any formal recognition that physicians might have a forensic role.[11]

When the barbarian kings created their own legislation, notably the collections of edicts known as the *Leges Barbarorum* (*Barbarian Laws*), which were written in Latin between the fifth and ninth centuries and used some of the technical terms of Roman law, they drew both on tribal tradition and Roman written and customary law, initiating a gradual process of integration and adaptation which ensured that elements of all three survived until at least the twelfth century. Early medieval justice therefore represented a fusion of barbarian and Roman law, which was further influenced by the rules, ideas and practices instituted by the universal Catholic Church.[12]

Legal procedure rested on two central planks, the *wergeld* and the irrational proofs, the former of which offered clear scope for the admission of medical knowledge to the legal process. *Wergeld*, which means 'man-price' in Old English, was a sum of money paid by the family of a killer to the victim's family in cases of murder or manslaughter, to avoid revenge in the form of blood-feud. This reflected the early medieval law's concern to penalize damage done to families rather than to protect individuals or society as a whole.[13] The amount payable varied with the gender and social status of the victim, so that a man was worth more than a woman or a boy and a priest more than a layman. A similar system of payments for physical wounding, the *bot*, was also used. The Visigoths, Franks and Anglo-Saxons specified fixed payments for bodily injuries that could impair the injured person's ability to pull his or her weight in the community, such as the loss of a limb, but in England at least the payments reflected only the seriousness of the injury, not the victim's rank.[14] Some form of medical inspection was required by law, notably amongst the Alemanni, Lombards and Franks,[15] but neither usual practice by these or other tribes, nor the steps taken in cases of internal injury, are known. The Anglo-Saxons, apparently recognizing the limitations of medical care, allowed a perpetrator to pay the *bot* in a way that would allow the money value of the wound to be counted towards the *wergeld* if the victim subsequently died.[16] Crucially for later developments, the Anglo-Saxon interpretation of the *bot* and *wergeld* evolved an understanding of the relationship between violence and social control, with the state gradually assuming more and more responsibility for punishing violent crimes.

During an era when writing was not widespread, normal judicial procedure in both civil (in the modern sense) and criminal cases relied on an accuser to bring a charge against another person and prove it, using oral eyewitness testimony to establish guilt or innocence. In cases where there was no accuser, or when the circumstances were particularly uncertain, as, for example, in accusations of rape, theft, poisoning and adultery, the courts turned to God's judgment, either in this world or the next. The irrational proofs on which early medieval justice relied included compurgation, or oath swearing, and the ordeals by hot water, hot iron or cold water, and trial by battle, all of which were sanctioned by the church. Relying on biblical passages and the writings of the Church fathers, particularly St Augustine, churchmen 'composed the texts and produced the liturgies suitable for the administration of ordeals', which became the province of the clergy.[17] Although legal historians have not always agreed with the propensity to define the ordeals as irrational,[18] the fact remains that they were modes of proof which were not based on human reason and critical enquiry but on an appeal to signs from an unseen, mystical world,[19] in which natural elements were required to behave in unnatural ways. Verdicts merely reflected the will of God: in many ways, the ordeals were as much a theological as a legal institution. Furthermore, in a reversal of the tenets of the *Corpus Juris Civilis*, ordeals shifted the burden of proof from the accuser to the defendant as, with the exception of trial by battle, it was he 'who underwent the unilateral ordeal or swore the purgatory oath proclaiming his own innocence'.[20]

Compurgation, or canonical purgation, was the most common method of proof used in the early medieval period. Solidly embedded in canon law, the law of the church, it introduced to criminal matters the same procedure used to prosecute those accused of ecclesiastical offences.[21] Compurgation required the accused to take a formal oath of innocence and to enlist a number of compurgators (oath helpers) to support the oath by swearing that they believed it. They swore 'not to the truth of the underlying facts, but to their belief in the trustworthiness of the oath of the accused',[22] thus offering a public and persuasive evidence of innocence that worked because it relied on the fact that the accused had a good reputation and that the oath takers understood and feared the theological consequences of perjury. A remnant of this religious institution remains in modern legal process, in the form of the oath that witnesses take to tell the truth in law courts.

When oath-taking was deemed inappropriate because the accused lacked suitable oath-worthiness, due to low status, prior bad reputation or inability to find oath-helpers, the legal system turned to ordeals as a way of resolving the most difficult cases, particularly those which involved slaves and serfs.[23] Ordeals were not therefore a common occurrence, but they were found throughout Europe from about 800 until the thirteenth century. Originally of Frankish origin, there were three forms of unilateral ordeal. The ordeal by hot water was the earliest, and involved plunging the hand into boiling water which had been blessed by a priest, and then pulling it out again. For more serious offences the person might have to pick something up from the bottom of the pot, which took more time, or put their whole forearm into the water. Then the hand and arm were bandaged. If an inspection three days later showed that the injuries were healing well, the accused was pronounced innocent; if the injuries were festering, they were guilty.[24]

The ordeal by hot iron was similarly religious in overtone: preceded by prayer, fasting and blessings, the accused had to pick up a red-hot iron bar, sometimes to carry it for a few feet, or walk over heated ploughshares. More serious charges involved a heavier bar or a longer path. The wounds were checked three days later, as with the hot water ordeal. Finally there was the ordeal by cold water, which was based on the assumption that water was a pure element which, when blessed, would refuse to accept the guilty. If the water received the accused when they were bound securely and thrown in – that is if they sank – they were innocent. If they floated, they were guilty.[25] The use of this form of ordeal in cases of suspected witchcraft survived into the early modern period in the form of the 'swimming' of witches in many parts of Europe.

While there may have been some small role for medical opinion in the ordeals by fire and hot water – regarding the determination of whether the wounds were healing well or not – there were no objective medical standards for what constituted healing, so that verdicts must have been subjective and influenced to some extent by compassion or politics.[26] Outcomes clearly depended on factors irrelevant to culpability, such as the temperature of the iron, calluses on hands, burn thickness, and the buoyancy of the human body, which is different for men and women. It may well be, therefore, that judicial ordeals were, at least on occasion, deliberately managed so as to give the accused a sporting chance.[27]

However, confidence in the unilateral ordeal was clearly beginning to fade as early as the twelfth century, due to the combined influence of resistance and criticism from a number of quarters. Rulers and townspeople distrusted their efficacy, lawyers doubted their legitimacy because the *Corpus Juris Civilis* ignored them, and theologians came to doubt them because they required God to perform miracles.[28] In 1215 the Fourth Lateran Council issued a prohibition forbidding clergy to take part in ordeals, at one stroke removing the religious foundation for the practice and thus its legal legitimacy. In areas where papal authority was strong or where unilateral ordeals had already lost some of their credibility, judicial ordeals were abandoned quickly, as in England and France; where papal power was weak or popular attachment to the practice strong, as in eastern Europe, they survived for longer.[29] Compurgation proved to be a good deal longer lived, continuing in Germany until the late medieval period and in England until the seventeenth century,[30] probably because it had not been condemned by the Church and offered a useful public means of clearing individuals of community suspicion.

Chance played a much smaller role in the third type of irrational proof, the judicial duel, also known as trial by battle. Used in both criminal and civil cases, particularly land disputes,[31] this method of proof also appealed to the will of God, though success relied to a very great extent on physical strength and training. Rules of engagement were rigorously adhered to, so that the combat itself was regulated, as also the sorts of people who could engage in it: lepers could not fight healthy people, bastards could not fight the legitimate, serfs could not fight freemen, women and children were not allowed to fight at all (though on occasion women did), and in 1140 the Pope forbade clerics to take part in such contests. The penalty for defeat was death or ignominy, but those who were legally barred from fighting had the option of hiring a champion.[32] In England, the parties in criminal cases fought in person but in civil cases were required to use champions,[33] who were found in all countries. Although champions were often servants or family members, a class of professionals existed, and criminals too might act as champions to avoid execution or banishment; in England they were known as 'approvers', the medieval equivalent of turning Queen's evidence.[34]

Trial by battle continued as a regular feature of the legal system all over the Continent until the fourteenth century, but had largely fallen out of favour by the fifteenth. The last judicial duel sanctioned by the Parlement of Paris occurred in 1386, when Jacques Le Gris was killed by Jean de Carrouges in a battle sparked by an accusation of rape made by the latter's wife against Le Gris.[35] Duels continued in France until 1482, but it was in the British Isles that the duel was to have a remarkable longevity, due to its legal status as a means of initiating a private prosecution for murder, as explained below. The last judicial duel in England occurred in 1492, and in Ireland a duel to the death was fought in 1583 with royal sanction; but the appeal of murder was not formally abolished until 1819, as a result of the cause célèbre of Ashford *v.* Thornton (Case Study 1.1).

Case Study 1.1: The abolition of trial by combat in England, 1819

Despite strong suspicion of guilt, in August 1817 Warwickshire bricklayer Abraham Thornton had been acquitted of the rape-murder of Mary Ashford. Evidence revealed after the trial undermined his alibi, however, and on the advice of a local solicitor the victim's brother, William Ashford, decided to prosecute him on an appeal of murder. This legal strategy had previously been used to secure convictions in cases where trial on indictment had failed,[36] but the person so appealed had the right to claim trial by battle, and Thornton did so when the case came before the Court of King's Bench in November 1817, 'conscious of the decided advantage which his uncommon personal strength would give him over the dwarfish and delicate frame of ... Ashford'.[37] Even though he could not have been unaware of this possibility, Ashford's barrister offered a weak counter-argument: 'it would appear to me extraordinary indeed, if the person who has murdered the sister should ... be allowed to prove his innocence by murdering the brother also'. He was quickly reminded by the judge that it was not murder but the law of England.[38] When the court ruled that Ashford had to accept the wager of battle or Thornton must go free, the appellant and his supporters realized that they had run out of options. Ashford declined to fight, Thornton was discharged from the appeal, and the government wasted little time in heeding calls for the immediate abolition of what by now was widely regarded as an undesirable remnant of the past.[39]

Sources: Sir J. Hall (ed.), *Trial of Abraham Thornton*, Glasgow: William Hodge, 1926, pp. 33–35; 'Abraham Thornton', *The Newgate Calendar*, http://exclassics.com/newgate/ng574.htm (accessed on 24 May 2010).

Medieval legal innovations

In addition to the admixture of barbarian and Roman law that governed the lives of the peoples of medieval Europe, there was another type of law, the law of the church, which applied everywhere in the Western Christian world. The word canon, from the Latin, means a rule or standard, and the collection of ecclesiastical laws that served as the source of church government became known as canon law. Influenced mainly by Roman law, as might be expected of a Church that had its centre at Rome, canon law continued to grow and expand following the fall of the Western Empire, to include decisions made by popes and Christian synods, as well as commentaries by various clerics written as guidance for the clergy, whose role in medieval society was deeply embedded in daily life. The boundaries between canon law and secular law were very porous, as church courts claimed jurisdiction over matters that would now come within the purview of civil courts, such as disputed wills and divorce, and also over criminal matters, especially sexual offences like adultery, incest and fornication and, during the medieval period, infanticide.[40]

By the eleventh century canon law had become a vast and complicated entity that was too difficult for most church courts to apply correctly. Attempts to systematize it and resolve the contradictions that had crept into it were made by scholars at the law school of Bologna, particularly by a cleric named Gratian during the twelfth century. His *Decretum* (*c.* 1140) provided an important conceptual step by insisting that judges should have jurisdiction over acts, not the sins of the accused, a point which gave canon law legitimacy independent of theology.[41] At the same time, the masters of Bologna were teaching Roman law, the *Corpus Juris*, and it was not long before traditional canon law had fused with it to create a new legal system common to scholars all over the Christian West. First defined around 1165, a key consequence of this fusion was the significant role that it gave to the secular authorities in the form of academically trained judges and judicial inquiry supported by written evidence.[42] This influence was felt early and strongly in Italy, the country where Roman and canon law had been born, and in both Italy and France laws and procedures developed as a result of astute combinations of judge-made, statute and professors' law, helped in large part by the existence of universities and strong municipal government.[43]

The first systematic treatise on the entire body of law, the *Decretum*, was followed in the thirteenth century by authoritative treatises on English, German, French and other systems of territorial secular law.[44] On the Continent, the law of proof which evolved from the fusion of Roman and canon law allowed for only two forms of evidence sufficient to convict a defendant: uncontradicted testimony from two eyewitnesses or confession by the accused. Such strict standards made it difficult to secure convictions in situations that, before 1215, would have led to the use of the ordeal, and it has been suggested that torture was introduced to the judicial apparatus to resolve this impasse. However there were other ways around it. Jurists and urban legislators allowed for judicial discretion to accept circumstantial evidence, reduced the standard of proof in certain notorious cases, and introduced new statutes to give judges more flexibility.[45] In England, where common law had developed through the influence of royal justice before the practical influences of Bologna could be felt, medieval justice took a much different course.

The Norman conquest of 1066 introduced centralized government and significant socio-cultural change to England, but not Roman law. Instead, a new body of Anglo-Norman law gradually evolved, based on Norman feudalism and long-established Anglo-Saxon customs. During the tenth century the law had been broadened to include innovations which reflected a growing acceptance that crime was an offence against society; declaring criminals to be outlaws and putting them beyond the protection of the law, confiscating their goods and inflicting physical punishments had all been added to the repertory of Anglo-Saxon legal sanctions. These were retained by the Normans, who added a few novelties of their own, particularly trial by battle, the use of written records, greater reliance on sworn testimony, and the removal of church-related cases from the customary law to the purview of the canon law, which was adopted by the English church in 1072.[46]

By the end of the eleventh century the Anglo-Normans were largely in step with developments found on the Continent, but there was one key difference: in England there is evidence for the existence of an early jury system at the time of the Domesday Book (1086). This early jury, not yet a feature of the legal system, was simply used to affirm the accuracy of the Domesday survey in a process known as an inquest. Such enquiries were carried out under oath, when witnesses were interrogated and verdicts given by a select group representing the community. A similar procedure was known on the Continent in a specifically criminal context, but with the adoption of Roman-canon process the juries were displaced by judges. In England, however, the jury was retained and, during the reign of Henry II (r. 1154–89), the institutional foundations of the English common law, so-called because, unlike feudal justice, it was common to all men in all regions of the country, were laid. Three interrelated factors underpinned the common law: strong monarchy; the growth of the jury system, which eventually replaced the ordeal as a method of proof; and a centralized royal court system staffed by professional judges and clerks.[47] The common law was made primarily by judges using precedent and common sense, rather than formal written enactments of law as on the Continent, but verdicts were given by juries.

Juries of 12 men, sworn to discover and declare facts in criminal matters, came into being in 1166 when the jury of presentment (or indictment) was established as a forerunner of what came to be known as the grand jury. This was made up of 16 local men of good repute, later 23 men drawn from the local magistracy, who were to formally establish and state the charges against any person accused of a criminal offence and who then still had to endure an ordeal to establish guilt or innocence. Trial by jury in civil cases came about soon after, mainly in cases of trespass, and following the abolition of trial by ordeal in 1215, the jury system was greatly extended into the criminal and civil areas of law. By the late fourteenth century it was an established legal institution taking much the same form as it has today: accused criminals would be confronted in court by their alleged victim (the accusatorial trial system) and would call witnesses to support their case before the judge and jury, the judge being bound to honour the jury's decision.[48]

The office of coroner was introduced by the Normans in 1194, to inquire into unnatural deaths and to determine whether the deceased was English or Norman and, if the community could not prove the former, to impose the *murdrum* or murder fine, a financial penalty designed to dissuade local people from murdering the foreigners. Coroners' inquiries, known as inquests, were held in a coroner's court, where the coroner sat with a jury of up to 21 local men.[49] This uniquely English institution existed nowhere else in Europe except in those nations where it was installed by a process of conquest and assimilation: Ireland in the early thirteenth century and Wales in the mid sixteenth century.

The key point to note about England, as regards the history of forensic medicine, is the crucial importance of the jury: the statement of 12 (or more, at an inquest) local men under oath was accepted as the authoritative judgment on questions of fact. Although English juries had by the late medieval period evolved from being self-informing due to their local knowledge, to being informed by hearing the testimony of eyewitnesses in formal proceedings, it remained the case that the court could, and for a long time did, assume that the jury's view superseded in value the opinions of all others, including medical professionals. As Crawford puts it, 'the English standard of proof was thus in effect lay consensus; jurors' unanimous opinion in favour of one party or the other was thought to provide an acceptable level of certainty'.[50]

In Germany political fragmentation acted to prevent the development of a uniform legal code, in contrast to the English, and also to the French and Italians, who had been quick to adopt the Roman-canon legal model not least because its hierarchical prince-centred organizational structure found favour among the leaders of states and city-states. What is now called Germany was then the Holy Roman Empire, which traced its origins to Rome on 25 December 800, when Charlemagne was crowned Emperor by Pope Leo III,[51] and which passed out of existence on 6 August 1806 when, as a consequence of Napoleonic pressure, the then Emperor renounced the crown and released all states from their oath of allegiance. The Holy Roman Empire was less an empire in the Roman sense than a loose federation of small states governed by dukes and princes aligned under a purely elective monarch. Hence it is not surprising that, given their strongly regional nature, these small states were strongholds of customary law. Although customary law was adequate for settling disputes between individuals, a much more broadly applicable law was needed to keep the territorial peace between states; in belated recognition of this fact, the Empire formally adopted Roman law in 1495.[52]

As a consequence, German criminal law and procedure underwent a substantial transformation during the sixteenth century: the culmination of what had been a slow process of reform. After the abolition of ordeals, princely and urban authorities had begun to take the initiative in prosecuting people charged with serious offences, and in such cases legal officials interrogated suspects before trial; in many areas of Germany official prosecutors were appointed. Mirroring developments elsewhere, the influence of the canon law had begun to grow in the twelfth century: it was applied first in church courts and then gradually adopted, with modifications, in the various territorial courts. Elements of an earlier Germanic 'accusatorial' model of criminal procedure, in which a trial was a 'contest between accuser and accused' and the outcome a manifestation of God's will, were thereby combined with facets of the canon law's 'inquisitorial' model, wherein trials were characterized by 'interrogation of the accused and witnesses by the court' and the outcome reflected reasoned human judgment. In the course of the fifteenth century the accusatory elements were subjected to far greater official controls, but remained important in non-capital cases.[53] For our purposes, the important point here is that fact finding became a central feature of the criminal trial in German lands, and one can see where this might influence the history of forensic medicine, if the legal system and the officials who served it were in the business of seeking the best evidence possible. Obviously, some of that evidence might well have had to come from medical practitioners.

The preceding survey of medieval innovations in European legal practice has sought to establish what they were and how they shaped the evolution of criminal process in different regions. In England, criminal matters were regulated by the common law of custom as interpreted by judges and juries, while in France and Italy criminals were dealt with by a mixture of written Roman and canon law interpreted by judges and legal scholars, and in Germany customary law was practiced in the light of procedures developed under canon law. The next question that the historian of forensic medicine must consider is how these legal systems actually functioned, and we will again find that there were key differences between England and the rest of Europe. To do this we need to examine the two main forms of criminal trial: the inquisitorial form, practiced on the Continent, and the accusatorial form, found in England and later exported to its colonies.

Judicial process: the inquisitorial and accusatorial systems

The earliest meaning of the Latin word *inquisitio* was simply 'the act of looking for something', but by the first century BCE it was being used in the narrower sense of enquiring into specific matters. Under Roman law, *inquisitio* came to mean a formal stage of legal procedure, the search for evidence to support an accusation, and although there was little of original Roman procedure in the process that survived into the early modern period, historians have, rightly or wrongly, come to describe it as Roman-canon inquisition process. Inquisition, as we can broadly translate the term, refers to the duty of the judge in a criminal case to discover the truth about any issue coming before his court, and may be contrasted with accusation, the duty of a private citizen to prove the case against someone who has harmed him.

Criminal trials carried out under the Roman-canon law tradition were dominated by the judge, who questioned witnesses, gathered evidence, formed an opinion, and acquitted or convicted accordingly. Beyond the church courts, where it originated, we find the procedure particularly early in southern countries, especially Italy and Spain, contemporaneously with the demise of the ancient methods of proof and often at about the same time as the establishment of Roman-derived law. Elsewhere, the spread of the procedure was slower. In France, a royal decree of 1260 substituted the inquisitorial procedure (*enquête*) for wager of battle, and trial by witnesses and oral or written pleadings became routine.[54] It then reached the Low Countries, and in the German lands the evidentiary inquest had become the dominant trial form by the fifteenth century, co-existing with compurgation.[55] In the trial by jury, as found in England, judges were bound by the jury's verdict, as formerly they were bound by the outcome of an ordeal.

Inquisitorial procedure is customarily contrasted with its accusatorial counterpart, most obviously in terms of the mode of initiation of a criminal prosecution. At the most basic level, we can think of the accusatorial system as one in which the injured party pursued his rights by instigating a private prosecution, in contrast to the inquisitorial system, in which the state received information about an alleged offence and prosecuted on behalf of the public good. The workings of the inquisitorial process also allowed for the private initiation of a prosecution, but it became the state's duty to carry it through to completion.[56] In England, prosecutors remained, in theory, responsible for organizing most or all of the proceedings by themselves until the nineteenth century,[57] although magistrates and coroners collected evidence in writing and committed individuals for trial. More importantly for our purposes as historians of forensic medicine, the English system offered no formal role to expert witnesses of any kind, and thus no incentive for a corpus of medico-legal knowledge to develop. Surgeons, apothecaries, midwives and occasionally physicians were called upon to testify in court and pre-trial proceedings, always orally and with no record kept,[58] though pre-trial depositions were written down at the discretion of the individual coroner or magistrate. This occurred on an ad hoc basis and without payment until the Medical Witnesses Act of 1836 authorized a fee of one guinea for attending at a coroner's inquest and a further guinea for performing an autopsy ordered by a coroner. This stands in stark contrast to Continental procedures, where under the impetus of the Roman-canon innovation, it had for centuries been normal practice for court-appointed and well paid medical professionals to submit written reports which offered an opinion, not merely a statement of observed fact. In England, recall, only juries could determine trial outcomes, guided by their own interpretation of the facts, and verdicts could not be appealed except on a point of law.

Another important feature of inquisitorial process which was not found in accusatorial process was the duty of the state apparatus of justice to investigate cases and establish the objective truth. The inquisitorial system embodied clear-cut ideas 'not only about who should conduct the criminal process, but about how he should go about it'.[59] An officer of the state, typically a judge, was responsible for investigating and assembling factual evidence upon which to base rational judgment about the guilt or innocence of individuals accused of criminal acts.[60] It was this need for certainty that fostered the resort to torture, in some types of cases, to induce a confession from the accused. The historiographical arguments about the medieval introduction of torture are complex,[61] and need not concern us here except insofar as to notice that, although there is as yet little scholarship on this subject in a medico-legal context, the use of torture under law required medical practitioners to assume a role in this aspect of legal procedure.[62]

By the middle of the sixteenth century, then, the western Continental legal systems exhibited common characteristics noticeably different from those found in England. In three countries there was especially important legislation to regulate criminal procedure: the *Constitutio Criminalis Carolina* of 1532 in the Holy Roman Empire; the *Ordonnance sur le fait de la justice* of 1539 in France; and the 1570 *Ordonnance criminelle* in the Spanish Netherlands. These were comprehensive codifications of criminal procedure and, as such, were designed to regulate the conduct of trials. That included securing the correct sort of testimony for all situations, to enable the judge to assemble a thorough case based on solid proof. The main point from our perspective is that such legislation incorporated space for medical testimony in circumstances where it seemed to be required. The most candid expression of this imperative is found in the Carolina, as it is usually referred to, which since its primary goal was the instruction of lay judges (*Schöffen*) in the principles of proof and techniques of investigation, had to include 'arrangements for securing expert advice for cases beyond the layman's capacity'.[63] It therefore included explicit mention of medical testimony in four of its 219 articles (Information Box), and specified the steps to be taken by judges who found

Information Box: The *Constitutio Criminalis Carolina* of the Holy Roman Empire

The Criminal Courts Ordinance of the Emperor Charles V of the Holy Roman Empire, 31 July 1532.

The Carolina, made up of a total of 219 articles, includes only four which specifically call for the intervention of medical men or midwives. They are:

Article 35: If a girl is suspected of having clandestinely given birth to a child and of having killed it, above all one must find if she has been seen in a very apparent state of pregnancy, and if then the swelling having diminished, whether she became pale and weak. If these kinds of signs and indications are found, and if the woman is such that one can suspect her, it is proper to proceed further and to have her examined in particular secretly by experienced, virtuous women. If this examination confirms the suspicion, and she nevertheless does not wish to admit the crime she can be put to the torture.

Article 36: When the child having been lately killed the mother has not yet lost her milk, it will be possible to draw the milk from the breast, and if it is good and perfect, this will be a strong and clear presumption to pass on to torture. However, as certain physicians teach that it can happen sometimes that milk, through natural causes, may occur in a girl who has never been pregnant, if such a fact is appealed to, it will be necessary to have a more thorough examination made by the midwives.

Article 147: If someone who has been struck and wounded dies after an interval so that it is doubtful whether or not it is the blows, or wounds which have caused the death, let surgeons experienced in these kinds of things be heard, who will understand if death could occur after the blows and wounds received and will indicate how long he has survived.

Article 149: In order that in the aforesaid cases there shall be means of recourse, once burial has taken place, to the examination and evaluation of the lesions and of the cause of the wounds, the judge, accompanied by one or by several surgeons, who will previously have taken an oath, must proceed diligently to the inspection of the cadaver before it is interred and have noted and recorded very exactly all the wounds, blows, marks, features, or contusions which they shall find on it each according as he shall perceive.

The following articles relate to offences which imply that a medical evaluation would be needed:

Article 37: Concerning sufficient indication of secret poisoning.

Article 59: When the miserable fellow to be examined has serious wounds.

Article 116: Punishment of immoral sexual relations against the order of nature.

Article 119: Punishment of rape.

Article 130: Concerning the punishment of one who clandestinely administers poison or toxin.

Article 131: Punishment of women who kill their children.

Article 133: Punishment of those who abort the children of pregnant women.

Article 134: Punishment of a doctor who kills by his doctoring.

Article 135: Punishment of suicide.

Article 137: Punishment of murderers and killers who can have no adequate excuse.

Article 179: Concerning criminals who, owing to youth or other reasons, lack understanding.

Article 219: Clarification from whom and in which places advice shall be sought.

Sources: R.P. Brittain, 'Origins of legal medicine: Constitutio Criminalis Carolina', *Medico-Legal Journal*, 1965, vol. 33, 124–27; J.H. Langbein, *Prosecuting Crime in the Renaissance: England, Germany, France* (1974), Clark, NJ: Lawbook Exchange, 2005, pp. 259–308.

themselves in doubt: they were obliged 'to seek advice from the nearest universities, cities, free cities, or others legally knowledgeable there where they think the information is obtainable at the least cost'.[64]

The French ordinance, of which 29 of 192 articles dealt with criminal procedure, was directed at a professional magistracy which had no need for detailed guidelines of the sort found in the Carolina. Instead, the main aim of the 1539 ordinance was to shorten lengthy proceedings, and it thus made no reference to special types of witnesses. But it is evident from brief references and extant medical reports that sworn experts, both male and female, had been known in the French courts since the medieval period. When the royal surgeon Ambroise Paré (1510–90), author of the earliest European medico-legal guide (1575), warned readers of the responsibility that doctors held, he was reflecting on a long-established practice.[65] A revised and expanded Ordinance of 1670 specified that the instructing judge, who supervised a case to judgment, was to order a medical report on any injured person or corpse.[66] In the Netherlands, the ordinance of 1570 was designed to do away with well entrenched local custom and replace it with statute and Roman law,[67] but it is clear that, in Amsterdam at least, tradition had not hindered medico-legal work, as court-ordered body inspections in cases of suspected homicide were a commonplace since the fifteenth century.[68]

The Continental inquisitorial system, with its reliance on proof, written evidence and fact-finding, stimulated the types of medico-legal writings that Crawford noted were abundant in early modern Italy, France and Germany but rare in England. The reason for this should now be evident: if medical practitioners were to be called upon to give evidence in court, they needed to know how that evidence should be collected and interpreted so as to enable judges to reach rational decisions. Medico-legal texts, then, performed the same function as legal texts in serving as guides to good legal practice. A system of referral to further medical authorities, linked in France to appeals against conviction, in Italy to the use of university scholars to clarify points of interpretation, and in Germany to the recourse that lay magistrates had to professors of law and medicine for guidance in resolving doubtful matters, led to the creation of a new type of legal literature, the *consilia*: published collections of opinions originally prepared for the court and appended to case dossiers.[69] In England, where recourse to experts was not sanctioned by law or legal practice, where trials were not adjourned to allow further evidence to be gathered (though inquests and magistrates' pre-trial hearings could be), and where juries did not have to provide justification for their decisions, there was a small medico-legal knowledge base on which to draw and little incentive for anyone to do so in a written form before the nineteenth century. There was one exception to this trend, however. The crime of infanticide, which was defined in law by a statute of 1624, was worded in such a way as to make medical opinion about live birth critically important to the prosecution case against the mother, and by the mid eighteenth century medical evidence had become a regular feature of inquests on dead infants.[70]

Conclusion

The evolution of European legal systems following the fall of the Roman Empire, the barbarian 'invasions' and the rise to prominence of written Roman and canon law culminated in a current of modernization in methods of proof that crossed medieval Europe from west to east. Two zones initially co-existed, characterized as in England by the predominance of the jury and analogous institutions, and by the prevalence of the style of trial derived from Roman procedure and canon law, as in Italy and France. The former zone shrank as the latter expanded to the point of dominating the whole of western Europe, leaving in place procedural systems which differed on either side of the English Channel. In England, the existence of an early form of jury was close at hand to replace irrational methods of proof, whereas elsewhere the crisis of the old methods coincided more closely with the introduction of legal procedure based on a fusion of Roman and canon law.

From our point of view as historians of forensic medicine, this process of legal change produced two key outcomes. The first was the emergence of two quite different trial procedures, inquisitorial on the Continent and accu-satorial in England. In the former process, judges conducted investigations that were based on written testimony, and in order to reach the truth they often sought the opinions of persons not directly involved with the alleged crime, such as medical doctors. This led, second, to a need for what we might consider expert opinion, and thus to a tradition of written medical opinions which formed but one strand of a growing body of legal literature on evidence and proof. To all intents and purposes medico-legal scholarship on the Con-tinent was fostered by the procedures stipulated by the criminal justice system. In England, by contrast, the common law and accusatorial system relied entirely on eyewitnesses who gave oral testimony before a lay jury, who then became the final arbiters of justice; judges controlled procedure and passed sentence, but did not decide the outcome of cases. Although coroners and magistrates could summon individuals who had not been eyewitnesses, they were under no obligation to do so. Nor were there any formal requirements governing the standards of proof presented in court, but rather a marked reluctance to privilege any sort of opinion above that of the jury. Thus, according to Crawford, before about 1800 'the contrasting state of medico-legal scholarship in England and continental Europe reflected nothing so much as the logic of their legal systems'.[71]

Legal innovation did not stop in the early modern period, of course. Old laws were abandoned or codified; the Carolina, for example, survived until 1870. Legislators refined trial procedures; in France, the Revolution of 1789 was a major turning point in the law and its processes as in all else. New nations emerged and adapted the laws of their former masters: the United States and Canada added additional layers of complexity to the common law in the form of local, state/provincial and federal courts. Everywhere scientific innovation has made its presence felt in the courtroom. In the rest of this book, however, we will be concerned with both medico-legal scholarship and medico-legal practice, that is, what it was that medical practitioners actually did in the service of the law, how they did it, and the influence that their actions had on society at large. The law itself will henceforth be of as much significance as legal procedure, as later chapters will consider how specific statutes influenced forensic practice at particular points in time, most notably after 1760 when the spirit of enlightenment ushered in the beginnings of important changes in attitudes to insanity, infanticide and suicide, thus furthering the acceptance of medical explana-tions for deviant behaviour. The next chapter will serve as a foundation for that discussion, as it surveys the history of forensic medicine in the pre-modern West.

Additional reading

The references for this chapter can be found in the Bibliography, and will allow you to expand on all of the issues discussed here. If you wish to do some further reading, you may also consult the publications listed below.

Carl Ludwig von Bar, *A History of Continental Criminal Law*, trans. Thomas S. Bell (1916), Union, NJ: Lawbook Exchange, 1999.

Catherine Crawford, 'Medicine and the law', in W.F. Bynum and Roy Porter (eds), *Companion Encyclopedia of the History of Medicine*, vol. 2, London and New York: Routledge, 1993, pp. 1619–40.

J.M. Kelly, *A Short History of Western Legal Theory*, Oxford: Oxford University Press, 1992.

2 Medico-legal practice before the modern period

An understanding of the history of forensic medicine must start with the activity itself: the practical business of providing medical knowledge in a legal context. This chapter surveys medico-legal practice from the ancient world – Western civilization is after all built on foundations laid in classical Greece and Rome, through the medieval period to the last decades of the eighteenth century, when recognizably modern states emerged in Europe and North America. The notion of professional expertise is typically associated with nineteenth and twentieth century science and medicine in the service of the state,[1] a connection which will be examined in Chapter 3, but it has long been evident that in many areas of critical importance to the state and its citizens, individuals possessed of specialized knowledge have assumed a privileged competence in public administration,[2] not least in the law courts. Medical practitioners, as a consequence of their professional experience and skill in interpreting the mysteries of the human body, have been among the most visible actors in this historical process, a fact which scholarship of the past 30 years has done much to emphasize. Physicians, surgeons and midwives were found in various legal forums, most notably in relation to death and injury investigations but also in civil procedures involving allegations of sexual delinquency. When legal officials required information about the hidden interior of the body, and the consequences on it of exterior actions, they turned to those who possessed medical knowledge. This stands in contrast to the history of attitudes to the mind where, for reasons to be discussed in Chapter 4, deference was by no means always accorded to the medical profession.

Historians of forensic medicine have long tended to refer to medical practitioners who testified in legal settings as 'expert witnesses', a term which is now used to refer only to someone who has attained a recognized professional skill and standing and, ideally, some court experience too, and who is therefore sufficiently qualified to give evidence of both facts and opinion. Following this definition, it is reasonable to ask to what extent a medieval physician or an early modern country surgeon could really be described as an expert? The next chapter will consider the early modern shift in the notion of expertise from 'practical experience' to 'intellectual understanding'; but in the medieval period, insofar as an individual to whom the community afforded status as a person skilled in medicine possessed knowledge that other members of the community did not have, he or she was to all intents and purposes an expert whose opinion deserved and carried an associated authority. This chapter will show how and why such expertise was used in pre-modern courts; the problems which arose when experts began to range themselves against one another will be considered in Chapter 3.

The ancient world

Physicians had a forensic role in the ancient world. In Athens, Rome and, following conquest and assimilation by first the Greeks and then the Romans, Egypt, medical testimony was not only used in a range of civil and criminal circumstances, but in medical matters it was given greater credence than other witness testimony. From classical origins a precedent emerged: pre-modern legal systems permitted medical practitioners to participate in legal fact-finding in certain circumstances, and accorded them special status as expert witnesses.

In Athens forensic practice was shaped by the private nature of the legal system: no one but the party affected could act as plaintiff or prosecutor unless the welfare of the citizenry as a whole was at risk, so the injured person had to bring a private suit. Even homicide was considered a private offence, with the kinsmen of the deceased bearing the responsibility for investigating, indicting and prosecuting an alleged killer. Thus, although Athens had a public medical service,[3] the physicians retained by the city to work for it had no specified forensic role. Nor does there seem to have been any city officer whose job it was to investigate cases of people found dead. Instead, by the fourth century BCE two areas of private forensic practice had been established: citizens called physicians as witnesses to give legal testimony regarding injury, death or disease; and to certify illness that would prevent a person from performing the functions of an office for which they had been chosen.[4] Although medical testimony was not mandatory in classical Greece, it was often thought to be useful by citizens engaged in legal disputes.

Cases in which assault victims took legal action show that the injured party believed that jurors would be receptive to the force of a physician's testimony because of his professional status, while both Plato (*c*.428–347 BCE) and his pupil Aristotle (384–322 BCE) assumed that, in medical matters, a qualified doctor's knowledge was greater than a layman's. In the civil arena, the law required those who sold slaves to declare in advance any physical disability from which the slave suffered or the buyer could return the purchase. If the buyer was a physician, however, he was not entitled to compensation, implying that physicians were able to detect ailments that most people would fail to notice and also that a successful claim for restitution would require medical testimony. Disabled citizens were entitled to a pension from the city, and there is evidence that in cases where the right of entitlement was disputed, the claimant could call a doctor to testify on his behalf if the nature of the disability was not immediately obvious. Finally, if a citizen elected to public office declined to serve for reasons of ill health, he could send his physician to bear witness to his illness. As this was not required by law, it offers a further indication that the value of a doctor's testimony depended entirely on professional skill and experience,[5] which is precisely the distinction that underpins the modern understanding of an expert witness.

In Rome, as in Athens, the law did not specify when medical testimony must be sought but referred to situations in which it might have been relevant, for instance in regard to the legitimacy of children born after the death of the mother's husband.[6] Illness and insanity were of particular interest to Roman jurists because of their relevance to the obligations of citizens to perform public duties: if a person was seriously ill he could be excused from appearing in court as a plaintiff, defendant, magistrate or judge. Illness or insanity exempted a person from acting as a guardian to a minor or from serving in the army; slaves could be returned to their seller for physical defect or disease; and varying degrees of mental responsibility were recognized. Although suicide was not a crime, the Emperor Hadrian decreed that a soldier who attempted it without good reason (disease, unbearable pain, weariness of life, insanity, fear of dishonour, grief) should be executed. Castration was punishable by death, unless performed as a cure for some illness, and poisoning became a serious offence under the *Lex Cornelia*,[7] a law introduced by the dictator Sulla in 82 BCE. In all of these cases people must have had to prove their claims of illness, insanity or poisoning, but the written law gives no guidelines on how such proof was to be obtained. The only reference in Roman legal literature to the need for a physician related to the military: if a soldier who had been medically discharged wanted to return to the army, he had to be examined by a magistrate and a doctor.[8]

Although it was the duty of judges and magistrates to investigate cases, they reached decisions based on their own opinions about the weight of the evidence; they did not have to seek advice on matters of fact. There were three exceptions to this rule, in relation to land surveying, the use of handwriting experts where there were accusations of forgery, and the employment of midwives to certify pregnancy. These were all legally mandated forensic functions, but in other cases where doctors were called to testify in a forensic capacity, it was almost certainly at the request of a defendant or a victim's family. After the assassination of Julius Caesar (44 BCE), a physician examined the body and determined that, of the 23 wounds he had suffered, only one was fatal; but we do not know why this examination was carried out, or who suggested it. Nothing prevented jurists from asking for medical advice, however, and although the lack of more than a handful of references makes it difficult to know for certain what normal procedure was, it seems to have been largely a matter of personal habit or plain self-interest on the part of judges, magistrates, plaintiffs and defendants.[9] In Rome, where a cohort of privileged, state-registered doctors existed, such practices may well have been more common than they were in the provinces,[10] but it is doubtful that they were wholly exceptional.

A much different and entirely unique situation pertained in another part of the ancient world. In Egypt, which was ruled by the Greeks following the conquest of Alexander the Great (332 BCE), and which became a Roman province in 30 BCE, the Greek law that the immigrants imported was personal, not territorial, so that physicians were summoned to court on individual initiative, as in Athens itself. During the Roman period, however, a new and distinctive role emerged for physicians, who were assigned specific forensic tasks in cases involving violent or accidental death or injury, as part of an investigation of a potentially criminal matter or to make an examination and provide a written certificate. Those who did the forensic work were called from among the ranks of the public physicians (*demosioi iatroi*), and by the middle of the second century CE they were writing medical reports (*prosphoneseis*) certifying death or the extent of injury.[11]

In Roman Egypt not only was it mandatory for magistrates to send public doctors to conduct medical examinations, but private individuals who were contemplating legal action sometimes requested a formal medical assessment. This differs considerably from a citizen asking their own doctor to appear as a court witness, as occurred in Athens and Rome, and begs the question of how the practice originated. A persuasive case can be made that it grew out of the vast bureaucracy that Ptolemaic Egypt inherited from the pharaohs, in which experts of various kinds were summoned whenever officials needed advice. This practice was modified by successive waves of conquest but, firmly established and with a proven tendency to ever greater complexity, under Greek influence and following Athenian custom some forensic medical practice was established. Then, the more intricate the bureaucracy became, the more its officials tended to delegate tasks and duties which were then written into procedural guidelines, so that forensic work acquired a formal role in law.[12]

At the end of the classical period, then, forensic medical testimony was not obligatory in any legal system other than that of Roman Egypt, but where it seemed to be in their own best interest the parties in civil and criminal cases, and also judges and magistrates, sought the opinion of a medical practitioner. After the fall of the Western Empire public medical service died out but the medical profession carried on, its members' conduct regulated by laws designed to standardize their activities and encourage responsible behaviour; the practice of medicine remained, as it had been in Greece and Rome, a craft taught by apprenticeship.[13] Thus, while literacy and consequently learned medicine fell into abeyance outside centres of Christian scholasticism,[14] medico-legal practice in a form oriented to the needs of barbarian law continued: its application shifted away from illness and insanity toward a clear focus on bodily injury.

Pre-modern criminal contexts

As we saw in Chapter 1, the personal and accusatorial nature of barbarian law led to the development of a system of monetary compensation for all forms of personal injury, called *wergeld*, whilst the irrational proofs of compurgation, ordeal and judicial battle were used to determine criminal guilt or innocence. Although there is no evidence that medicine played a role in evaluating the physical effects of ordeals, for *wergeld* it was a different matter. The principle of financial recompense meant that barbarian law-givers became dependent on medical advice for the assessment of wounds which their laws, promulgated between the fifth and tenth centuries, classified and described in meticulous detail.[15] The law of the Alemanni tribe, in present-day Germany, gave precise anatomical details of wounds and discussed the value to be assigned to them depending on their location and gravity, requiring this to be assessed by a competent physician.[16] The Visigothic Code enacted a system graded according to the wealth of the offender as well as the serious-ness of the wound.[17] The Franco-Germanic Salic Law Code of the early sixth century was much more gruesomely detailed:[18]

> If any person have wished to strike another with a poisoned arrow, and the arrow have glanced aside, and it shall be proved on him; he shall be sentenced to 2,500 denars, which make 63 shillings.
>
> If any person strike another on the head so that the brain appears, and the three bones which lie above the brain shall project, he shall be sentenced to 1,200 denars, which make 30 shillings.
>
> But if it shall have been between the ribs or in the stomach, so that the wound appears and reaches to the entrails, he shall be sentenced to 1,200 denars – which make 30 shillings – besides five shillings for the physician's pay.
>
> If any one shall have struck a man so that blood falls to the floor, and it be proved on him, he shall be sentenced to 600 denars, which make 15 shillings.

In a clear break with Roman law, which did not grant human status to a foetus, the Christian barbarians strengthened laws against abortion, enacting legislation which increasingly reflected church policy. Thus, there was special provision for pregnant women. The Salian (northern) Franks allotted a *wergeld* of 28,000 denars for the death of a pregnant freeborn woman, but only 8,000 for the killing of a woman past child-bearing years,[19] while the Visigoths made abortion a crime subject to execution or blinding.[20] In all cases, wounds were to be assessed by those competent to do so.

The barbarians were responsible for a further – remarkably long-lasting – innovation which can properly be considered to be part of the history of medico-legal practice. In the event of a suspicious death, the victim's body presented one obvious starting point for investigation, and some form of body inspection was as we have seen not unknown in the ancient world. But between a simple viewing of the body and the modern medico-legal autopsy there was an intermediate stage known as cruentation, from the Latin *cruentare*, to make bloody or to spot with blood. Also known as the ordeal of the bier (a sign of its origins as a species of irrational proof), cruentation was a simple test used to reveal a murderer. Of Germanic origin and largely confined to northern Europe, it was considered to be a judgment of God manifested by the 'indignation' of a corpse when its killer was nearby. Standard procedure called for the suspected murderer to approach the dead body, call it by name, walk around it two or three times, and stroke its wounds. Evidence of guilt was revealed if during the process fresh bleeding occurred, the body twitched or foam appeared at the mouth. Theory held that a sympathetic action between the cadaver and its murderer would occur,[21] but any positive outcomes were almost certainly due to natural post-mortem effects.[22]

Cruentation occurred in medieval Britain, France, Germany, Italy and the Netherlands, apparently for two quite different reasons. In England and Scotland, it provided a form of proof to legal officials who did not have recourse to the Continental procedures of torture and formal medico-legal investigation to provide evidence against suspects; in Italy and France, the bleeding of a corpse in the presence of a suspect was thought to supply evidence sufficient to justify torture.[23] Cruentation probably survived for so long because the reactions of the guilty person could often be as revealing as anything that the corpse might do: if witnesses believed that the dead body might reveal its murderer, the killer was likely to yield to psychological intimidation and give himself away. It had become much less common by the seventeenth century, but there is a record of it being used in France as late as 1639. It was considered conclusive evidence in two cases tried at the English assizes in the first third of the seventeenth century, and in a Scottish case of 1688 cruentation was adduced as a link in the chain of evidence against a parricide. It was used in support of a case tried at Marburg in 1608, and seems to have continued in use in some German states during the early eighteenth century, as it was the subject of a book by Michael Alberti (1682–1757), the professor of forensic medicine at Halle: *On Haemorrhages from Corpses and the Principle of Cruentation* (1726).[24] In a case of infanticide that took place in Wales in 1753, the men who retrieved the infant corpse from a pond fetched the presumed mother

> in order to prevail with her to take the said infant out of the pool (this examinant imagining that if it was her child and she had any wise occasioned the death of it, the corpse would bleed afresh on her touching it) but when [she] was brought ... she would not be persuaded to touch the said corpse or come near the pool in which the said infant lay.[25]

The surprising vitality of this popular belief is reflected in nineteenth-century references in England and the United States, where Mark Twain alluded to it in *The Adventures of Tom Sawyer* (1876).[26]

For a brief period during the early medieval era the barbarian reliance on irrational proofs was displaced by the thoughtful system established by Charlemagne (742–814) during his 14-year reign as Holy Roman Emperor. In his Capitularies, a compilation of Germanic, Roman and Frankish law codes, he insisted that judges should not condemn without being confident of the fairness of the judgment, which should be based on clear and relevant proofs.[27] Judges were therefore mandated to seek medical evidence, most especially in questions of blows and wounds, infanticide, suicide, rape, bestiality and divorce on the grounds of impotence.[28] The extent to which the Capitularies can be viewed as a short-lived attempt to create an early type of medico-legal practice is at best doubtful, as it is by no means evident that these formal exhortations ever took the form of concrete action; and, in any case, at Charlemagne's death central control of his vast empire vanished and local customs favouring private arbitration over public judgment reasserted themselves. It would not however be unreasonable to suppose that vestiges of the ideal remained in a form suited to the needs of the feudal societies that succeeded the empire, so that when public justice and legal scholarship re-emerged in the twelfth century – stimulated by communal government in Italy, strong monarchs in England, Sicily, Germany and France, and the papacy – some of the practices suggested by Charlemagne could be revived.

The legal codes enacted for the Frankish states established by crusaders in the Latin East (1099–1291), known collectively as the Assizes of Jerusalem, indicate that some Carolingian norms survived in France, from where the crusaders imported the feudal laws and customs utilized in the Holy Land. The most important work, for medico-legal purposes, was the *Livre des assises et des usages et des plais de la haute cort dou reiaume de Jerusalem* (*The Book of Assizes, Customs and Pleas of the High Court of the Kingdom of Jerusalem*, dating from the mid thirteenth century), which specified the use of physical examinations by medical practitioners on behalf of the legal system when a man claimed to be too ill to appear in court to plead, and thus possibly be subjected to trial by combat. In such instances, three members of the court (that is, other vassals) were to establish this with the aid of a doctor (*miege, fisisien*), who would examine the man, take his pulse and inspect his urine; or a surgeon (*selorgien*), who would examine his wound. If they were not convinced, he had to go to court.[29] In cases of alleged murder, three persons were to examine the body but the Assizes did not specify that they must be medically trained; it seems unlikely, however, that no medical opinion would have been sought.[30]

Medico-legal examinations appear to have been reasonably frequent in medieval France and were, importantly for the development of forensic medicine, formalized in legal practice. The bishops of Maine and Anjou had medical experts (*médecins jurés*) in their service from the eleventh century, there were surgeon-experts in Paris from the twelfth century, and when Louis IX suppressed ordeals and judicial combat in 1260, replacing them with written witness statements, he established a link between sworn medical testimony and legal procedure. Louis's successors Philip III and Philip IV provided for sworn surgeons in legal matters, and at the Châtelet (the main Parisian municipal court), sworn physicians, surgeons and midwives were regularly required to provide written reports on the injured, people found dead in public places, and in matters of pregnancy and sexual offences. Norman laws of the thirteenth century similarly ordered medical inspections by 'expert men and reliable women' in cases of disease, injury and rape. These reports were intended to provide a diagnosis, prognosis for recovery, and an indication of whether a death was due to criminal causes, but judicial records suggest that examinations were external only. Although the quality of the medical information provided by an exterior examination may have been deficient, the recognition that medical practitioners had a valuable forensic role to play is of great significance;[31] it created a formal need for written reports and appointed medical experts who, by means of repetition, gained a level of practical expertise.[32] Later, it provided a ready market for textbooks and guides designed to aid those who served the courts.

The degree to which medico-legal practice was embedded in French legal procedure, and the way in which it was conducted, is vividly portrayed in the criminal records of the Provençal town of Manosque. With a population of 3–4,000 between 1262 and 1348, the inhabitants were well served by the medical profession: 41 physicians and surgeons, three apothecaries and a number of midwives practised in the town, with approximately four to five practitioners active in any given year. It was these individuals who provided expert opinions 'à la demande de la cour ou des personnes intéressées'.[33] Sometimes the doctor was selected because he had attended the victim of an assault who subsequently sued their attacker, but in cases of serious wounding or death a judge would order one or more practitioners, some of whom held court accreditation, to examine the victim and write a report. The earliest of these documents (1285) pre-dates the earliest surviving Italian medico-legal reports (1289; see Case Study 2.1), to which manosquin practices can be

---

Case Study 2.1: The death of Jacobus Rustighelli, Bologna, February 1289

One of the earliest extant medico-legal reports was written at Bologna in 1289, when two physicians were sent by a judge to view the corpse of a man lying dead in a church, to which the body was presumably carried by the first finders. The case is indicative of medieval medico-legal procedure, including the directing role of legal officials and the general lack of autopsy.

Master Albertus Malevoda and Master Amoretus, physicians, who, on the injunction of Albertus of Gandino, judge, have seen and examined Jacobus Rustighelli in the Church of St Catherine of Saracocia, wounded and dead, state in concordance, after having seen and examined, to have found the following: in the thorax, seven deadly wounds; in the neck, one deadly wound; in the middle of the forehead, two deadly wounds; in the occiput, one deadly wound; in the upper jaw, one non-fatal wound. Sworn to be true on Saturday 12 February.

Source: E.H. Ackerknecht, 'Early history of legal medicine', in C.R. Burns (ed.), *Legacies in Law and Medicine*, New York: Science History Publications, 1977, p. 265.

compared,[34] suggesting that in both Italy and France forensic testimony was well established in urban centres by the second half of the thirteenth century. Geographical proximity to one of the host of universities founded during the Middle Ages was surely a significant contributory factor: Salerno (10th century), Bologna (1088), Paris (1150), Montpellier (1220), Padua (1222), Naples (1224) and Toulouse (1229) were all institutions built on strong traditions of teaching in medicine and law.

In Italy, the thirteenth century proved to be a watershed, as the papacy began to extend its power over worldly authorities in matters of justice. Reflecting on the separate cases of two Italian clerics who had been involved in the untimely deaths of men struck on the head during melees, Pope Innocent III (1198–1216) demanded medical evidence to help him determine how to apportion blame. His decisions were recorded in decretals issued in 1209, which provided a foundation in canon law for the formal appointment of doctors to the courts to give evidence about cause of death and the nature of wounds, at which time such practice seems already to have been established.[35] Canon lawyers had by now expressed the principle of expertise: 'Quaecumque in arte peritis credendum est' (Whatever those skilled in an art find worthy of belief),[36] and it can be no coincidence that prior to his election as pontiff, Innocent received legal training at Bologna, the most prominent centre of legal learning in Europe since the twelfth-century fusion of Roman and canon law. Thus endowed with the authority of the church, secular authorities soon turned to dissection in the cause of justice. In 1249 the surgeon Hugo of Lucca (*c.*1160–1257) took an oath to act as medico-legal consultant to Bologna, the first city in Europe to make statutory provision (1252) for medical evidence in criminal cases and to permit autopsy, and which in 1292 founded an elected college of paid experts.[37] Yet, although Bolognese doctors performed some of the earliest known medico-legal autopsies, on an alleged victim of poisoning in 1302, and on a woman who died of internal bleeding in 1307,[38] the use of autopsy remained relatively infrequent and highly localized: French doctors measured and probed wounds but did not regularly open bodies in the interests of criminal justice, while those in Bologna and Venice were far more likely to do so.[39]

Venetian statutes were similar to those of Bologna. To enable public officials to take control of violent incidents and prevent private acts of vengeance, a city ordinance of 1281 required doctors – who had to register with and meet standards set by their guild and the government – to inform the municipal police of wounds that seemed to result from violence. Even more importantly, medico-legal autopsy was common in Venice: it was required in all murder cases and whenever the cause of death was unclear, and fourteenth-century criminal records show that its use was not infrequent.[40] As evidence of the myth of medieval resistance to human dissection, the use in Italy of autopsy for both judicial and educational purposes spread to several northern cities during the fourteenth century,[41] and within two hundred years all the principal Italian city states had made formal provision for the use of medico-legal witnesses.[42] The Italians did not share northern European religious beliefs about bodily integrity or related taboos against opening corpses, nor did they acknowledge a papal prohibition against autopsy: in 1299 Boniface VIII prohibited the boiling of flesh off human bones, but not dissection. It is this that explains their readiness to perform autopsies during a period when the practice was unusual outside Italy and, to a lesser extent, southern France.[43]

In 1234, under the terms of the *Nova Compilatio Decretalium* of Pope Gregory IX (1227–41), doctors acquired the unpleasant task of overseeing the application of judicial torture by ecclesiastical tribunals (the nascent Papal Inquisition, charged with rooting out heresy), an undertaking that was soon imitated by other courts.[44] The details of what medical practitioners actually did in this regard are not extensive, as medieval legal records are often silent about the grisly particulars, but doctors were present to treat the victims' physical injuries and to ensure that they did not die.[45] In early modern Spain medical men looked after the health of suspects held in the prisons of the Inquisition, advised on their mental state, and determined whether prisoners were in a fit condition to undergo torture or non-capital punishments. In cases of men accused of being Jews, surgeons had to confirm whether they were circumcised.[46]

The papal edict of 1234 also specified a number of offences which required medical evidence to support a charge, including affairs that normally concerned the Church, such as marriage, abortion and sexual transgressions, but also witchcraft, concealment of pregnancy and infanticide.[47] Leprosy was of medical, legal and social importance, and canon law called on physicians to diagnose the disease so that lepers could be banished from society.[48]

Medico-legal reports were commonplace in Paris between 1300 and the late sixteenth century,[49] when the king's surgeon Ambroise Paré published his *Traité des rapports* (*Treatise on Reports*, 1575), but the degree to which the practice was regularized in Paris or elsewhere is unclear. The Châtelet had both expert surgeons (*chirurgiens jurés*), who held a monopoly on providing judicial reports,[50] and expert midwives (*matrones jurées*) from the fourteenth century, but we do not know how magistrates elsewhere generally obtained expert medical testimony, though the evidence from medieval Manosque is suggestive. Some method was clearly in place, however, for Paré's work, the first of its kind in Europe, offered advice to surgeons on what he saw as the key problems of legal medicine (violent death and disputed sexual relations),[51] provided examples of medico-legal reports, and reminded readers of the responsibility they bore because judges relied on their opinion.[52]

Some regularity was imposed in 1606 when Henri IV gave his chief physician the right to appoint by warrant, in all towns within the royal jurisdiction, two experienced and well-reputed persons from the disciplines of medicine and surgery to hold the exclusive right to provide medico-legal reports to the courts on all victims of wounding and homicide; in Paris the king himself appointed the sworn experts.[53] The criminal ordinance of 1670 reaffirmed the duty of judges to order medico-legal reports from an officially-appointed physician, surgeon or midwife – municipal posts created in 1662 (for an example of such a report, see Case Study 2.2), gave injured victims the right

---

Case Study 2.2: The death of Jeanne Souchet, Mantes, February 1683

Jean Devaux (1649–1729), a master surgeon of Paris, recorded this case in his guide to writing surgical reports for legal purposes (1703). An unspecified number of royal doctors were ordered by the *Procureur du Roi* (crown prosecutor) of the town of Mantes (50km west of Paris) to examine the body of a woman found dead in a nearby village. The case is typical of Continental medico-legal practice at this time: the body was opened on site, selectively, to allow the surgeons to form conclusions based on direct observation. They then offered an opinion about the manner and cause of death: a murder (by stabbing) had been staged to look like a suicide.

> We have found the corpse of a woman, aged about 50 years, hanging from a rafter which we were told was the body of a certain Jeanne Souchet. As this corpse had the face in no way discoloured, nor any foam at the mouth, no black tongue, no nostrils filled with mucous excrement nor even the slightest redness, wound or other change of colour round the neck at the place where the cord by which it had been suspended had made its impression we have decided to make an exact examination of all the other parts of the corpse. Whereupon we have found a very small wound at the anterior right part of the thorax, hidden under the breast and where a small probe could hardly enter. Having dilated this opening

we have found that it penetrated between the sixth and fifth rib. Whereupon we have opened the thorax in order to study the progress of the said wound. We have found that this little wound has been produced by a round, very narrow piercing instrument and traversing the heart from one side to the other had caused a great, very extensive haemorrhage into the thorax. In summarizing all these observations we conclude that the wound in the thorax has preceded the suspension of the corpse of the said Souchet woman and has been the only and true cause of her death. (23 February 1683.)

Sources: E.H. Ackerknecht, 'Early history of legal medicine', in C.R. Burns (ed.), *Legacies in Law and Medicine*, New York: Science History Publications, 1977, pp. 269–70; J. Devaux, *L'art de faire les raports en chirurgie*, Paris: Laurent D'Houry, 1703, pp. 518–20.

to seek a medical examination from any other doctor for use in court, and required midwives to examine women under sentence of death who claimed or appeared to be pregnant. In the early 1690s the right to appoint experts was transferred to local corporations of surgeons and physicians. Appointments were made on payment of a fee to the government and the offices consequently acquired a hereditary and venal nature that did little to promote the interests of the best qualified candidates. Corrupt or not, however, the system remained in place until it was abolished in 1790.[54]

In contrast to the French and Italians, the English and Germans 'came almost to the end of the Middle Ages with a native, customary legal tradition substantially undisturbed by Roman law', with laymen entrenched in the administration of the criminal justice system.[55] Notwithstanding structural similarities, however, very different medico-legal imperatives existed in the two countries, differences which must in my view be ascribed to the Carolingian inheritance. In the German states, ruled by Charlemagne's heirs and successors, the laws and practices instituted by the 'father of Europe' lived on, while the inhabitants of Anglo-Saxon Britain went their own way, at a clear remove from the European legal tradition found in the lands that Charlemagne had dominated.[56] While both countries relied on accusatorial legal proceedings and placed judicial power in the hands of lay officials, the English inquest and trial obviated the need for medico-legal evidence (the jurors were the fact-finders), whereas the Germans, harking back to the barbarian focus on private compensation, retained an interest in establishing the severity of wounds and thus preserved a forensic role for medicine in the public prosecutorial system that developed during the medieval period.

The key distinction between the history of legal change in Germany from that in France and England was the lack of central direction;[57] municipalities and territories followed their own local procedures in matters of law and, for that matter, medicine, and our knowledge of those practices is shaped by the greater survival rate of municipal records. These show that medieval town physicians – some of whom were actually surgeons – included among their duties the writing of forensic reports on injuries,[58] as in Italy and France. The evidence from medieval Freiburg shows that from 1275, those who had been wounded had to establish that it was 'durch hut und durch braten', through skin and flesh, in order to take the case to the town's high court, suggesting that it was from this date that medical evidence became formally desirable. A city law of 1218–20 had required each of the 24 court judges to inspect the victim of a homicide, and by 1293 three members of the lower court were to inspect the wounded. In 1361 the Emperor gave the high court the right to bring criminal charges if the victim could or would not do so, and it may have been this shift to a form of public prosecution which led to the city's high court ordinance of *c.*1407–17, which was the first to require that two members of the high court together with the surgeons or barber-surgeons 'that belong to the commission' – almost certainly the town surgeons – should be sent to inspect the wounded or dead.[59] By the early sixteenth century surgeons had become dominant in the medico-legal sphere and in Freiburg, the founding of the university and medical school in 1457 did much to advance the quality of the medical expertise that the courts could draw upon.

Other cities, including Magdeburg, Freising, Basel and Memmingen, had similar laws, generally designed to use medical evidence to determine the degree of seriousness of a wound and thus which court, lower or higher, the case should go to. The procedure in Freiburg may have been the most meticulous; surgeons were specifically mandated to decide, in tandem with two judges, whether the wounds had caused death and, if so, whether the circumstances warranted a high court case. Only in Freiburg was there no requirement to present physical evidence (part of the body, a bloody garment, hair) as a material representation that a crime had been committed. The Capital Court Statute of the prince-bishopric of Bamberg near Bavaria (the Bambergensis, 1507), on which the Carolina was closely modelled,[60] finally abolished *wergeld* and compurgation but still required the presence in court of physical proof of a crime in order to initiate a case. The Carolina substituted protocol (article 149) and written documents for this last remnant of the medieval legal tradition.[61]

Medico-legal practice was thus clearly an established part of the judicial procedure in Germany for centuries before the Carolina made it compulsory throughout the Empire. Going further than the previous city codes, which had sought to establish whether there was a case to answer but had not built medical testimony into the judgment process, the new criminal code appreciated that many questions could not be settled by purely legal methods and, in cases of doubt and difficulty where death had resulted from violence or suspicious means, whether criminal or accidental, it compelled the judges to seek the evidence of medical men. They were sworn in advance, and more than one could be consulted. Knowledge of anatomy became essential, especially as so many of the cases involved surgical issues, and there was a correlation between the date of the statute, the rise of the study of anatomy and the growth of a new area of intellectual medical study. The old medical hierarchy soon asserted itself, however, and in Germany physicians with specialized anatomical and physiological knowledge of the body tended to become responsible for writing medical reports, rather than lowlier surgeons and midwives. In a system called *Aktenversendung* (despatch of the *Akte*, the written case record), German courts referred entire case dossiers to external specialists, particularly university faculties of law and medicine, for discussion and expert advice. In capital cases, of which there were many, these collective decisions were especially important and were therefore periodically published for instructional purposes, the first such volumes appearing within a few years of the promulgation of the Carolina.[62] Soon those who were involved with them began writing their own monographs on subjects of related interest, triggering the creation of a recognizable discipline of forensic medicine. It became a subject for special instruction in the eighteenth century with the creation of professorships in most German universities.[63]

The situation in England was the least satisfactory so far as forensic medical activity is concerned, largely because of the key role played by the coroner in the investigation of sudden and unnatural deaths. Of Norman origin, the office was formally created in 1194 to take on some of the duties previously performed by legal officials known as justiciars (essentially judges at the town or county level), sheriffs (county officials responsible for administering justice and collecting revenues) and their subordinates the serjeants; and also to safeguard the financial interests of the crown.[64] As independent officials elected for the whole county, coroners served for life, had to hold land and high social status, were obliged to keep written records, and assumed responsibility for a wide variety of functions of potential pecuniary concern to the monarch. These included the appraisal of the goods and chattels of outlaws, felons and suicides; and the assessment of deodands. These were god-gifts, the value of a moveable object or animal that had caused a death, originally payable to the church in expiation of the 'sin' but usually forfeited to the crown and abolished as late as 1846. By far the most important and frequent duty of the coroner was to enquire into the death of anyone who died suddenly, in prison, in suspicious circumstances, or from anything other than natural causes. This was done in a procedure known as an inquest.[65]

When a death occurred the coroner was summoned by the person who found the body, or by the sheriff's bailiff, and then assembled a jury of 12 to 21 men from the four neighbouring townships. The jurors and coroner together inspected the naked body which, if it had been buried, was exhumed, examining it for injuries and signs of violence with the aim of establishing the identity of the deceased, the time and place of death, and the cause and manner of death (by what means and whether natural, suicidal, accidental or homicidal). Jurors reached their conclusions on the basis of their external inspection of the body, information provided by the first-finder and other local people, and their own knowledge; there was no requirement to consult a doctor. Records of medieval and early modern inquests, which survive in large numbers, tend to record decisions and bare case outlines rather than deliberations,[66] however, so despite the extensive historiography which draws upon these manuscripts – investigating everything from the office of coroner to the incidence of and public reaction to suicide, infanticide and murder – little is known about the participation of medical professionals in English inquests prior to the seventeenth century. All the available evidence suggests, however, that medical testimony did not become usual in English inquests until after the middle of the eighteenth century.[67]

The principal reason for this delay in the introduction of medical evidence to inquests was financial. The office of coroner was unpaid until 1487, when a fee of 13s for each inquest into a homicide (murder, manslaughter or suicide) was permitted, plus 4d from the goods of the guilty man, at last providing an incentive for neglectful coroners to perform their duties. That this did little to encourage the investigation of accidents was acknowledged in 1509 when any coroner who failed to hold an inquest or demanded a fee in cases of mis-adventure could be fined 40s, though the reason for this was not the forensic need to exclude homicide but the fact that such bodies remained unburied![68] More importantly, the Act of 1509 (1 Hen VIII c.7) gave justices of the peace – unpaid part-time officers of local government and justice established by statute in 1361 – the power to enquire into coronial defaults, thus confirming their administrative power over coroners. A new law of 1751 finally sanctioned the payment of £1 to coroners for each inquest 'duly held' plus travel expenses of 9d per mile (one way only), but the justices often assumed that inquests were unnecessary except in cases of obvious violence and refused to pay, leaving coroners and witnesses out of pocket. Even the Medical Witnesses Act of 1836, which for the first time authorized coroners to obtain medical evidence – an autopsy and toxicological analysis could be carried out for a maximum fee of £2.2s – did not prevent interference by the justices, and coroners were not freed from this constraint until 1860, when they became salaried officials. A further boost to their authority and autonomy was provided by the Coroner's Act of 1887, which gave them the power to hold inquests whenever they felt it appropriate, and in the following year the office became one held on appointment by a city or county council. By this time most coroners tended to be either solicitors or doctors, though no formal educational standards were set until 1926, when the Coroner's Amendment Act made it compulsory for coroners to be qualified in law or medicine. The earliest known medically qualified coroners were surgeons elected during the second half of the eighteenth century.[69]

Female practitioners

The forensic activities of female practitioners known as midwives, matrons or *sages-femmes*, were more limited in scope than those of male physicians and surgeons but were nonetheless significant to pre-modern European justice systems. As the principal providers of birth assistance until the eighteenth century, midwives were valued for their familiarity with female bodies, the processes of pregnancy and childbirth, and the stages of child development, and it was for their expertise in these matters that legal officials sought them out. The criminal courts required midwives to examine the victims of rape and infanticide, women under sentence of death who claimed pregnancy, and even on occasion suspected witches; the civil courts asked their opinion in cases of disputed pregnancy and virginity; and the ecclesiastical courts mandated them to examine men and women suspected of being impotent. Midwives took oaths as medical practitioners and expert witnesses just as men did, were licensed to practice and paid by the courts, and had to be trustworthy and reputable in order to keep their jobs.[70] They were throughout the early modern period the normal attendants at childbirth, but they did not have a monopoly on knowledge about birth or women's bodies: the process of professionalization that began in western European medicine in the thirteenth century was dominated by literate men, so that when gynaecology emerged as a specialized medical discipline in the sixteenth century, its practitioners looked to male authorities, not to midwives, as experts on obstetrics.[71] This led to a gradual lessening of midwives' sphere of expertise, from the bodies of both mother and baby, to a more restricted focus on the pregnant female body or the external appearances of birth or rape; male doctors assumed responsibility for overseeing their work.[72] The masculinization of obstetrics was most extreme in Britain and the United States,[73] but midwives were eventually supplanted in the Western courtroom by more scientifically trained doctors, a process which began during the sixteenth century, gathered pace during the eighteenth and was largely complete by the end of the nineteenth century.[74]

This decline in the status of the midwife followed centuries of relative autonomy. They held positions of respect in the ancient world, being among the first medical personnel to appear as court witnesses; in Rome this was tied to the legal definition of the duration of pregnancy (ten months) and the prohibition against the execution of pregnant women. Midwives provided opinions on the presence or absence of virginity, pregnancy and female impotence, and on trauma or infection of the female sexual organs. They seem to have had a relatively high status in ancient Rome, but we have little information about their activities between the fall of the Western Empire and the later Middle Ages. What is known of barbarian law in the period implies that male physicians assessed injuries to both males and females, but it is likely that midwives were responsible for examining women when rape or pregnancy were involved: in the moral climate of the time, it was improper for a man to see and touch a woman's genitals.[75]

Our knowledge of midwives in a medico-legal setting resumes in the thirteenth century, when the Roman legal tradition was reflected in an order made by Gregory IX in 1220 that women should be examined by midwives in divorce proceedings: impotence was almost the only legal ground for dissolution of a marriage, so canon law judges had to be certain of its existence and causes.[76] The proof in such cases had previously relied on compurgation, but this was replaced first by inspection of the woman to establish her virginity, and then by inspection of the man. We will return to the curious institution of trial by congress, which evolved from this practice, in Chapter 5.

French court archives contain numerous examples of midwives' forensic testimony, mainly in cases of rape, assaults on pregnant women, and doubtful pregnancy. Female virginity was important in allegations of rape and male impotence, and pregnancy could delay torture and execution. It tended to offer a temporary respite, however, not a permanent escape, and it is likely that until alternative punishments were put in place, women sentenced to death simply remained in prison until they had given birth and were then executed, though some may have been pardoned, as is known to have happened in seventeenth-century England. The role of the midwife as a medico-legal expert was fixed in German law by the Carolina of 1532, and the same provision was included in a Swiss law of 1530: as in Italy and France, midwives were to provide written reports.[77]

This procedure was made problematic by the fact that many midwives were unable to write, and from the sixteenth century onward physicians and surgeons launched attacks on their competence. One form this took was controversy over the female hymen; medical men denied its existence because evidence of an intact hymen was one of the foundations of the midwife's diagnosis of virginity. Regardless of professional rivalry, however, midwives continued to carry out important medico-legal functions in Europe until the eighteenth century. Abortion and infanticide were within their purview, and criminal justice records show that midwives often testified in trials for newborn child murder and rape in France, England, Italy, Holland, Germany and Spain. In France, midwives were required by law to ascertain the father of the children they delivered, to ensure that men paid for the upkeep of their offspring, and to notify local authorities of possible secret births; English midwives performed a similar role.[78]

In England, always a little different from its European neighbours, a unique institution known as the jury of matrons came into existence in the thirteenth century. Unlike the formal procedures followed by Continental judges and court-appointed midwives, English judges would when necessary select, in a fairly ad hoc manner, 12 matrons, married women who had borne children but who were not necessarily or even probably midwives, to carry out forensic tasks. In civil cases they decided whether a widow was pregnant by her dead husband, a question affecting inheritance, or if a woman was a virgin; and in criminal cases they determined whether women sentenced to death were pregnant with a 'quick' child, a foetus old enough to be felt moving inside its mother, or if a woman had recently given birth. This function of women in English courts migrated to the colonial United States and survived in both countries until the late nineteenth century, when male obstetricians and gynaecologists had achieved dominance as experts on pregnancy and child-birth and the courts had grown accustomed to the use of medical expertise. As in so many other areas of medico-legal practice, then, the English were out of step with their European counterparts as a direct consequence of their legal system: the jury of matrons, though clearly a specialty jury of a kind known since the seventeenth century,[79] in no way possessed the expertise, in training or experience, that midwives had. There was no requirement for them to do so: the role was established in legal practice well before English courts grew amenable to the use of expert witnesses and abandoned the ideal of the self-informing jury.[80]

Conclusion

An apparently straightforward pattern of forensic activity emerges when medico-legal practice in Europe during the pre-modern period is considered, characterized by three key features. Most important, and the point that goes furthest in explaining the obvious differences between England and her Continental neighbours, is the determining role of the law; wherever the law and its officers recognized that medical practitioners could be useful to the maintenance of an orderly society, and were mandated to seek out medical advice and assistance, medico-legal activities were fostered and supported, leading by the early modern period to the development of a new and recognizably academic field of study. In the absence of a clear legal directive, as in ancient Athens or early modern England, however, forensic practice was at best ad hoc and at worst non-existent. The development of forensic medicine as an academic discipline was thus largely due to stimulating factors external to medicine. In the German lands the Carolina spurred the creation of an academic literature devoted to medico-legal problems, and this was soon followed by the creation of university posts. In Italy, canon law and cultural beliefs about the dead body sanctioned activities that civic authorities swiftly appropriated to their own needs, as the interpersonal violence endemic during the medieval period was brought increasingly under state control. In France a mixture of feudal, canon and royal law, together with a strong tradition of medical learning, enabled civic authorities to retain sworn experts of both sexes, although of course Parisian practices may not have been replicated in the provinces. In England, by comparison, where jurors were long held to be the principal fact-finders in both criminal and civil cases, there was little to encourage medico-legal practice or scholarship until new laws and changing perceptions of old ones began to impact on investigative procedures, most obviously in relation to infanticide and suicide (see Chapter 5).

Second, until the twentieth-century introduction of a host of forensic techniques that took things like bullets, insects and fibres as much as people as a focus of interest at the scene of a crime, the victim's body offered the only starting point in the investigation of interpersonal offences. Bodies were thus the main source of evidence in medico-legal work of all kinds, not just in death investigations but in any case that involved questions of identity, or where individuals were alleged to have engaged in criminal practices that might leave bodily traces (witches, homosexuals, infanticidal mothers), and subsequent chapters will suggest how medico-legal interest in the human body can reveal changes in social attitudes and practices. Lastly, the extensive history of medico-legal practice in pre-modern Europe shows that even though the medical practitioners called upon by the law may not always have been particularly distinguished, nor their testimony privileged above that of other witnesses, legal tribunals accepted that their knowledge in medical matters was superior to that of the average person, and therefore accorded them a status as experts which other witnesses did not have.

Additional reading

The references for this chapter can be found in the Bibliography, and will allow you to expand on all of the issues discussed here. If you wish to do some further reading, you may also consult the publications listed below.

Helen Brock and Catherine Crawford, 'Forensic medicine in early colonial Maryland, 1633–83', in Michael Clark and Catherine Crawford (eds), *Legal Medicine in History*, Cambridge: Cambridge University Press, 1994, 25–44.

Tatjana Buklijaš and Stella Fatović-Ferenčić, 'Medico-legal practices in the fifteenth century Dubrovnik', *Croatian Medical Journal*, 2004, vol. 45, 220–25.

Esther Fischer-Homberger, *Medizin vor Gericht: Gerichtsmedizin von der Renaissance bis zur Aufklärung*, Bern: Hans Huber, 1983.

T. R. Forbes, 'Early forensic medicine in England: the Angus murder trial', *Journal of the History of Medicine and Allied Sciences*, 1981, vol. 36, 286–309.

—— 'A jury of matrons', *Medical History*, 1988, vol. 32, 23–33.

Malcolm Gaskill, 'The displacement of providence: policing and prosecution in seventeenth- and eighteenth-century England', *Continuity and Change*, 1996, vol. 11, 341–79.

David Harley, 'The scope of legal medicine in Lancashire and Cheshire, 1660–1760', in Michael Clark and Catherine Crawford (eds), *Legal Medicine in History*, Cambridge: Cambridge University Press, 1994, 45–63.

Mary Lindemann, 'The body debated: bodies and rights in seventeenth- and eighteenth-century Germany', *Journal of Medieval and Early Modern Studies*, 2008, vol. 38, 493–521.

Cathy McClive, 'The hidden truths of the belly: the uncertainties of pregnancy in early modern Europe', *Social History of Medicine*, 2002, vol. 15, 209–27.

Paul F. Mellen, 'Coroners' inquests in colonial Massachusetts', *Journal of the History of Medicine and Allied Sciences*, 1985, vol. 40, 462–72.

Camille Molinier, 'La torture judiciaire vue à travers un Traité médical à Montpellier au XVIIe siècle', *Recherches & Travaux, Mélanges DEA* (Faculté de Droit de Montpellier, Cahiers de l'École Doctorale), 2007, vol. 6, 119–33.

Alessandro Pastore and Giovanni Rossi (eds), *Paolo Zacchia: alle origini della medicina legale 1584–1659*, Milan: FrancoAngeli, 2008.

Michel Porret, 'Viols, attentats aux moeurs et indécences: les enjeux de la médecine légale à Genève (1650–1815)', *Equinoxe: Revue romande de sciences humaines*, 1992, vol. 8, 23–43.

Julia Rudolph, 'Gender and the development of forensic science: a case study', *English Historical Review*, 2008, vol. 123, 924–46.

Laurel Thatcher Ulrich, *A Midwife's Tale: The Life of Martha Ballard, Based on her Diary, 1785–1812* (1990), New York: Vintage Books, 1991.

3 Experts and expertise

The term 'expert witness' has a long history, and is today defined much as it was at the end of the eighteenth century, when it first came into use. An expert witness is one who, in a court of law, is permitted to give evidence of both facts and opinion, to help judges and juries come to accurate decisions. This is very different from other witnesses, who give evidence solely about the facts of which they have direct knowledge. Furthermore, the term is associated for the most part with science, medicine and technology,[1] so that 'expertise' is considered largely in relation to these fields. This chapter surveys the history of the role and influence of medico-legal experts and expertise before using six national case studies to explain how states supported the professional development of forensic medicine by formalizing the connections between medical education and legal procedures for investigating deaths and criminal offences, thereby helping to create a cadre of expert witnesses in the modern sense. The final section considers the expert witness in action, taking as its subject toxicology and trials for criminal poisoning, for it was the toxicologist 'who emerged as the leading representative of the growing field of nineteenth-century medico-legal expertise'.[2] The subsequent development of various fields of medico-legal expertise will be addressed in Chapter 6.

In its focus on the period before the twentieth century, the chapter is concerned to show what it was that enabled medical practitioners to offer testimony in particular circumstances, to what degree they could be considered experts, and how this changed over time. In other words, how did forensic medicine come to be 'a body of knowledge or experience which is sufficiently organized or recognized to be accepted as reliable by a court'?[3]

The expert witness: history and theory

In Chapter 2 we saw that medical practitioners who testified in legal settings prior to the modern period were often referred to as 'experts'. Today, the more accurate term for an individual who gives specialized evidence in court is 'expert witness', referring to an authoritative specialist who is professionally qualified to give evidence of both facts and opinion. The 'expert' has in essence undergone a change in definition, so that although the words (expert, expertise) remain the same, the competence that they now connote is different from that understood in the pre-modern period. Though always centred on the notion of skill or experience, as suggested by the Latin root *experior* (to test or prove), by the seventeenth century the expert was distinguished as an individual who possessed a greater intellectual competence and broadly-applicable knowledge and skill than had hitherto been the case; previously, expertise had been based on limited personal know-how.[4] In England, skill often implied experience, but 'one did not necessarily need to have done something over and over again (experience), in order to be able to do it well (skill)'.[5] In France, the *expert* was considered specifically in relation to justice, and *expertise* was the procedure by which the *expert* gave their opinion, grounded in a technical competence.[6] Probably the closest early modern equivalent to the modern expert witness was the role played by German and Italian university staff: the written opinions that they supplied at the request of legal officials were indeed expert, drawing on specialized medical skills and reasoning to interpret facts provided by others; but they had not seen these facts for themselves, nor did the law necessarily privilege their opinions above those of lay witnesses.[7]

Appeals to experience and skill fit with what we know of the medieval understanding of expertise in relation to forensic medicine: thirteenth and fourteenth century Italian legal texts, the earliest to discuss the role of medical witnesses in court, accepted that doctors were *peritus* (skilled, expert), so that their evidence was both factual and subjective. Thus, medical witnesses offered an interpretation of the facts together with the facts themselves, at a level not accessible to the average witness or indeed the judge, assuming a function clearly different from that of other witnesses. Medieval legal commentators recognized that the medical expert (*medicus peritus*) might adopt a role akin to that of the judge: the written reports they produced were more than a series of answers to questions but autonomous statements of fact and opinion that judges might accept without hesitation.[8] Medical witnesses routinely appeared as experts in medieval and early modern European courtrooms, mainly in relation to violent death and issues concerning sex and generation, and judges sought specific expertise 'where general consensus placed it' – in the knowledge held by midwives, physicians and especially surgeons. Expertise was assessed on the basis of practical skills rather than academic credentials, and social legitimacy was associated as much with membership in a corporation as with social rank.[9] Pre-modern experts were certainly 'expert', but they were more like judges than witnesses, making assertions in court only about matters of which they had direct experience, or offering written opinions based on their study of other written documents.[10] The expert witness in the modern sense appeared only in the eighteenth century, and the term itself is clearly derived from English legal procedure.

When forensic medicine emerged as a distinct discipline at the intersection between medicine and law during the seventeenth and eighteenth centuries, concern about the role played by experts was rising: lawyers were uneasy about their potential to usurp the role of the judge; physicians and surgeons clashed over discrepancies between autopsy results and the teachings of traditional medical doctrine; and the new cadre of medico-legal writers were acutely aware of the uncertainties that the human body could present. These factors provided grounds for possible friction between medical practitioners, and between doctors and jurists.[11] In essence, the question became one of authority linked to professional competence: it was increasingly necessary to identify who was qualified to give expert evidence and thus to be an expert witness, and to know what it was that distinguished them from other medical witnesses.

How then should we define the modern expert witness, and how did the role develop? It is surprisingly difficult to specify what precisely the expert witness is and does without referring to what they do not do: they rely on specialized knowledge developed during the course of a professional career in an academically recognized discipline in order to interpret facts using their expertise, but notwithstanding their professional status, they do not give eye-witness evidence or factual evidence based solely on their experience.[12] The distinction is best understood in relation to science, medicine and technology, and it was in a scientific context that the term arose.

Intellectual scrutiny of the expert witness is Anglo-American in origin, and has had two main academic priorities since the 1980s. Historians of science working primarily in the area of sociology of scientific knowledge,[13] criminal justice scholars interested in the current use of expert evidence in the judicial system,[14] and legal historians have all been concerned to show that modern misgivings about the partisan nature of scientific expert testimony are far from new.[15] Controversies regarding the proper scope of expert evidence can be traced back at least two centuries. Historians of medicine, on the other hand, have concentrated on the role played by medical practitioners in the legal system, as representative of historical trends concerning professional authority in and service to society.[16] French contributions to the debate about the role of expert witnesses in history have focused especially on their importance to the decision-making process in both legal and political environments,[17] while recent German scholarship has confirmed the importance of the late eighteenth century in the emergence of modern scientific expert witnesses and their significance in public administration.[18]

The concept of an expert witness arose in England as a result of a procedure used mainly in civil cases, when people with special expertise were appointed as advisers to the court, or to serve on special juries.[19] Originally they did not appear on the witness stand, but during the seventeenth century they began to be called into court to present their testimony before a lay jury. Many of these possessors of specialist knowledge were asked to give advice on technical questions.[20] Another important development occurred at about the same time. Until the seventeenth century, English criminal trials were almost entirely lawyer-free, being primarily a direct confrontation between the accuser and the accused. However the scandal of perjured testimony during a series of treason trials in the last quarter of the century led to significant changes in practice, most notably the introduction of defence counsel into treason trials and then, by the 1730s, the extension of the same benefit to felony trials.[21] This set the stage for the adversarial criminal trial now typical of common law jurisdictions, a system which was firmly in place by the end of the eighteenth century and which modern legal scholars hold to blame for the partisanship which now infects criminal trials and expert witnessing.[22]

Legal texts cite the 1782 case of Folkes *v.* Chadd as the precedent for the acceptance of expert opinion testimony. This civil action concerning the decay of a harbour led the chief justice to conclude that the opinion of scientific men upon proven facts may be given by men of science within their own science.[23] Such individuals have been described as 'expert witnesses' ever since: the first explicit discussion in a legal text was published in 1791, noting that they were a growing class of witness whose personal opinions on medical and scientific matters were, exceptionally, of evidential value to the court.[24] This decision, along with the increasing use of lawyers in criminal trials, led to a shift in position: experts were no longer impartial advisers or medical practitioners who testified about what they had seen, but hired consultants dependent on the side which engaged their services.[25] The problems spawned by the new system were rapidly exported to the United States, and numerous studies have shown that the growth of industrial society gave doctors and scientists a highly profitable market for their expertise; in civil cases, the 'hired gun' analogy was frequently accurate.[26]

The expert witness was required to draw inferences that 'went beyond describing the current state of affairs with the benefit of a particular skill', as had been standard practice in the medieval and early modern periods, and to form opinions on causation based on a complex interpretation of past events.[27] By the 1790s this understanding was also common in France: 'the proof from the attestation of persons on their professional knowledge, we may properly, with the French lawyers, call proof by experts'.[28] The changed understanding of what an expert (witness) did was far more subtle in France, where the *expert* had always been defined in relation to legal practice, but by the late eighteenth century the word *expert* was being used as a legal noun, replacing its use as an adjective to refer to a person of practical experience. The *expert* had become the expert witness, a person who used knowledge that they possessed as a result of their professional training, separate from what they had seen or heard in the case at hand,[29] to assist the legal process. By 1870 the French defined expertise as 'l'opération à laquelle procèdent des personnes possédant la connaissance spéciale d'une science, d'un art, d'un métier, en vue de résoudre une question qui leur est adressée par le juge. On appelle *experts* les personnes chargées de cette opération, et l'acte ou le procès-verbal qui la constate se nomme *rapport*'. The definition is reminiscent of the duties of the early modern *chirurgiens jurés*, but in 1791 lawmakers specifically sought to redefine the relationship between the state and the medical profession, laying a foundation for the emergence of the modern expert witness.[30]

After the middle of the nineteenth century most European languages reflected the use of 'expert' and 'expertise' in relation to 'technical or scientific competence in the service of a public administration',[31] often the law, and the expert witness became a noticeable figure in the law courts. The controversy associated with them was a largely Anglo-American phenomenon, because the adversarial system tended to polarize rather than reconcile differences between experts. Key attributes of the effective expert witness in a common law courtroom included the ability to testify about complicated issues in terms that a jury could easily understand, and to withstand vigorous cross-examination by opposing counsel. However, these attributes had a drawback: one of the major weaknesses of the adversarial system's use of expert witnesses was the potential for jurors to rely on the experts' personal credibility rather than a proper scrutiny of their evidence, while experts may have been tempted to tailor their testimony to suit the needs of the side that hired them. The inquisitorial system's judge-led investigations meant that for the most part judges commissioned written evidence from approved lists of experts, so there was less scope for an Anglo-American style battle of experts to occur. The main limitation was that the experts on an approved list may not have been the best qualified persons to undertake the work. The solution to this problem went hand in hand with the growing professionalization of medicine and science during the nineteenth century, as groups of experts came together in professional associations that guaranteed the qualifications of their membership. The next section looks at this process in six national contexts, before the chapter concludes with a study of one of the earliest and most controversial venues for expert evidence, the nineteenth-century trial for criminal poisoning.

Institutionalization of the medico-legal expert witness

Medicine is today organized through systems of teaching, examination and certification which give the profession considerable autonomy under state protection. These systems crystallized in the nineteenth century, prior to which a very different situation pertained. By the late medieval period European medical practitioners had achieved self-regulation and a corporate identity: physicians studied at universities to earn an academic degree, followed by membership in a medical faculty or college endorsed by the monarch or municipal government; the lesser ranks (surgeons, apothecaries and provincial practitioners) were apprenticed for five to seven years and then admitted to a guild, which conferred a license to practice.[32] Both paths provided professional prestige and the right to practice within a defined region, but national differences began to emerge in the eighteenth century, and determined the differing paths of development for forensic medicine in the West.

France

In *ancien régime* France, medical practice was regulated by a corporate structure, with physicians at the top. Only members of the 40 or so local colleges of physicians could practice medicine in the largest towns, while incorporated communities of surgeons and apothecaries (roughly 300 each) monopolized the practice of surgery and pharmacy in smaller towns.[33] In the 1690s the right to appoint forensic experts was given to the local corporations, who had to pay a government fee, but as soon as money became involved, corruption gained a foothold. Although legal procedure allowed problematic decisions to be referred for higher legal and medical review, thus stimulating specialized work on forensic medicine, medico-legal institutions simply reflected the weaknesses of old regime France: offices became mercenary, permanent and hereditary, and thus closed to innovation. It was not long after the Revolution that the official experts were abolished (1790), and the whole system of medical education was reorganized (1794) along lines that stressed hands-on experience and the use of anatomy to establish knowledge about pathology, or so-called pathological anatomy. The removal of the public hospitals from clerical to state control facilitated this new form of learning: medical teachers and their students now had access to vast numbers of patients for clinical study.[34]

Crucially, the reorganized system recognized the importance of medico-legal learning by creating chairs of legal medicine at all French medical schools in December 1794.[35] The French state dictated that forensic medicine should be amongst the compulsory subjects in a medical degree, and the Paris Morgue pioneered practical methods of instruction in forensic medicine; its directors became leading medico-legal experts (Information Box).[36] Furthermore, a law of March 1803 required judges to appoint medical experts who were graduates in medicine, who had attended a course and passed an examination in forensic medicine.[37] This instituted a formal relationship between the police service and medico-legal experts, replacing the previous system and improving upon it by requiring those who acted as medico-legal witnesses to have a common and certified standard of knowledge. This state support helped the French to assume dominance in nineteenth-century medico-legal research.

The police in every region were generally organized into two groups; those who preserved order and attempted to prevent crime through visible patrols, and those who investigated crime: the judicial police, known as the Sûreté.[38] The Paris Sûreté could call upon three different services for specialized support in criminal investigations: 'Physicians and technicians evaluated the evidence of forensic medicine through the Laboratoire de toxicologie, which tested for poisons and drugs, and the Institut Médico-légal, where autopsies were performed.' Each major district began the practice of retaining scientists and physicians for this assistance early in the nineteenth century. The third service that the police could call upon was the Identité judiciare, which was founded in 1888 under the leadership of Alphonse Bertillon (1853–1914), a pioneering criminologist who developed a system for identifying criminals based on bodily measurements, known as bertillonage, which was eventually supplanted by fingerprinting.[39]

The French system as it developed after the Revolution seemed well disposed to the reception of medico-legal expertise. Summoned by the investigating magistrate, as required under the inquisitorial system, they presented their reports as servants of the court, and thus of the state; a decree of 1811 fixed their fees and set the limits of their intervention. In 1868 the Société de médecine légale de Paris was founded, and soon metamorphosed into a national association which aimed to advance science and offer disinterested support to justice.[40] However, despite a growing professionalism, medico-legal experts had to contend with criticism from a variety of sources, particularly public prosecutors, defence attorneys and the media. This was for the most part a problem in poisoning crimes and cases where a defendant's sanity was in question, the two main areas of controversy in nineteenth-century medico-legal practice (see Case Study 3.1 and Chapter Four).

Case Study 3.1: Trial of Marie Lafarge for the arsenic murder of her husband (Tulle, France, 1840)

Marie-Fortunée Cappelle (1816–52) married iron industrialist Charles Lafarge in 1839 because she needed a husband and he appeared to be wealthy. However, when she arrived at his country estate in Corrèze she got a shock; he was heavily in debt, and the house was dilapidated and rat-infested. This was a union destined to fail, and at the beginning of 1840 Lafarge died after a short illness characterized by violent vomiting, stomach pain and delirium. His doctor diagnosed cholera, but when white powder was found in food his wife had given him, she was suspected of poisoning him with arsenic, the poison most commonly used for criminal purposes in the nineteenth-century West because it was cheap, easily available, colourless, odourless and largely tasteless. There was a new chemical test for it, however. In 1836 the English chemist James Marsh (1794–1846) published his eponymous and very sensitive test, which involved boiling a sample of suspect matter with arsenic-free zinc and sulphuric acid to produce hydrogen and arsine gas. When the arsine was ignited it decomposed into hydrogen and metallic arsenic which formed a mirror-like deposit on a cold glass or porcelain plate. The examining magistrate asked Lafarge's doctors to perform a post-mortem and, having heard that Parisian experts were using a new test for arsenic, asked them to apply it to samples from the victim's body. However they did not know how, and instead used older tests which relied on reactions between arsenic and various reagents to produce colourful precipitates indicative of the presence of arsenic.

At her trial in September 1840 Mme Lafarge's defence lawyer realized that the case hinged on the tests made by the local doctors. Coincidentally, he also acted for the country's highest authority on toxicology, Mathieu Orfila, and asked him to confirm the results; but in a written affidavit Orfila denounced them as careless and meaningless since they had been done so inexpertly. The prosecutor agreed to have the Marsh test performed and invited two well known local apothecaries and a chemist to do it; they attempted the test without the slightest previous experience, and failed to find any arsenic in the stomach or its contents. The prosecutor, who had been studying Orfila's books, suggested that further tests be performed on other internal organs, which were known to absorb arsenic. The local doctors and chemists tested six different organs, again with negative results, but the chemists then reported finding an enormous amount of arsenic in eggnog the accused woman had given her husband. This time the court called upon Orfila to settle the matter: he performed the Marsh test using the same samples and reagents that had been used in the earlier experiments, and his conclusions produced a sensation: he had found arsenic in Lafarge's body that could not have come from any source other than ingestion. It was not the test that gave erroneous results, but the fact that it had been performed incorrectly. Mme Lafarge was convicted and imprisoned for life; released in June 1852, she died soon after.

This trial attracted worldwide attention, and the contemporary controversy about the use of the Marsh test resulted in intense scrutiny of toxicological methods, including how samples should be collected, analyzed and presented in court. The test's sensitivity offered legal officials a new way to thwart the rising incidence of secret poisoning, a phenomenon mainly of the 1830s to 1850s, but its sensitivity made it difficult to use outside controlled laboratory conditions. This encouraged a stricter standard of evidence preservation and a higher level of skill than previous tests had required, so favouring the intervention of experts above the general practitioner. Once a protocol for its use had been established by the Academy of Science (1841), controversy disappeared and the Marsh test for arsenic became one of the most reliable of all nineteenth-century medico-legal innovations.

Sources: J.R. Bertomeu-Sánchez, 'Sense and sensitivity: Mateu Orfila, the Marsh test and the Lafarge Affair', in J.R. Bertomeu-Sánchez and A. Nieto-Galan (eds), *Chemistry, Medicine and Crime: Mateu J.B. Orfila (1787–1853) and His Times*, Sagamore Beach, MA: Science History Publications, 2006, 207–42; J. Thorwald, *Proof of Poison*, trans. R. and C. Winston, London: Thames and Hudson, 1966, pp. 11–18, 29–43.

The nation's most competent experts were located mostly in Paris, Lille and Lyon, but this small elite was often undermined by the inadequate training of provincial colleagues. They were also unhappy with the low rates of pay: in the 1890s the fee for an autopsy in Paris was raised to 25 francs from six, while the fee for a mental assessment remained at ten francs for a three-hour session. However, they were in positions of some power, and could clearly influence the course of justice. Socially, their appearances in court brought public recognition, intriguing clinical material and publications which served to advance their careers.[41] Some of the *fin-de-siècle* problems with qualifications were addressed by the institution in 1913 of a formal diploma for chemical experts (*chimistes-experts*), while lists of medico-legal experts (*médecins légistes*) were drawn up annually by the regional courts in the light of suitable medical accreditation.[42] Today, French medico-legal experts are accredited by diploma following two years of training in a medico-legal institute or hospital forensic department. In cities they work mainly in university hospitals, but in rural areas the work is done by GPs for whom medico-legal activity represents only a marginal part of their practice.[43]

In many respects a laudably fair arrangement, the French inquisitorial system is not without its faults. Expert evidence is commissioned mainly by investigating judges and the police from lists of official expert witnesses which are still compiled by the courts and reviewed annually; however, in some areas quality is mediocre, and experts who are not on the list are consulted. Defence lawyers can in theory challenge expert evidence, but this rarely happens so there is little critical examination of expert reports.[44] One of the key weaknesses of the accusatorial system – the tendency to rely more on the experts' character and personal authority than on the content of their evidence – may thus be found also within the inquisitorial system.

Germany and Austria

Medicine in Germany was regulated by a system of academic qualifications: leading physicians and medical professors typically belonged to a medical college attached to the royal court, and licenses were granted by the state college of physicians. Chains of command and responsibility existed between the state colleges and city councils and descended to town and village doctors, especially the district medical officers, who had administrative obligations including attendance at the law courts (for relatively small fees).[45] Forensic medicine became a subject for special instruction in the seventeenth century due to the influence of the Carolina, and the first lectures were given at Leipzig by Johann Michaelis (1607–67) in 1650. By the middle of the eighteenth century professorships of forensic medicine were being created in German universities, Zacchia's text had been superseded by German works, and a periodical literature was developing.[46] Obligatory and complete autopsies became law in 1720, and a formal medical role in prisons was instituted.[47] Germans dominated research in forensic medicine during the eighteenth century, for reasons touched upon in Chapter 2: trial reports had to be written, and the law courts submitted these to the medical faculties of the universities for discussion. Decisions were published for instructional purposes, and led those who were involved with them to write their own monographs on subjects of related interest, including suicide, infanticide, virginity, drowning, hanging and wounds.[48] University professors published influential text-books,[49] and advances in sciences like physiology, histology and toxicology were applied with success to medico-legal problems including time of death, blood-stain analysis and poisoning. When the first meeting of the Deutsche Gesellschaft für Gerichtliche Medizin (German Society for Forensic Medicine) was held in 1905, its members were told that 'Nothing will serve more to raise our professional standing than the increase of our scientific output'.[50]

During the early modern period most German states developed formal rules to guide medical jurists in conducting post-mortem examinations, and when Germany was unified in 1871 the Prussian rules of 1858 were adopted for the new nation. A Royal Scientific Commission for Medical Affairs drew up a revised protocol in January 1875, and it was soon accepted by the ministry which oversaw both education and medicine. The new rules stipulated that a medico-legal examination was to be done by two people, usually a court-accredited district physician (*Gerichtsarzt*) and a district surgeon, in the presence of a magistrate. Autopsies had to be performed within 24 hours of death, and there were special instructions for dealing with newborn children. The magistrate was to write, in easily understood language, a protocol of all the details on the spot, and the cause of death had to be specified.[51] The standard autopsy procedure was created by the renowned pathological anatomist Rudolf Virchow (1821–1902), whose extremely productive and wide-ranging academic career attested to the strength of the German university system and its links with the state. Government support for forensic medicine during the twentieth century enabled five new institutes to be founded after World War I, and 11 new institutes after World War II, bringing the total at the end of the century to 32. Forensic medicine is now a compulsory part of the medical curriculum, and institute staff undertake a wide range of medico-legal work for a variety of clients; but only a *Gerichtsarzt* may perform autopsies for the courts.[52]

After a slow start relative to France and Germany, by the late eighteenth century the situation in the Austrian empire compared favourably with that elsewhere. The earliest official decree on the use of a forensic autopsy dated from 1734, and was included in the Criminal Code of 1768; like the earlier Carolina, the criminal code promulgated by the Empress Maria Theresa (r. 1740–80) was largely concerned with criminal procedure, not expert evidence. There were thus no medical experts permanently employed by the Austrian judicial system until the end of the eighteenth century, when the task was given to the public physicians. Previously, forensic examinations were carried out by the two youngest members of the guild of barber-surgeons, in the private rooms of the deceased, for no fee. When the General Hospital opened in Vienna in 1784, the two youngest hospital doctors were expected to carry out autopsies; later they were replaced by a court-appointed doctor (*Beschaumeister*) who had sole authority to carry out post-mortem examinations.[53]

Licenses to practice medicine were conferred by the universities of Vienna and Prague, and forensic medicine entered the medical curriculum in 1775, when it was included in the surgery courses taught at Vienna; ten years later lectures on forensic medicine began at Prague. In 1804 a professorship of *Staatsarzneikunde* (state medical research) was created in Vienna, with responsibility both for forensic medicine and for hygiene or public health, and with this new post forensic medicine became a compulsory part of the medical programme. In 1807 another professorship was established at Prague, where the teaching emphasis was on autopsy, and composing and writing official medico-legal reports.[54]

In 1815 the Vienna city council united the post of official court dissector with that of the professor of forensic medicine, and made the morgue at the General Hospital the principal location for medico-legal post-mortems. The entire medico-legal system was linked to the state's inquisitorial investigative procedures and, as a consequence, Vienna became the site of the world's first university institute of forensic medicine; by the late nineteenth century it was acknowledged as the best in Europe.[55] Further expansion came in the form of a professorship at Graz (1863) and institutes of forensic medicine at Innsbruck (1894) and Salzburg (1967), with teaching responsibilities for both doctors and lawyers and a mandate to carry out medico-legal autopsies and research.[56]

United Kingdom

In eighteenth-century England medical practitioners outside London were free to practice as they wished, with no ties to any overseeing body. The London Colleges of Physicians and Surgeons did not act as teaching bodies, though the College of Surgeons and the Society of Apothecaries set examinations for their members. Until the early nineteenth century the universities of Oxford and Cambridge were the only English institutions to award medical degrees, but many students studied at Leiden, or in France, Italy or Scotland, especially at Edinburgh, where a medical school was founded in 1726. There was no regional system of medical licensing because there were no regional medical faculties,[57] nor was there any formal system for obtaining or remunerating medical expertise.

Innovations in medical education took place entirely outside the universities, where two types of medical instruction emerged to meet students' needs. Private anatomy schools grew in number, mainly in London, throughout the eighteenth century, and it was there that famous surgeons and medical lecturers like William Hunter (1718–83) were based, teaching core courses in anatomy, medicine, and chemistry and specialist subjects like obstetrics. The other new site for medical teaching was the hospital. In 1700 London had three hospitals, by 1750 there were eight, and similar institutions were founded in the provinces, where no genuinely medical hospitals had previously existed; by 1800, 33 English provincial towns had a general hospital.[58]

During the 1820s rules enacted by the College of Surgeons discriminated against private medical schools and increased the hospital elite's control of teaching, while training in human anatomy was difficult because so few bodies were available until the Anatomy Act of 1832 ensured a regular supply.[59] Those who wished to reform medical education in England used forensic medicine as a platform to further their claims for formalizing and standardizing medical instruction, by pointing out that uninformed medical witnesses could easily make fools of themselves and harm others through their ignorance, while the properly trained medical witness could advance the public importance and utility of medicine in a modern state. The idea of forensic medicine thus exemplified some of the goals of the medical reformers, though medico-legal activity illustrated serious defects, including the ineffective regulation of medical practice and the inadequate training of practitioners in dissection and pathological anatomy.[60]

Change came after 1831, when the Society of Apothecaries began requiring medical students in London to attend courses on forensic medicine in order to qualify for its licence, the main qualification that most general practitioners held. This guaranteed teachers of forensic medicine a sizeable audience of fee-paying students even though no examinations were held, so some of the London hospitals appointed lecturers in the subject.[61] In the second quarter of the century, 11 provincial medical schools were founded; these new institutions also taught forensic medicine. The academics who filled the new posts variously wrote textbooks, published original research, and carried out medico-legal investigations on behalf of local coroners and other legal authorities, particularly the police (established as a national force only in 1856), becoming a recognized group of experts who could be called upon by the authorities or defence lawyers when special expertise was needed.[62] By 1875 each of the 23 medical colleges in Britain taught forensic medicine, with special degrees in state medicine available at Cambridge, Oxford, Edinburgh and Dublin.[63] Additionally, doctors took on roles as police surgeons, who were paid an annual salary to look after members of the police force, but who also treated the victims of physical assaults and carried out autopsies, forming a second tier of professional medical witnesses, though not necessarily expert witnesses, within which differences in practical experience and training existed until 1962, when a diploma in medical jurisprudence was instituted.[64]

University lecturers and police surgeons were joined in the witness box by a far larger number of general practitioners and hospital doctors to whom local coroners turned for medical evidence at inquests. The Medical Witnesses Act of 1836, which assumed that all doctors were equally competent, set the fee for an autopsy or toxicological analysis at one guinea,[65] but the fees demanded by university lecturers and acknowledged experts were usually higher, a factor which acted to restrict the use of recognized medico-legal experts to all but the most suspicious cases. Coroners' inquiries into mysterious deaths were a public duty, however, and Thomas Wakley

(1795–1862), a surgeon, coroner, MP and founding editor of *The Lancet*, urged the use of all means, including autopsy, to reach clear-cut answers, advocating shared responsibility between medical experts and the inquest jury, but with limited success until coroners gained administrative autonomy from local magistrates.[66] The Medico-Legal Society, founded in London in 1900 as a cooperative organization between doctors and lawyers, set about lobbying for a London based medico-legal institute under Home Office control, to serve as a teaching centre and a resource for coroners, but after World War I government interest turned to forensic science, leading in the 1930s to the creation of the Forensic Science Service.[67] Although the Coroner's Amendment Act of 1926 gave coroners broad powers to order post-mortem examinations, so that England consequently has the highest autopsy rate in the West,[68] the current standard of post-mortems is nationally inconsistent.[69]

The progress in Scotland has been very different. The first lectures on forensic medicine were offered at Edinburgh around 1790 by Andrew Duncan senior (1744–1828), and his son Andrew Duncan junior (1773–1832) was appointed to a professorship of medical jurisprudence and medical police (public health, which gained its own chair in 1898) founded within the faculty of law in 1807, where it remained until 1825 when it moved to the medical school. Probably the most famous holder of the chair was Sir Robert Christison (1797–1882), who shifted the focus more firmly onto forensic medicine and developed an international reputation as an expert on toxicology. Until the early 1830s the University of Edinburgh was the only medical school in Britain to offer systematic instruction in forensic medicine, which was already a popular subject when it became compulsory in 1833.[70]

In Glasgow, an interest in forensic medicine developed outside the university, within the city's administration, where there had long been a tradition that the surgeon to the town gaol acted as an expert witness in criminal trials. During the 1830s the incumbent, James Corkindale (d. 1842), a powerful figure in the local medical hierarchy, supported the creation of a chair in forensic medicine, as did the procurators fiscal, the lawyers responsible for investigating suspicious deaths and acting as public prosecutors. The Glasgow chair in forensic medicine was created by the government in 1839 with the aim of stimulating university reform and local political interests; it provided no salary in its early years, and appointments were based largely on political patronage. The professors were relatively undistinguished until the late nineteenth century, when John Glaister the elder (1856–1932) was appointed. He and his son and successor John Glaister the younger (1892–1971) dominated academic research and teaching in British forensic medicine until the 1960s, becoming household names as 'medical detectives',[71] a soubriquet generally reserved for a select group of medical experts, most of whom were located in London, Edinburgh and Glasgow, to whom the police turned in every large-scale murder investigation in interwar Britain (Information Box).

Information Box: Notable medico-legal experts and expert witnesses 1820–1990

France

François-Emmanuel Fodéré (1764–1835), professor of legal medicine (1814–35), Strasbourg (the founding father of French legal medicine).

Mathieu Orfila (1787–1853), dean of the faculty of medicine (1830–48) and professor of medical chemistry (1823–53), Paris (the founding father of toxicology).

Alphonse Devergie (1798–1879), professor of medicine (1840–67) and medical inspector of the Morgue, Paris.

Ambroise Tardieu (1818–79), professor of legal medicine (1861–79) and Morgue pathologist, Paris.

Paul Brouardel (1837–1906), professor of legal medicine and director of the Morgue (1879–1906), Paris.

Alexandre Lacassagne (1843–1924), professor of legal medicine (1880–1921), Lyon (a founding father of criminology).

Edmond Locard (1877–1966), Police Scientific Laboratory (1912–54), Lyon (founder of forensic science and first police laboratory).

Germany and Austria

Joseph Bernt (1770–1842), professor of forensic medicine (1813–42) and Staatsarzneikunde (1815–42), Vienna (founder of the first medico-legal institute).

Johann Ludwig Casper (1796–1864), professor of forensic medicine (1839–64) and forensic physician to the justiciary court (1841–64), Berlin.

Eduard von Hofmann (1837–97), professor of forensic medicine (1875–97), Vienna.

Richard von Krafft-Ebing (1840–1902), professor of psychiatry, Graz (1873–89) and Vienna (1889–1902) and court expert (pioneering sexologist).

Hans Gross (1847–1915), examining magistrate and professor of criminal law (1905–15) and founder of the Criminological Institute, Graz (the founding father of criminalistics).

United Kingdom

Sir Robert Christison (1797–1882), toxicologist, professor of medical jurisprudence (1822–32) and materia medica (1832–77) and medical officer to the Crown (1822–66), Edinburgh.

Alfred Swaine Taylor (1806–80), toxicologist, lecturer and professor in forensic medicine (Guy's Hospital, 1831–77) and medico-legal expert, London (author of leading English-language textbooks on poisoning and forensic medicine).

Sir Thomas Stevenson (1838–1908), lecturer in forensic medicine (Guy's Hospital, 1878–1908) and Home Office analyst (1872–1908), London.

Henry H. Littlejohn (1862–1927), professor of forensic medicine and chief police surgeon (1906–27), Edinburgh.

Sir Bernard Spilsbury (1877–1947), lecturer in pathology (St Mary's Hospital, 1907–19) and morbid anatomy (St Bartholomew's Hospital, 1919–47) and Home Office pathologist, London.

Sir Sydney Smith (1883–1969), professor of forensic medicine (1928–53), Edinburgh.

John Glaister junior (1892–1971), professor of forensic medicine (1931–62), Glasgow and medico-legal examiner to the Crown.

Keith Simpson (1907–85), reader and professor of forensic medicine (1946–73) and Home Office pathologist, London.

United States of America

Theodore George Wormley (1826–97), professor of chemistry and toxicology (1877–97), University of Pennsylvania.

Rudolph August Witthaus (1846–1915), professor of chemistry and toxicology (1898–1911), Cornell University.

William Scott Wadsworth (1868–1955), coroner's physician (1899–1955), Philadelphia.

George Burgess Magrath (1870–1938), lecturer in legal medicine, Harvard University (1907–37) and medical examiner, Boston (1906–35).

Milton Helpern (1902–77), chief medical examiner (1954–73), New York City.

Thomas Noguchi (b. 1927), chief medical examiner and coroner (1967–82), county of Los Angeles.

Michael Baden (b. 1934), office of the chief medical examiner, New York City (1961–86), currently co-director, New York State police medico-legal investigation unit and private medico-legal practice.

Sources: E.H. Ackerknecht, 'Early history of legal medicine', in C.R. Burns (ed.), *Legacies in Law and Medicine*, New York: Science History Publications, 1977, 249–71; E.A. Cawthon, *Medicine on Trial: A Sourcebook with Cases, Law, and Documents*, Indianapolis, IN: Hackett Publishing, 2004; M.A. Crowther and B. White, *On Soul and Conscience.*

The Medical Expert and Crime: 150 Years of Forensic Medicine in Glasgow, Aberdeen: Aberdeen University Press, 1988; J. Johnson, 'William Scott Wadsworth: an appreciation of an anomalous career', *Transactions and Studies of the College of Physicians of Philadelphia*, 1990, vol. 12, 335–46; H.A. Kelly and W.L. Burrage, *American Medical Biographies*, Baltimore, MD: The Norman, Remington Company, 1920; J.C. Mohr, *Doctors and the Law: Medical Jurisprudence in Nineteenth-Century America*, Baltimore, MD and London: Johns Hopkins University Press, 1993; K.D. Watson, 'Medical and chemical expertise in English trials for criminal poisoning, 1750–1914', *Medical History*, 2006, vol. 50, 373–90.

In 1856 knowledge of forensic medicine became a prerequisite for admission to the Faculty of Advocates, the professional association for Scottish lawyers, thus further integrating the subject into the national educational structures for both medical and legal professionals.[72] This link has helped to ensure its survival; today, although it is no longer compulsory, forensic medicine is taught in three Scottish universities (Dundee, Edinburgh and Glasgow) with financial support from the devolved government, and the staff provide medico-legal expertise to the police and procurators fiscal. In England, the Home Office maintains a register of forensic pathologists and is responsible jointly with the Royal College of Pathology for developing national standards for forensic pathology, but since World War II forensic medicine as a discipline has had little government support, university teaching has declined inexorably in favour of forensic science, there is no institutional focus, and research is isolated from the mainstream of medicine and pathology.[73] Contrary to the well established institutes and university departments in Scotland and on the Continent, where groups of regionally or nationally accredited experts work together, English medico-legal experts are today located in a bewildering range of NHS, private and government laboratories and departments, so that expertise is largely an individual attribute associated with personal credibility and one's standing with lawyers and the police.

United States of America

In the United States prior to the nineteenth century medicine and law were distinct specialities that did not often mix in practice, nor was medicine an important element of many trials.[74] When doctors did appear in court, American law considered them to be experts in any aspect of medicine, regardless of their actual training or experience, but forensic pathology began to emerge as a specific occupation during the last quarter of the nineteenth century, as both population and crime rates rose.[75] Benjamin Rush (1745–1813) is credited with first emphasizing the significance of the relationship between law and medicine with his published lecture 'On the study of medical jurisprudence', delivered to medical students in Philadelphia in 1811, and he was followed by a select group of forensic practitioners who became immensely influential. The first American physician to gain an international reputation, Theodric Romeyn Beck (1791–1855), did so on the strength of his *Elements of Medical Jurisprudence* (1823), a text which dominated the field for 30 years. The first professorship was established at Columbia Medical School in 1813, but by 1876 medical jurisprudence was taught as a special subject in fewer than a quarter of medical schools and had little state support.[76] Even though the Medico-Legal Society, the first of its kind in the world, was organized in New York in 1867,[77] by the end of the nineteenth century most American doctors had withdrawn from legal processes, and relations between doctors and lawyers were strained, with setbacks after 1850 due to professional and political disputes as well as highly public disagreements in cases of insanity (see the trial of Charles Guiteau in Chapter 4) and poisoning (Case Study 3.3).[78]

Forensic medicine was relegated to a position as an occasional subject taught outside the mainstream,[79] but from about 1950 the increasing authority of some of the most active practitioners of forensic medicine – pathologists – particularly in helping to solve murder cases, has been a noticeable change, as has their rise to hero status.[80] Despite well publicized limitations such as the botched autopsy of President Kennedy in 1963, professional progress was made when national organizations devoted to issues at the interface of medicine and law were established in 1955 (the American College of Legal Medicine) and 1972 (the American Society of Law and Medicine). Teaching in forensic medicine has expanded in both law and medical schools; the American Board of Legal Medicine administers examinations to professionals who hold both legal and medical degrees, certifying over 250 individuals since 1982.[81] However, forensic pathologists are regarded as 'a cadre of expert technicians, with very little professional power outside their own sphere'. With the exception of some of the individual 'heroes', whose failings have famously been displayed in controversial trials such as that of O.J. Simpson (1995), forensic pathology has an inferior position in the medical hierarchy because of its status as a lawyer-controlled – rather than an intellectual – discipline.[82]

Many of the problems in the United States stemmed from the coroner system, which was imported from England in the seventeenth century and suffered to a large extent from a lack of professionalism, organization and coordination. Often, local undertakers served as coroners; in other jurisdictions coroners were elected in partisan contests and had no training in the examination of dead bodies, or were reluctant to order autopsies because they perceived them as unpopular with voters. In the second half of the nineteenth century and the beginning of the twentieth, several US states and localities sought to reform the system by making it independent of juries, but the more successful option was to replace coroners with a medical examiner (ME) system; in 1877 the first ME was appointed in Massachusetts, and the system established by New York City in 1918 became a model for subsequent reforms elsewhere. Medical examiners were expected to have expertise in pathology and were responsible for investigating deaths, but their lack of legal training and relationship with the police and district attorneys, who respectively investigate and prosecute crime, could be problematic. By the 1980s the ME system was widespread, but coroners still serve about half the US population. The fame of some forensic pathologists (there are about 300 full-time practitioners) is akin to that of the British medical detectives and has generally been linked to their role as a district ME.[83]

In the United States, intervention in and regulation of the activities of medico-legal practitioners are mediated not just by the national government but also local governments, the electorate, and the medical and legal professions; there are so many different jurisdictions and competing professional claims that it is unlikely that a single system can prevail. The influence of the American legal profession, particularly prosecutors, has led to a tendency for the courts to favour expert witnesses who work closely with them, leading to accusations of bias, error, lack of disclosure and a cult of personality on the part of some expert witnesses. To counter this problem, judges now attempt to restrict the introduction of expert testimony to that which is sufficiently recognized or organized – professionally and empirically – to be accepted as reliable; but since the nineteenth century it has usually been the criminal defendant's expert witnesses who have faced the harshest scrutiny.[84]

The expert witness in action: toxicology and trials for criminal poisoning

With a few noteworthy exceptions – ancient Rome and seventeenth-century France and Italy being probably the most well known instances – criminal poisoning has never been common in the West, but its secrecy and typically domestic setting have always caused a frisson of horror in the public imagination, an evidentiary dilemma for legal officials, and a serious scientific challenge to doctors and scientists. How did one render visible that which by its very nature was invisible? Prior to the eighteenth century those crimes that were revealed owed more to informants and the use of torture to extract confessions than to the ability of doctors or chemists to accurately detect and identify poisons,[85] but by the end of the century it was clear that poisoning crimes, jointly with insanity, would require specialized forensic knowledge of the type that only an appropriately qualified expert could provide. During the nineteenth century these experts brought the fledgling science of toxicology to public prominence and, in so doing, became household names.

Poisoning was unlike other crimes of violence because of the difficulty in discovering that a crime had occurred at all. Although not a painless process, death by poison did not involve blood-letting, and so might possibly go unrecognized. There was also a real risk that it would be mistaken for natural disease, and it tended to happen behind closed doors, with no direct witnesses. The early modern medico-legal approach to poisoning focused mainly on the bodily changes that it was thought to cause: external blackening and intestinal excoriation; the symptoms exhibited before death and substances found in the stomach were also important indicators. If an animal perished after eating suspect food, vomit or matter removed from the corpse, that was accepted as indirect evidence. However, superstition and poor observation could undermine attempts to prove that poison was the cause of death: the ordinary phenomena of decay could be confused with the signs of death by poison, chemical tests were rudimentary or non-existent, and there was almost no way to prove how the victim had really died unless the poisoner was practically caught in the act.[86]

The nature of poisoning crimes meant that proof had to be both medical (cause of death) and chemical (identity of the poisonous substance). For centuries the main poison used for criminal purposes was arsenic, because it was cheap, tasteless, odourless, colourless and quite deadly in small doses. In 1755 a Frenchman was executed on the strength of a medico-legal investigation which purported to have found arsenic in his dead wife, but it is unclear how the surgeons demonstrated that the substance they found was indeed arsenic.[87] During the celebrated trial of Mary Blandy, an Oxford woman hanged in 1752 for the murder of her father, chemical evidence was given by the physician who had attended the deceased and performed the autopsy. He made a variety of experiments on a powder found mixed with food given to the victim by the defendant, and compared the results to the same tests made on a sample of pure arsenic. The correspondence was so close that he swore the suspect powder was arsenic; his results were corroborated by 'an experienced chemist'. A second doctor confirmed the obvious conclusion: 'Is it your real opinion that those symptoms and those appearances were owing to poison? – Yes. And that he died of poison? – Absolutely'.[88] Although no tests were made on the body itself, this case is thought to be the first in which credible scientific proof of poisoning was presented in an English court. It was not, however, presented by expert witnesses in the sense described previously in this chapter.

One of the earliest known English trials in which a medical practitioner was called as an expert was that of John Donellan in 1781, but in this instance a great doctor failed to be an adequate expert witness. Donellan was accused of poisoning his brother-in-law with cherry laurel water, which contains cyanide, and the renowned surgeon John Hunter (1728–93) agreed to act as a defence witness. He had not been present at the autopsy and was therefore obliged to express an opinion based on the prosecution medical evidence: but he could not determine the cause of death because the symptoms suggested either poisoning or apoplexy and the brain had not been examined for signs of stroke. The judge and jury were unimpressed and Donellan went to the gallows, but Hunter's encounter was typical of 'the difficulties experienced by a really expert witness in conveying the uncertainties of a case to a legal audience'.[89]

From the mid eighteenth century until about 1836 and the Medical Witnesses Act, the autopsy and the analysis were often carried out by the same surgeon, many of whom were also apothecaries and thus had some experience with chemical analysis. However, it was not uncommon to find that the surgeon, coroner or magistrate requested that an apothecary or professional chemist be brought in to carry out the analysis. Most of those who had the necessary training were medical men or chemical entrepreneurs, as there were then few academic chemists.[90] If surgeons were prepared to state that the poison identified by the analyst had killed the victim, juries tended to believe them. Since defence counsel was so rare, there was usually no one to attempt to rebut their claims, and judges were satisfied when the balance of all the evidence proved guilt beyond reasonable doubt.[91]

The scientific approach to solving poisoning crimes was stimulated by the work of the founder of toxicology, Mathieu Orfila, a Spaniard who made his career in Paris and established the first modern forensic science on a firm quantitative basis by introducing new, primarily chemical, experimental methods of proof of poisoning. His monumental *Traité des poisons* (1814–15), the first systematic attempt to correlate chemical and biological information about poisons, was intended for use by forensic witnesses and family doctors.[92] Orfila's British counterpart was the Scot, Robert Christison, whose *Treatise on Poisons in Relation to Medical Jurisprudence, Physiology and the Practice of Physic* (1829) was the first of its kind in English.[93] Both works were widely read and translated, and both men became quintessential expert witnesses: Orfila was most famed for his role in the conviction of Marie Lafarge for the murder of her husband (Case Study 3.1), while Christison was consulted by legal officials throughout Scotland and in England also. Americans acknowledged both as internationally renowned experts and, following the European lead, devoted a significant proportion of their own texts on legal medicine to poisons and toxicology.[94] Medical jurists everywhere recognized poisoning as a growing menace, and became increasingly concerned to develop accurate tests for the most common poisons of the Victorian era: arsenic and compounds of other heavy metals such as iron, mercury and antimony; alkaloids such as strychnine; opiates; acids; and, in France especially, phosphorus.[95] The two most important tests were undoubtedly the Marsh (1836) and Reinsch (1841) tests for arsenic, as the lethal white 'inheritance powder' accounted for 42 per cent of known criminal poisonings in France, 47 per cent in England, and 57 per cent in Belgium.[96] Experts regularly appeared in court with test tubes full of colourful precipitates, arsenical mirrors produced by the Marsh test, and solid extracts of substances recovered from victims' bodies. The invisible was rendered visible through the medium of science.

The modern expert witness thus emerged fully into public view during the 1830s, as a consequence of the growing number of poisoning crimes caused by poverty, publicity and ease of access to cheap poisons, the increasing ability to detect them quantitatively, and rising numbers of academic chemists and toxicologists employed in the universities, teaching hospitals and medical schools which began to proliferate.[97] They expressed their opinions as part of their evidence, and testified about experiments made and their significance to the case. By mid century, 'scientists could isolate the tiniest traces of some poisons from the corpses of murder victims and produce them for all to see in court'.[98] It was not all plain sailing, of course. 'Scientists who appeared as witnesses quickly learned that the transfer of knowledge from the laboratory to the courtroom was fraught with difficulties',[99] and the adversarial structure of British and American trials had an unfortunate tendency to lead to unseemly and contradictory displays by hired experts. Among the most prominent examples of trials affected by such problems were those of William Palmer (Case Study 3.2) and Robert Buchanan (Case Study 3.3), both of which involved then poorly understood vegetable alkaloids. Indeed, some of the most complicated trials for poisoning concerned alkaloids.[100]

Case Study 3.2: Trial of William Palmer for the strychnine murder of John Parsons Cook (London, England, 1856)

Few trials attracted as much attention as that of Palmer (1824–56) – a surgeon addicted to women, drink and gambling who became a serial poisoner to fund his bad habits – for the murder of his horse-racing associate Cook (28), who died in agonizing convulsions at Palmer's house in Rugeley, Staffordshire, in November 1855. Five local doctors, including Palmer, were present at the post-mortem, and despite his efforts to disrupt the proceedings, the stomach contents were removed and sent to Alfred Swaine Taylor – then the most eminent toxicologist in England – for analysis. Taylor detected only a small amount of antimony, however, and was unable to state the cause of death at the inquest until he heard the testimony of a maid who had seen Cook suffer painful spasms; this prompted Taylor to conclude that in the absence of any wounds that might have caused tetanus, death must be due to strychnine, a vegetable alkaloid that was known to cause tetanic spasms and which Palmer was shown to have purchased. The only problem was that no strychnine had been detected in the body, and this was to prove a major source of controversy in the ensuing trial – held at the Old Bailey in May 1856 because of adverse local publicity. There were 60 witnesses who testified during the 12-day trial, the first in England for a strychnine murder: the financial motive and circumstantial evidence were compelling, but the key scientific question was whether Cook had died from strychnine, for which an extraction method had been introduced in 1851 by the Belgian chemist Jean Servais Stas (1813–91).

A large number of expert witnesses lined up for each side: Taylor, his colleague Owen Rees, Professor Brande of the Royal Institution and Christison testified about the chemical analysis and their conclusion that enough strychnine had been given to kill the victim, but not enough so that a residue remained to be discovered in the stomach contents; seven surgeons testifying as experts on tetanus stated that Cook had not died from any natural form of that disease. Taylor in particular was closely cross-examined and had to admit that his experimental knowledge of strychnine was limited to tests performed on rabbits years earlier. There were 13 scientific witnesses for the defence, all of whom testified on the basis of second-hand knowledge; they assigned five or six different diseases as the possible cause of death and suggested that if Cook had been poisoned with strychnine, Taylor should have been able to find it. The judge's summing up defended Taylor's impartiality while intimating that some of the defence witnesses had acted as partisan advocates for the prisoner; Palmer was convicted and hanged despite lingering doubts about his guilt. Taylor was forced to defend himself in print and acknowledged the damage that the conflicting scientific testimony had done to the medical profession.

The chemical tests failed because although Taylor had extracted the poison using the Stas method, he had not got a large enough sample to test by the methods then in use. It was because strychnine deaths were so unusual in 1856 that the case caused such rancour, and strychnine soon became one of the easiest of the alkaloids to detect because it killed so quickly that it could not be entirely eliminated from the body. The toxicological dispute displayed in the Palmer case made it clear that in poisoning crimes, conclusive evidence of guilt could not be supplied only by chemical analysis but must rely on a balance of medical, chemical and circumstantial evidence, and that the proper way for a jury to evaluate opposing scientific evidence was by cross-examination to determine which of the expert witnesses had the authority of established science on their side. This concern still pervades Anglo-American discussions of expert witness testimony today.

Sources: G. Lathom Browne and C.G. Stewart, *Reports of Trials for Murder by Poisoning*, London: Stevens and Sons, 1883, pp. 85–232; I.A. Burney, 'A poisoning of no substance: the trials of medico-legal proof in mid-Victorian England', *Journal of British Studies*, 1999, vol. 38, 59–92; T. Ward, 'A mania for suspicion: poisoning, science, and the law', in J. Rowbotham and K. Stevenson (eds), *Criminal Conversations: Victorian Crimes, Social Panic, and Moral Outrage*, Columbus, OH: Ohio State University Press, 2005, 140–56.

Case Study 3.3: Trial of Dr Robert Buchanan for the morphine murder of his wife Anna (New York City, 1893)

Everything about this case was bound to attract attention. New York doctor Robert Buchanan divorced his first wife in November 1890 and was remarried within days, to a wealthy brothel-keeper 20 years his senior whom he had first persuaded to make a will in his favour. In April 1892 his second wife, Anna, lapsed into a coma shortly after taking medicine he gave her. Two doctors agreed that her symptoms were those of narcotic poisoning, kidney disease or cerebral haemorrhage, and decided on the latter after Buchanan helpfully told them that was what her father had died of. When she died the story might have ended had Buchanan not remarried his first wife within weeks: Anna's body was exhumed for autopsy and toxicological analysis. The analyst, Rudolph Witthaus, who had recently testified at the trial of Carlyle Harris for the morphine murder of his secret wife, confirmed the presence of a fatal quantity of morphine in the Buchanan case. Two morphine murders in the same city within six months did not seem like chance and, indeed, were not. Buchanan had followed the Harris trial, boasting that it was possible to successfully murder with morphine. The prosecution surmised what he meant: it had been clear from the outset that Harris's wife had died from morphine because of the unmistakeable contraction of the pupils which it caused. Anna's pupils had not contracted because Buchanan had countered the effects of morphine by giving her atropine eye drops, which had a dilating effect.

The defence attacked the autopsy evidence as incomplete and the chemical evidence as outmoded and unreliable. Each side relied on courtroom demonstrations to try to persuade the jury of the truth of their claims, stressed the professional and educational qualifications of their expert witnesses, and attempted to undermine the opposing experts' credibility. The fiercest battle was fought over the question of whether Anna had died from morphine poisoning or natural causes. Witthaus described the colour reaction and physiological (frog) tests he had used, all of which indicated the presence of morphine. To rebut his evidence, the defence called Victor Vaughan, Dean of the University of Michigan medical school and an expert on ptomaines, alkaloid-like compounds produced by decaying cadavers. Vaughan performed the colour tests in court on a sample of morphine mixed with ptomaines and on ptomaines alone, to claim that the results were more indicative of ptomaines than morphine. Under cross-examination, however, he had to admit that evaluating the colours produced was a subjective process. Witthaus then performed his own tests before the jury, leading to further arguments about his methods.

Buchanan was eventually convicted and died in the newly invented electric chair in 1895, two years after Harris, but it was not because of the scientific testimony. Rather, contemporary media analysis, supported by comments made by a juror, indicate that the jury based its decision on Buchanan's bad character, motive and circumstances, but did not take the toxicological evidence into consideration. The classic adversarial courtroom 'battle of experts' had revealed one of its greatest flaws: juries might ignore the scientific evidence altogether.

Sources: J. Thorwald, *Proof of Poison*, trans. R. and C. Winston, London: Thames and Hudson, 1966, pp. 85–99; M. Essig, 'Poison murder and expert testimony: doubting the physician in late nineteenth-century America', *Yale Journal of Law and the Humanities*, 2002, vol. 14, pp. 192–204.

By the last quarter of the nineteenth century, the toxicological experts who regularly appeared in poisoning trials were drawn largely from the academic sphere, as in the United States. In England, the position of Scientific Analyst to the Home Office was created in 1872, and post-holders, all of whom held appointments at teaching hospitals, acted as the prosecution's principal scientific witness in the most complicated poison trials until the 1950s.[101] Regional public analysts, who were mainly concerned to ensure food and drug standards, also carried out chemical tests in cases of suspected poisoning. In France, where the world's first police laboratory was founded in 1912, the toxicological work in criminal cases could be done by staff from regional laboratories, or academics in hospitals or universities. In Germany, Austria and Italy, toxicologists attached to medico-legal institutes acted as expert witnesses. In all Western nations, expert evidence in poisoning trials, no matter how apparently straightforward, can be subject to rigorous contestation by the defence – as occurred in the three case studies – because experts do not always agree on the implications of their scientific findings.

Conclusion

Recent studies on the evolution of the term 'expert' and changing meanings associated with the word 'expertise' have largely considered the matter from the point of view of science and technology, to try to account for the growing influence of expert evaluation in decision-making processes stimulated by public administration, or to explain the rise – particularly evident in the Anglo-American sphere – of a distinct class of witness whose influence in the courtroom has become powerful and controversial. Moreover, historians have identified a shift in the notion of 'expertise', from the pre-modern practical hands-on experience of 'how to do things' to the intellectual under-standing of 'how and why things work' which emerged in the eighteenth century. In other words, the proliferation of experts, while not a new phe-nomenon, has led to changes in the role, importance and definition of experts and expertise in Western society, and to the expansion of their field of activity most especially during the nineteenth and twentieth centuries. The modern medico-legal expert witness was recognized earliest and most clearly in rela-tion to the two areas of forensic interest that were the most difficult for the non-expert to penetrate: insanity and poisoning. Toxicologists used increas-ingly sophisticated chemical tests to prove the presence of poison in a manner impossible for anyone not properly trained in the requisite techniques. We will see in the next chapter that physicians of the mind also adopted elaborate professional theories concerning human agency and responsibility.

On the European continent and in Scotland, modern medicine since the eighteenth century has been closely linked to the state, and doctors have used medico-legal expertise as a means of establishing their claim to a special knowledge and authority in society; they connect their professional ambitions to the state in a collaborative effort designed to reform and improve the functioning of a modern society in which regulated medical education interacts favourably with socio-legal ideals. In England and the United States, govern-ments failed to integrate medicine and to specify a single means of entry to it as a profession until the mid nineteenth century, and took a hands-off approach to medico-legal expertise until quite late in the nineteenth century, so that forensic medicine as both an academic discipline and a practical pursuit languished in the Anglo-American world while it flourished on the Continent. Forensic pathology emerged in twentieth-century England and America as the successor to nineteenth-century forensic medicine, while the adversarial system brought the expert witness into the glare of public scrutiny.

Additional reading

The references for this chapter can be found in the Bibliography, and will allow you to expand on all of the issues discussed here. If you wish to do some further reading, you may also consult the publications listed below.

Elisa M. Becker, 'Judicial reform and the role of medical expertise in late Imperial Russian courts', *Law and History Review*, 1999, vol. 17, 1–26.

Abraham Blinderman, 'The coroner describes the manner of dying in New York City, 1784–1816', *American Journal of Medicine*, 1976, vol. 61, 103–10.

Ian A. Burney, 'Testing testimony: toxicology and the law of evidence in early nineteenth-century England', *Studies in History and Philosophy of Science*, 2002, vol. 33, 289–314.

Ian A. Burney, 'Bones of contention: Mateu Orfila, normal arsenic and British tox-icology', in J.R. Bertomeu-Sánchez and A. Nieto-Galan (eds), *Chemistry, Medicine and Crime: Mateu J.B. Orfila (1787–1853) and His Times*, Sagamore Beach, MA: Science History Publications, 2006, 243–59.

Anne Crowther, 'The toxicology of Robert Christison: European influences and British practice in the early nineteenth century', in J.R. Bertomeu-Sánchez and A. Nieto-Galan (eds), *Chemistry, Medicine and Crime: Mateu J.B. Orfila (1787–1853) and His Times*, Sagamore Beach, MA: Science History Publications, 2006, 125–52.

Louise Ellison, 'Closing the credibility gap: the prosecutorial use of expert witness testimony in sexual assault cases', *International Journal of Evidence and Proof*, 2005, vol. 9, 239–68.

M.A. Green, 'Dr Scattergood's case books: a 19th century medico-legal record', *The Practitioner*, 1973, vol. 211, 679–84.

G.I. Greenwald and M.W. Greenwald, 'Medicolegal progress in inquests of felonious deaths, Westminster, 1761–1866', *Journal of Legal Medicine*, 1981, vol. 2, 193–264.

Julie Johnson-McGrath, 'Witness for the prosecution: science versus crime in twentieth-century America', *Legal Studies Forum*, 1998, vol. 22, 182–99.

E. Lignitz, 'The history of forensic medicine in times of the Weimar republic and national socialism – an approach', *Forensic Science International*, 2004, vol. 144, 113–24.

A.K. Mant, 'A survey of forensic pathology in England since 1945', *Journal of the Forensic Science Society*, 1973, vol. 13, 17–24.

——, 'Milestones in the development of the British medicolegal system', *Medicine, Science and the Law*, 1977, vol. 17, 155–63.

Virginia A. McConnell, *Arsenic Under the Elms: Murder in Victorian New Haven*, Westport, CT and London: Praeger Publishers, 1999.

Christelle Rabier, 'Defining a profession: surgery, professional conflicts and legal powers in Paris and London, 1760–90', in Christelle Rabier (ed.), *Fields of Expertise: A Comparative History of Expert Procedures in Paris and London, 1600 to Present*, Newcastle: Cambridge Scholars Publishing, 2007, 85–114.

Roger Smith, 'Forensic pathology, scientific expertise, and the criminal law', in Roger Smith and Brian Wynne (eds), *Expert Evidence: Interpreting Science in the Law*, London and New York: Routledge, 1989, 56–92.

Stefan Timmermans, *Postmortem: How Medical Examiners Explain Suspicious Deaths*, Chicago and London: University of Chicago Press, 2006.

Sacha Tomic, 'Alkaloids and crime in early nineteenth-century France', in J.R. Bertomeu-Sánchez and A. Nieto-Galan (eds), *Chemistry, Medicine and Crime: Mateu J.B. Orfila (1787–1853) and His Times*, Sagamore Beach, MA: Science History Publications, 2006, 261–92.

Bettina Wahrig, 'Organisms that matter: German toxicology (1785–1822) and the role of Orfila's textbook', in J.R. Bertomeu-Sánchez and A. Nieto-Galan (eds), *Chemistry, Medicine and Crime: Mateu J.B. Orfila (1787–1853) and His Times*, Sagamore Beach, MA: Science History Publications, 2006, 153–82.

Katherine D. Watson, 'Criminal poisoning in England and the origins of the Marsh test for arsenic', in J.R. Bertomeu-Sánchez and A. Nieto-Galan (eds), *Chemistry, Medicine and Crime: Mateu J.B. Orfila (1787–1853) and His Times*, Sagamore Beach, MA: Science History Publications, 2006, 183–206.

4 Criminal responsibility and the insanity defence

From the earliest times in Western jurisprudence there has been a tension between the law's recognized duty to expose and punish the guilty, and those medical, philosophical and psychological theories concerning the determinants of human conduct. The ancient courts took the criminal act itself as evidence of mental capacity and saw to it that damages were compensated, crimes punished and society protected against the deeds of the mad. Ancient Greek and Roman law made specific provision for the insane, and Roman law had precise terms for insane defendants: *non compos mentis, fanaticus, ideotus, furiosus*. It even recognized that a *furiosus* might not be mad at the particular time an act was committed, thus accepting that some forms of madness are episodic. However Roman law never defined insanity: rather, it regarded it as a matter of fact, to be settled according to community custom. In practice, however, the insane could not be held accountable for their deeds.[1] References to the insane in Justinian's sixth-century *Digest*, the part of the *Corpus Juris Civilis* intended for judges and magistrates and which included selections from classical jurists, noted that uncontrollable lunatics and murderers who were insane at the time of the crime, and not merely feigning, should be imprisoned or confined in their homes, but not punished; insanity was itself punishment enough.[2]

Ancient Greek law dealt with madness as a practical matter, accepting that some actions were controlled by the gods or by factors beyond individual control, but others by a person's own deliberate choices. Insane people who committed offences were therefore required to make restitution to the victims or their families, but on a lesser scale than someone who was sane.[3] The most influential medical writers of the classical period, the members of the Hippocratic school, argued for naturalistic theories of disease, including mental disease,[4] and by the beginning of the Common Era Greek medicine fully accepted that insanity could be expressed in many ways, and that the violently insane could be either impulsive and fairly obviously mad, or rather more cunning and able to hide their madness.

Although ancient medical theory clearly encompassed a sophisticated understanding of insanity, the subject was not routinely included in legal discussions because the mad were irrational, unfit for citizenship and unable to be improved by punishment. Since the insane could not take responsibility for their actions they were excluded from the affairs of state, and there was thus no need for legal theory to acknowledge them. Their status was equivalent to that of a wild beast, perhaps of interest to doctors but irrelevant to the law.[5]

The emerging Christian world of early medieval Europe accepted the equivalence of the insane and wild beasts, but connected mental illness to personal fault and ultimately to sin. Thus, although the insane were not held accountable for their actions except during periods of lucidity,[6] they were yet great sinners deserving of some form of penance; a mental illness was itself evidence of God's displeasure and thus of social unworthiness. Religious beliefs made the issue of insanity and diminished capacity more complicated than it had been in the ancient world, and placed a new and unique hardship on insane defendants: they were at risk of being thought to be demonically possessed. Although the insane could not be considered guilty of a crime if they had not knowingly committed the offence, any persons whose ravings led to a suspicion of demonic possession were subject to the strongest penalties.[7] The insanity defence could not therefore be used in witchcraft trials before a growing understanding of melancholia and delusion in the sixteenth and seventeenth centuries began to offer alternative explanations for the phenomena associated with witches.

Medieval European medico-legal views on insanity evolved largely from the Roman model, which equated madness with a form of infancy, so that criminal responsibility depended on rationality and consent. Barbarian laws recognized a difference between violent actions that were premeditated and those that were spontaneous, or carried out on a sudden impulse, and the latter were not subject to customary punishments because a crime could not exist if no wilful desire to harm was present. Later medieval thinking on the subject reflected the fusion of Roman and canon law, accepting that the madman should not be punished but allowing that actions were reflective of inner intentions. As soon as the interior state of the actor came into play, a subtler understanding of insanity became possible and it is perhaps unsurprising that, given their Roman heritage and the intellectual vigour that surrounded the canonists, it was Italian lawyers who showed the greatest concern for the subtleties of madness.

Medieval canon lawyers accepted three versions of the insanity defence, pointing to three distinct notions of insanity: as a defect of knowledge (the individual did not know what he was doing); as an inner compulsion (the individual was compelled or forced by some inexplicable necessity); and as a defect of rational capacity (the individual was not capable of reason because of intellectual impairment). All three categories implied, to a greater or lesser extent, a lack of free will, reducing the madman in essence to the status of a beast having no freedom and no capacity to sin. The insane and those with mental disability, in other words, lacked the freedom of will required to form a criminal intent and thus could not be subject to full punishment even if they were guilty. According to canon law 'affliction should not be heaped upon the afflicted',[8] and thus legal thinking and Christian theology, to the near exclusion of medical opinion, shaped the medieval approach to mentally ill wrong-doers.

Law, medicine and the early modern insanity defence

By the late medieval period the essential elements that would afterwards come to be systematically assessed in cases of insanity were being progressively identified. First, whether offenders were of sound mind or insane had to be determined. If they were insane, jurists had to decide whether they should be free from blame. Second, social interests had to be safeguarded and the problems of custody resolved. In legal provisions for the insane, there was generally less concern for their care than for the public order. If insane persons killed or harmed someone, they were imprisoned and their families made to provide for their upkeep. If they had not committed a serious crime but were considered likely to do so, they were placed in the care of those around them and kept locked up if necessary. By the fourteenth century the legal status of the insane was well-defined in most European countries, and separate facilities for their seclusion had begun to develop. Among the earliest of these were the Montpellier Hospital in southern France, which was run by a religious order, and the famous Bethlem Hospital founded in London in the thirteenth century, which remained the only major public asylum for the insane in England until the early eighteenth century.[9]

Ecclesiastical and secular courts routinely acquitted defendants judged to be insane or mentally deficient. In medieval Italy murderers who were held to be insane were not executed but released into the custody of their families or sent to prison.[10] In thirteenth-century England mentally deranged offenders were normally acquitted and those found guilty were usually pardoned; where pardons failed it may well have been because their families chose not to continue caring for them.[11] French inquisitorial procedure did not permit accused persons to bring witnesses on their own behalf but did allow them to offer facts supportive of their innocence, including evidence of their own insanity at the time the act occurred.[12] Quite how a mentally unbalanced defendant would have been able to do this is unclear, but almost certainly other witnesses, though probably not doctors, would be questioned about the appearance of any signs of insanity in the weeks leading up to the act: medieval jurists generally took the view that insanity was evident to those who knew the sufferer and did not require medical expertise to diagnose.[13]

A further indication of the relative sophistication of medieval judicial attitudes to the insane is shown by the concern of canon lawyers with the question of whether an offence was committed during a lucid interval, if madness was not persistent. How could a judge know the state of mind of criminals at the time of their act? This was very difficult to do, but by the fifteenth century established scholarship on the insanity defence, the *De maleficiis* by Angelus Aretinus (1472) suggested that a previous period of madness should shift the burden of proof to the accuser to prove that the offence occurred during a period when the culprit's sanity had returned.[14]

A somewhat different situation existed in Germany where, as we saw in Chapter 1, Roman law was slower to penetrate. Although German legal writers seem to have followed their Italian and French counterparts in absolving the insane from responsibility, this was not always the case in practice: the statutes of late medieval German towns specifically held mad people to be accountable for their actions, and certainly some criminal lunatics were executed in the fifteenth century. Change came in the early sixteenth century, when Roman law began to make real inroads into criminal practice, first via Johann von Schwarzenberg (1463–1528), the legal scholar who wrote the influential Bambergensis of 1507, and then via the Carolina of 1532, which was heavily modelled on the Bamberg code. Both codes returned to the ancient Roman perception of madness in equating it with the state of childishness, in which malicious intention was assumed to be lacking. However, there was a problem inherent in the analogy: the Carolina (article 179) allowed that cunning and understanding in a child could make up for age, which opened the door to punishing lunatics who seemed to show enough malice to be treated as legally sane.[15] Nonetheless, legal commentators in the Holy Roman Empire began to consider elements of the actual mental and physiological condition of those accused of crimes, suggesting that there might be limits to the insanity defence connected to the seriousness of the crime and the extent of the mental derangement. Drunks, for example, could not be held accountable for libelling someone, but drink would probably not be a full excuse for physically harming someone.[16]

Although medicine did not produce any new mental insights during the sixteenth century, the insanity defence was pushed in a new direction by the controversy surrounding the Dutch physician Johann Weyer (1515–88) and his book *De Praestigiis Demonum* (*On the Deceits of the Demons*). Then personal physician to the Duke of Cleve, Weyer's masterpiece was first published in Latin in 1563, then later translated into French and German and published throughout Europe.[17] Considered the first medical treatise to deal with mental disorders in connection with the law, it reflected Weyer's lifelong fascination with witchcraft, Lutheran belief in the devil's power to deceive, his profound uneasiness with the way in which theology linked witchcraft to heresy and demanded the execution of witch-heretics, and contemporary medical ideas about melancholy and hallucinatory drugs as explanations for the wild claims of supposed witches.[18] The book began with a description and classification of demons that tended to attribute women (the stereotypical witch was a single or widowed elderly woman) with a melancholic disposition that allowed demons to trick them into engaging with them, though illusions could also be creations of the imagination. Black bile, one of the four Hippocratic humours, thought to be responsible for melancholy madness, had a direct influence on the imagination, and an excess could result in disorders such as those seen in witches. It should therefore be left to the physician to

decide whether a given case involved true possession or a complication
brought about by melancholia:

> But we have shown that our *Lamiae*[19] are so totally deprived of their
> senses by reason of their decrepit age, the despair that results from their
> misery, the corruption of their imagination, drugs that induce madness,
> and the efforts of the demon, that they confess to things which they did
> not do and could not have done, and they voluntarily leap to a certain
> death. No sane person, however brave, would do such a thing, because
> his will is as it should be.[20]

Weyer thus neatly removed witchcraft from the legal–theological sphere to the
medical sphere by declaring it to be a disturbance of the mind.

One of the most important transformations in the history of the European
witch-hunt had occurred in the late medieval religious and legal redefinition
of witchcraft as heresy, emphasizing sin and denial of faith rather than harm
by magical means, as earlier laws had understood the crime.[21] Instead of
repudiating the common Bible-based assumptions of his day, Weyer rear-
ranged them into an account of witchcraft in which the crime, but not spirits
and demons, disappeared. A man of enormous theological, legal and medical
learning, he scrutinized the Bible for what it interpreted witchcraft to mean,
and concluded that it had nothing to do with pacts with the devil but was
more to do with causing harm to others, often through poison; poisoners,
Weyer believed, should be prosecuted to the full extent of the law. The activities attributed to witches, on the other hand, had often not occurred at all, or
could be explained by natural phenomena, or were simply the product of a
gullible imagination;[22] his own medico-psychological interventions in several
cases had proved the efficacy of his approach to mental illness.[23] Weyer
therefore argued that the only possible crime committed by old women
accused of witchcraft was the mental crime of heresy, for which no one
should be executed. Witchcraft itself was impossible, and the proper remedy
for a spiritual crime was a spiritual penance.[24]

This could be a dangerous argument, not least because it was not the place
of a physician to comment on the laws of the land or on the Church's teachings,
merely on the medical status of the defendant, and Weyer was immediately
accused of exceeding his professional authority; both Catholics and Protestants
took a stand against him. Although lawyers found it easy to ignore his views
on witchcraft per se, because he had interpreted Roman law in an unorthodox
manner, they could not ignore his medical claim that those accused of witchcraft were usually mad. The issue of melancholia in relation to witchcraft
became one in which medical advice became directly relevant: prosecutors
accepted that witches could make pacts with the devil, but it became important
to sort out the ones who had actually done so from those who were simply mad.[25]

Thus, the insanity defence took on an additional medical quality that had
been lacking before the sixteenth century. Weyer's discourse, if not his

conclusions, began to affect legal arguments, as the sort of thinking he advocated could be extended to other types of crime, like murder (and especially infanticide), where legal officials recognized that a criminal 'might be melancholy and desperate and therefore not fully culpable, but also not entirely innocent either'.[26] Conversely, as treatises on forensic medicine multiplied during the seventeenth century, physicians were forced to deal with abnormal behaviour and its legal significance, most especially in the wake of the pioneering medico-legal treatise of the Italian papal physician Paolo Zacchia (1584–1659).[27]

Felix Platter (1536–1614), dean of the medical faculty at the University of Basel, devoted a section of his *Praxis Medica* (*The Practice of Medicine*, 1602) to mania and insanity as causes of violence and crime, but it was Zacchia who published the first full medical discussion of the insanity defence. In his great work *Quaestiones Medico-Legales* (*Medico-legal Problems*, 1621 and expanded in editions of 1630, 1634, 1651 and 1654) Zacchia declared that 'physicians should have exclusive competence in the field of pathological mental states', and proposed a classification based on a mixture of ancient medical tradition and modern legal principles. Within the group of what he called the 'fatuous' he distinguished three categories of patients: (1) the *ignorantes*, who had some civil privileges and were punishable for criminal acts; (2) the *fatui* who could occasionally carry out civil functions like marrying or making a will; and (3) the *stolidi*, who were 'like stones' and could not enter into civil obligations or be held criminally responsible. For legal reasons he distinguished melancholia characterized by intervals of lucidity from mania with partial delirium. Finally, *insania* and *phrenitis* denoted altered mental states caused by delirium (intermittent or constant). In setting out the case for medical distinctions between different types of mentally deficient people, Zacchia's text laid down new considerations for the courts, and showed the importance of the law's needs to the development of medical interpretations of mental illness.[28] One other key feature appeared in his work: Zacchia accepted that the melancholy could be as chaotic in their reasoning as the furious, but that they were often mad in only one respect or on only one subject and could therefore be tried for their crimes.[29] In the German-speaking lands this disorder was known as 'melancholia without delirium'.[30] It was an issue of both will and intellect, as first outlined by the medieval canon lawyers, and this distinction was to remain an important element in the nineteenth-century debates about monomania.

At this point we can begin to see a potential source of discord between medical diagnosis and legal interpretation. A doctor can recognize the symptoms of insanity, but is not necessarily trained to translate that thinking into legal categories of responsibility and freedom of will, as there are differences in language and interpretation that are not always easy to overcome, problems that continue to trouble jurists and psychiatrists today. We can also find here the origins of the need for medical testimony in cases involving insanity. Once melancholia was accepted as a possible cause of crime, judges had to worry about the possibility that madness might be feigned, and were thus forced to seek a medical opinion, as insanity was possibly the easiest disease to imitate. If the insanity defence was now based on medical symptoms, how else could the legal system ensure that only the mad were protected by it?[31]

The principle that the mad and some mental defectives should not be tried for criminal acts, and that those who became mad after conviction should not be executed, was accepted in English common law and in legal practice, but decisions about criminal culpability were of course made by juries. The *furiosus* (raving mad) was usually easy to recognize, but might have lucid intervals, and the feeble-minded were considered as dumb animals (*brutus*).[32] Both the insane and the diabolically possessed were shown a degree of leniency under the Tudors because they lacked the ability to form the criminal intent which the law required to render a guilty verdict in a capital case. However in 1591 controversy was stirred by the execution of a convicted traitor whom many believed to be mad. William Hacket, an illiterate maltster, was condemned for preaching sedition in London, while one of his followers was merely imprisoned for a year on the grounds of diminished responsibility. Henry Arthington later claimed that he had been a demoniac but not insane, as he could recall his actions, while the officials who hanged Hacket had to overlook his mania by claiming that since he knew what he was saying, he must be sane. Prior to this event, the distinction between the insane and the possessed, who were well known to share medical symptoms, had not been one that English law had been required to make, and Arthington was forced to craft an apology that avoided any hint that he might have been temporarily insane, as that would have left him open to further punishment.[33] The English were thus grappling with issues of feigned insanity, partial insanity and criminal intent in much the same way as the Germans, French and Italians, but on the case by case basis favoured by the common law.

At around the same time that Zacchia was writing his *Quaestiones Medico-Legales* in Rome, England's great common law scholar Sir Edward Coke (1552–1634) was working on his *Institutes of the Laws of England,* which was published in four volumes between 1628 and 1644. This work shaped the legal profession's view of its past and thus its priorities for the future, but unlike Zacchia, who drew on medical theory, Coke's approach to insanity called on the weight of past traditions. Thus, it was in the tradition of the common law that individuals who had diseased minds should be considered *non compos mentis.* Rather than developing various categories like those Zacchia used or which had been inherent in Roman law, Coke considered anyone who was of unsound mind to be *non compos mentis,* but then distinguished degrees of culpability encompassed by the term. Where the Romans and Continental Europeans used terms like *furiosus, lunaticus, fatuus* or *stultus,* he thought that *non compos mentis* was the most certain and legal term. An idiot, some-one of unsound mind from birth, was *non compos mentis,* as was someone who lost his memory and understanding through grief, sickness or accident. Equally, a lunatic who was sometimes lucid and sometimes not was only *non compos mentis* in the latter circumstance, while someone who became of unsound mind through his own choice, like a drunkard, was also *non compos mentis* but could gain no legal exculpation by it.[34]

Coke used loss of memory and loss of understanding interchangeably in identifying the degree of mental weakness worthy of the law's attention, but the important point is that the traditional understanding of legal responsibility defined it in terms of the nature and quality of the act. The common law had always insisted upon the presence of *mens rea*, the guilty mind of the accused, in order to convict, so although temporary insanity was potentially exculpatory, those who successfully planned and executed a crime could not legally be regarded as insane.[35]

Later in the century one of England's most famous judges, Sir Mathew Hale (1609–76), personified the dichotomy that still existed between natural and religious explanations for deviant mental states when he sentenced two widows to death for witchcraft in 1662.[36] However his belief in witches was not reflected in his legal interpretation of criminal responsibility, which was highly cogent and influential. Hale's unfinished work of legal history, *Historia placitorum coronae* (*History of the Pleas of the Crown*, 1736), devoted Chapter 4 to 'the defect of idiocy, madness, and lunacy, in reference to criminal punishments'. He acknowledged the existence of melancholia (along with disease or brain injury) as a cause of partial or total madness, but did not link it to witchcraft. Idiocy was a 'question of fact triable by jury, and sometimes by inspection' (by the judge or a special jury). He accepted that insanity could be partial and limited, just as Zacchia did: a person could kill with guilty intent yet coincidentally be insane in an irrelevant respect. He does not seem to have considered the alternative: that an individual might appear sane in most respects but kill as a direct result of a limited defect of the mind, an issue which entered debates on criminal responsibility only in the nineteenth century.[37] Voluntary drunkenness offered no privilege unless it was habitual, foreshadowing the nineteenth-century interpretation of alcoholism as a disease, and no legal excuse was offered to those who killed in a sudden drunken passion.[38] Here, though, the power of the English jury seems to have weakened this legal tenet, as numerous examples of the seventeenth and eighteenth centuries indicate that juries regularly acquitted in such cases, a form of leniency which diminished only during the nineteenth century as a growing intolerance for both drunkenness and violence took hold.[39]

Most importantly, Hale introduced the concept of knowing the difference between right and wrong, by identifying mental disability with the intellectual capacity of a child of 14, the age of discretion. Below the age of seven children were deemed incapable of distinguishing between good and evil, but between seven and 14 although children might know the difference, they were assumed not to appreciate the full significance of their actions; the mentally ill were accorded the same status. Nigel Walker has suggested this indicates an understanding that although a lunatic might conceive a criminal intent, they could still lack full understanding of its consequences. By the second quarter of the eighteenth century the 'right-wrong test', as it came to be called, had progressed a long way towards becoming part of the Anglo-American test of criminal insanity, and also part of the element of malicious intention crucial to the designation of guilt, which was to receive its abiding legal expression in the 1840s following the trial of Daniel McNaughtan.[40]

In summary, then, the insanity defence in Europe was derived largely from Roman law, which in Italy and France was modified by canon law and its Christian interpretations of madness and sin. In Germany, Roman legal thinking was influenced by Johann Weyer's belief that melancholia could explain odd behaviours. Medicine therefore entered legal discourse on criminal responsibility by two routes: the general and ancient concept of the mad beast, on which laymen and jurists could comment as well as physicians; and the more specifically Renaissance medical concept of melancholia, which only doctors possessed the knowledge to correctly identify. In England, the central role given to the jury meant that although varying degrees of insanity and responsibility were recognized in law, there was no need for medical evidence in the courtroom. No need, that is, until a growing lay understanding of the influence that external circumstances could exert on the will and thus on behaviour gave medical testimony a new, powerful and potentially subversive importance in determining criminal responsibility.

Criminal responsibility and the development of forensic psychiatry

The late eighteenth and early nineteenth centuries were marked by trends that were to have a lasting impact on the Western approach to criminal responsibility. A humanitarian and utilitarian way of thinking about criminal justice, rooted in Enlightenment ideals of individual rights and social justice, and spearheaded by Cesare Beccaria's (1738–94) *Dei delitti e delle pene* (*On Crimes and Punishments*, 1764), led gradually to a movement away from the death penalty and physical punishments, as jurists and politicians began to develop a more sophisticated view of the nature of deterrence. Rather than a general use of terror, the aim was to impose a system of penalties, each a known and certain consequence for a different type of crime, with the intention of rehabilitating and reintegrating the criminal.[41] Although legal changes were implemented more slowly in some countries, such as England,[42] than in others, once the idea that punishment should be adapted to the offender rather than to his offence took hold, concern shifted from crimes to criminals and their 'motives, moral attitudes and instincts', and medical science was called upon to study, describe and explain criminal behaviours. The insane provided a focus of medico-legal interest, while insanity came increasingly to be seen as a natural and potentially curable disease.[43]

The effects of these currents were felt in the courtroom as, during the second half of the eighteenth century, medical witnesses began to make an appearance in trials involving claims of insanity. In London between 1760 and 1843, 322 trials for capital crimes against both persons and property involved an insanity defence, and medical participation in these trials rose from one in ten to one in two. Prior to the 1840s, when the psychiatric expert witness had become an established figure, doctors tended to testify less as experts in mental medicine than as character witnesses; they, and the accused themselves, spoke about states of mind, rather than mental disease. Although acquittal rates cannot be tied directly to medical testimony, mad prisoners became more understandable to jurors, who were told about constraints on behaviour that operated independently of the will.[44] Dana Rabin has shown what this meant in practice, by studying the mental criteria that were deployed to mitigate criminal acts. English defendants constructed pleas of diminished responsibility based on lay perceptions of mental distress, a version of madness that differed significantly from legally defined exculpatory insanity. The reasons employed included necessity, passion, compulsion, emotional distress and drunkenness: defendants argued for their lives using emotional terms and descriptions, elaborating their psychological circumstances in ways that juries were increasingly willing to consider positively.[45] By the early decades of the nineteenth century, lay and legal assessment of mental debility came to rely more and more on medical evidence to support claims of distracted mental states, evidence which drew upon a science of the mind pioneered by a new group of medical experts, the psychiatrists.

A similar phenomenon occurred in eighteenth-century Germany, and Doris Kaufmann has traced the origins of the controversies which dominated the relationship between criminal justice and psychiatry during the nineteenth century to the Enlightenment. In the eighteenth century lay witnesses were, as in England, more important than medical ones in criminal cases involving the insanity defence, and judges tended to request medical reports only when they suspected that a person was simulating madness. However, Enlightenment ideas about rationality and free will led to a revision in the way that a criminal's soundness of mind was assessed, so that the principle of free will became the highest criterion for determining culpability. Crime was interpreted as a failure of the human will to triumph over its own animal passions, so that to determine a suspect's degree of guilt, both the circumstances of the crime and the defendant's psychological state had to be investigated. Whilst judges had long been accustomed to doing exactly this, the medical profession began to question their proficiency, and to suggest that they themselves were more competent to do so.[46]

This new understanding of mental competence can also be linked to medical discoveries of the eighteenth century, when interest in the psychology of deviant individuals began to appear as part of the Enlightenment movement towards naturalistic and deterministic explanations for human behaviour. Criminal compulsion began to draw attention as the research of Giovanni Battista Morgagni (1682–1771) in pathological anatomy and Albrecht von Haller (1708–77) in neurophysiology suggested an organic origin for some mental symptoms.[47] In 1797 Ernst Platner (1744–1818), dean of the medical faculty at Leipzig University, described *amentia occulta*, a disease characterized by a defect of feeling which impelled the sufferer to commit acts of violence. As crime was its only symptom, doctors could presume authority to intervene in the course of justice, most especially in cases where the hidden nature of the abnormality made it difficult for all but the experienced practitioner to detect (Case Study 4.1).

The term *psychiaterie* appeared for the first time in 1808, coined by Johann Christian Reil (1759–1813), professor of medicine at Halle and a leading advocate of a mind–brain relationship that assumed a physiological basis for mental illness. The word was derived from the Greek for 'soul' or 'mind' (*psyche*) and 'physician' (*iatros*), heralding the fact that its practitioners intended to cure, not just to study; the suffix 'ology' indicates the 'study of the mind or soul', psychology. Psychiatric medicine 'made it first common, then routine, and finally almost inescapable, for the mentally ill to be treated in

---

Case Study 4.1: Trial of Johann Christian Woyzeck for the murder of Johanne Christiane Woost (Saxony, 1821)

Woyzeck, aged 41, was rejected by his lover Woost and turned to drink, becoming increasingly jealous and aggressive; eventually he stabbed her to death. Quickly apprehended, he willingly confessed and rumours of his insanity began to circulate. However, a medical report by the Leipzig public health officer J.C.A. Clarus, professor of medicine at Leipzig University, found that although Woyzeck had been emotionally agitated and indifferent to his fate, his mental state was not such as to diminish his free will or responsibility for the crime. He was convicted and sentenced to death. Efforts to save him failed: the courts would not accept that delusion caused by jealousy was a form of mania or mental disorder, and Woyzeck was executed in 1824. The case gained worldwide fame as a result of Georg Büchner's eponymous drama. No German state ever formally recognized syndromes which denied free will (monomania, *manie sans délire*, *amentia occulta*) as grounds for declaring a person *non compos mentis*, but when the German Criminal Code was adopted following unification in 1871, offenders whose mental illness or unconsciousness prevented them from making a free, voluntary choice were exempted from punishment.

Sources: H. Steinberg, A. Schmidt-Recla and S. Schmideler, 'Forensic psychiatry in nineteenth-century Saxony: the case of Woyzeck', *Harvard Review of Psychiatry*, 2007, vol. 15, 169–80; H. Oppenheimer, *The Criminal Responsibility of Lunatics: A Study in Comparative Law*, London: Sweet and Maxwell, 1909, pp. 46–48.

what were successively called madhouses, lunatic asylums and then psychiatric hospitals, where they increasingly fell under the charge of specialists'.[48] It was from among the ranks of these specialists that theories of mental illness of critical import to the notion of criminal responsibility emerged.

In 1801 Philippe Pinel (1745–1826), chief physician at the Salpêtrière (the main Paris asylum for women), introduced a new way of classifying the forms of insanity. The ideas found in his *Traité médico-philosophique sur l'aliénation mentale ou la manie* – which was translated into German and English (*Medico-Philosophical Treatise on Mental Alienation or Mania*, 1806), suggested that insanity was not merely a lack of intellectual capacity but could also have a psychological basis, mental delirium but no loss of intellect, and its ideas spread widely throughout Europe and the United States. Pinel, for whom insanity involved a range of symptoms related to insane persons' mental awareness of themselves, had made extensive clinical observations of the asylum inmates and noted how much variation there could be in their symptoms and how frequently their derangement could be linked to mental rather than physical causes. The mental alienation referred to in the book's title explains the derivation of the nineteenth-century name for a psychiatrist, 'alienist', reflecting the growing medical understanding of insanity as a mental alienation from reality, or in the worst cases a complete disassociation from reality.

In contrast to previous classifications, which had identified entirely distinct types of insanity, Pinel perceived the various forms of alienation to form a connected continuum and classified them in order of decreasing distance between the patients and their insanity. At one end lay melancholia, delirium with a single focus, while idiocy, a complete lack of intellect and emotion, was at the other. His most innovative type came after melancholia: *manie sans délire*, mania without delirium, designated those patients who retained their intellectual powers but could not control their emotional and often violent impulses; this was in effect a partial insanity in which the personality but not the intellect was warped. Delirious mania and dementia completed the list.[49]

Pinel's *manie sans délire* was called 'moral derangement' by Benjamin Rush in the United States (1811) and 'moral insanity' by the English doctor James Cowles Prichard (1786–1848) in 1835, denoting uncontrollable and repeated criminal behaviour by offenders conscious of wrongdoing but who had no remorse. By the late nineteenth century, American neurologists and psychiatrists had given this diagnosis yet another name, moral imbecility, the emotional equivalent of arrested intellectual development which today would be categorized as an antisocial personality disorder.[50] Those who studied moral insanity conceived of criminality as a natural phenomenon which could be explained by scientific means, and Pinel's widely-adopted classificatory system was accepted by psychiatrists as an explanation and justification of diminished responsibility. Lawyers, however, were resistant, wary of any theory that did not recognize free will as the main criterion of criminal culpability.[51]

Lack of free will was thrust into the centre of medico-legal evaluations of violent crime when Jean-Étienne Esquirol (1772–1840), a student of Pinel, sidestepped *manie sans délire* and proposed his theory of homicidal monomania (1819, 1827), in which the intelligence and the will could be independently diseased. His intentions in relation to the law were clear: he wanted to alert judges to the fact that some crimes were committed by people whose abnormal mental state meant that they lacked free will.[52] Although the afflicted might seem normal and reasonable in all aspects of everyday life, they nonetheless suffered from a mental disease which compelled them by some irresistible force to commit certain actions. The key differences between homicidal monomania and the types of insanity the law had always recognized as exculpatory were its hidden nature and role in premeditated killing, and it offered a meeting point, albeit controversial, for psychiatrists and jurists concerned by the problem of what to do with these dangerous offenders.

Criminal lunatics and the problem of dangerousness

Once mental disorders without outward manifestations had gained clinical credibility, largely as a result of Pinel's work, the legal and medical professions were faced with the problem of how to distinguish potentially dangerous lunatics and what to do with them. Across Europe, the violently insane had for centuries been subject to ad hoc measures of confinement in hospitals, gaols and workhouses, but there was no formal legal provision for their detention. In England, mentally ill offenders were sent to Bethlem Hospital by royal warrant, but such confinement was of dubious legality and it was not until Hadfield's case of 1800 that the law was forced to address the issue (Case Study 4.2).[53] In France there was no attempt to legislate for the

---

Case Study 4.2: Trial of James Hadfield for the attempted murder of George III (England, 1800)

Hadfield (1771/2–1841) was a soldier who received serious head wounds in action against the French in 1794, as a consequence of which he developed millenarian beliefs that led him to think he had to die to save the world but must not kill himself; he decided to shoot the king, imagining that he would swiftly be put to death. Clearly delusional but well aware of the consequences of his actions – in effect suffering from partial insanity – Hadfield was charged with treason and ably defended by barrister Thomas Erskine (1750–1823), who rejected the wild beast and right-wrong tests, and urged the jury to acquit because Hadfield was labouring under a delusion at the time of the offence and so believed his act was right. So persuasive was the evidence given by a series of lay and medical witnesses, including Dr Alexander Crichton of Bethlem Hospital, that the judge directed the jury to find a verdict of 'not guilty ... being under the influence of insanity at the time' and remanded Hadfield to Newgate Gaol. His detention was however illegal, and because he was obviously a danger to himself and others, the government swiftly brought in retrospective legislation, the Criminal Lunatics Act 1800, which created a new verdict of not guilty on the grounds of insanity and required individuals thus acquitted, or found mentally unfit to be tried, to be kept in strict custody. Hadfield was transferred to Bethlem, where he remained for the rest of his life. The Act of 1800 created a new category of offender, the criminal lunatic, who gradually came under central government control.

Source: R. Moran, 'The origin of insanity as a special verdict: the trial for treason of James Hadfield (1800)', *Law and Society Review*, 1985, vol. 19, 487–519.

detention of the dangerously insane before the nineteenth century; a law of 1790 ordered lunatics gaoled for crimes to be medically assessed and either released at the end of their sentence or cared for in a hospital, but took no account of their potential dangerousness.[54] Nor did the Penal Code of 1810 rectify this lacuna, though later piecemeal legislation allowed the police to incarcerate lunatics in one of a growing number of hospitals, the precursors of the lunatic asylums that were finally established in 1838.[55] In German states, the question of legal responsibility and punishment of the insane 'coalesced into a subject of ongoing discourse for the general public and the specialist legal and medical fraternity' in the early nineteenth century, when the criminally insane had either to be acquitted and released or convicted and punished.[56] As a consequence of several major trials which took place during the nineteenth century, however, Western governments were compelled to confront the question of what to do with the criminally insane, and alienist physicians began to address themselves to the problem of dangerousness.[57]

By the 1830s, apparently motiveless homicides like that committed by Henriette Cornier (Case Study 4.3) best expressed the problems inherent in

Case Study 4.3: Trial of Henriette Cornier for the decapitation murder of a child (France, 1827)

Cornier, a domestic servant aged 27, had been melancholic since 1825 but found a job in Paris, where she became close to a neighbour's 19-month-old daughter. She suddenly and inexplicably murdered this child, having convinced the mother to allow her to take the girl for a walk, and made no effort to deny the crime, even admitting that she had planned the murder. Showing no remorse, she said only 'J'ai voulu le tuer' (I chose to kill it). She was repeatedly examined by alienists, and at her trial Esquirol testified that she suffered from homicidal monomania, the first use of this defence in a criminal trial. The case proved that insanity did not necessarily involve an impairment of the intellect, and Cornier was convicted of voluntary unpremeditated homicide and sentenced to life imprisonment with hard labour. An immediate focus of public debate, the monomania diagnosis remained controversial until the 1850s.

Source: J. Colaizzi, *Homicidal Insanity, 1800–1985*, Tuscaloosa, AL and London: University of Alabama Press, 1989, pp. 141–42.

the form of insanity called homicidal monomania, and offered psychiatrists a way to intervene in the legal process and seize a place for themselves both in the courtroom and in the service of the state, as experts skilled in the detection of a form of insanity that common sense could not diagnose.[58] Doctors and lawyers agreed that the dangerously mentally ill should not be set free, Esquirol noting with surprise that no country had a law which allowed the confinement of a mentally ill person for the good of society.[59] On 30 June 1838 just such a law came into effect in France, the *Loi sur les aliénés*, the result of collaboration between administrative, judicial and medical organisations. Confinement was subject to three conditions: medical certification, notification to the judiciary, and regular visits by an administrative commission;[60] crucially for the psychiatric profession, isolation of the insane on medical grounds displaced judicial control of the process, further entrenching the alienists' medico-legal importance.[61] The French legislation subsequently served as a model for most European countries, only the English having already begun a national programme of public asylum building.[62]

In the United States 1838 was also an important year, as it marked the publication of Isaac Ray's (1807–81) *Treatise on the Medical Jurisprudence of Insanity*. Ray was a general practitioner with no legal training or clinical experience of insanity, but his book established forensic psychiatry in America as a professional discipline, and shaped debate in the field for half a century. Ray's ideas were influenced by both Esquirol and Prichard, among other French and English alienists; like them, he believed that the brain of a homicidal monomaniac was diseased, but he went further in hypothesizing that there were precise physical spots in the brain that were damaged in some way. The greater the amount of damage, the more extreme the violent behaviour would be.[63]

Ray's linking of insanity to damage done to specific parts of the brain had some intellectual foundation in concepts associated with phrenology, a set of techniques for making psychological diagnoses and predictions. Developed by the Austrian doctor Franz Joseph Gall (1758–1828) in the early nineteenth century, phrenology held that the brain was the organ of thought and will, that it determined character, and that its physical configurations revealed personality. The brain was a patchwork of separate 'organs' (acquisitiveness, destructiveness, etc.) occupying specific surface areas of the brain and thus shaping the personality. The functional power of a given organ was correlated with its size and peripheral expansion, so that a large cerebral organ of amativeness, for example, would tend to be found in people displaying strong sexual proclivities. Gall claimed the contours of the skull indicated the brain configurations beneath, so that an observer could read the innate mental character from head shape, because the overall balance of the external bumps on the skull's surface determined personality. Based on anatomical research, Gall initially identified 27 faculties, and more were later added.[64]

Gall's work was translated into English by his assistant, the German doctor Johann Spurzheim (1776–1832) in the 1820s and proved immensely popular in Britain and America, where alienists recognized that the clinical features identified by phrenology seemed to match their own experiences with asylum patients. Phrenology explained crime and mental disorders by either deficient or excessive development of the cerebral organs, so that homicidal insanity was the result of derangement of the organ of destructiveness. Further, the theory postulated that over-activity of that organ could cause delusions, an explanation for homicidal monomania which, though too simplistic even by the medical standards of the 1830s, made a link between the brain and mental illness that added further support to the alienists' claims to expertise in the varying forms of insanity. The phrenologists' belief that deficient or excessive development of an organ could be countered by exercising or resting its use, in much the same way as muscles could be developed or allowed to waste, gave a theoretical basis to the moral and educational system of management of mental patients advocated by the Western asylum movement. By 1840, doctors and the Anglo-American public associated insane homicide with distinct mental phenomena, so that more and more asylum doctors were called upon by the courts to make judgments about whether a killer was a homicidal lunatic or merely a criminal (Case Study 4.4).[65]

Case Study 4.4: Trial of Abraham Prescott for the murder of Sally Cochran (New Hampshire, 1833)

Prescott, aged 18, killed his employer and immediately confessed, giving a variety of reasons for his act; finally he offered a defence of insanity on the grounds that he was in a somnambulistic state, a claim supported by the fact that he had, allegedly, been sleepwalking when he attacked the victim and her husband with an axe six months earlier.

Expert medical witnesses included Dr Rufus Wyman, superintendent of an insane asylum, and Dr George Parkman,[66] who had kept a private asylum in Massachusetts. They testified that Prescott suffered from monomania which resulted in a sudden paroxysm of violence, and his defence lawyer argued that the crime itself provided evidence of insanity and diseased intellect, as Prescott's violent nature emerged only when he was unconscious and not in control of his own will. Prescott was nevertheless convicted and executed. Leading alienist Isaac Ray later concluded that Prescott was an imbecile motivated by financial gain, not mania, but that his limited intellect meant that he should not have been hanged. The case was indicative of the problems of determining the mental capacity and thus culpability of mentally deficient defendants.

Sources: K. Halttunen, *Murder Most Foul: The Killer and the American Gothic Imagination*, Cambridge, MA and London: Harvard University Press, 2000, pp. 88–89, 228–30; I. Ray, *A Treatise on the Medical Jurisprudence of Insanity*, London: G. Henderson, 1839, pp. 100–7.

The association between insanity and criminality was strong in the public imagination, making the distinction between the criminally insane and the insane criminal essential. The criminally insane were those whose criminal acts were directly attributable to their insanity. Once recovered, they would again be respectable law-abiding members of the community. Insane criminals were those whose insanity was not a contributory factor in their criminality, so that even if recovered from insanity, they would still be a threat to society. This distinction was based on the cause of an individual's criminal behaviour, and was tacitly accepted in the McNaughtan Rules of 1843, adopted in the United States as well as in England, which stressed not only the understanding of right and wrong but a causal relationship between an insane person's delusions and the crime they committed (Case Study 4.5). Each case had to

Case Study 4.5: Trial of Daniel McNaughtan for the murder of Edward Drummond (England, 1843)

McNaughtan (1802/3–65), a Glaswegian, had for years suffered from a mental illness that would today be diagnosed as paranoid schizophrenia. His delusions were directed against the Tory government, and had become so strong by January 1843 that he decided to kill the prime minister; his careful plans went awry when he shot Drummond (the PM's private secretary) instead, believing him to be Sir Robert Peel. Charged with murder, McNaughtan's defence was that although he committed the act and knew it was a crime, his delusions had driven him to it and thus relieved him of responsibility. The prosecution countered that although he might not be wholly sane, McNaughtan was responsible unless he was totally incapable of knowing right from wrong. Nine medical experts appeared for the defence, the prosecution offered no testimony in rebuttal, and the judge practically directed a verdict of 'not guilty on the grounds of insanity'. This decision was immediately attacked, the Queen herself expressing her displeasure in a letter to Peel, so the government sought the opinion of a panel of five common law judges, in the form of answers to five questions. Their replies constituted the so-called McNaughtan Rules, which directed that a successful insanity defence had to prove 'at the time of committing the act, the party accused was labouring under such a defect of reason, from disease of the mind, as not to know the nature and quality of the act he was doing; or, if he did know it, that he did not know he was doing what was wrong'. McNaughtan was sent to Bethlem, then to Broadmoor on its opening, where he died a forgotten man. The McNaughtan Rules were the only test of criminal responsibility in England until 1957 – when the Homicide Act replaced them with the Scottish concept of diminished responsibility, though only in murder cases – and in the United States until 1954, where some version of the Rules still remains in effect in most legal jurisdictions. The concept of diminished responsibility, first used in Scotland in 1867, is less controversial than a verdict of not guilty by reason of insanity because it acknowledges the defendant's guilt but accepts the existence of extenuating mental circumstances. Before capital punishment was abolished in 1965, this verdict allowed judges to reduce the punishment from death to a lesser sentence associated with convictions for manslaughter. Depending on the circumstances, people convicted under this verdict are sent to prison or a secure hospital.

Sources: R. Moran, *Knowing Right from Wrong: The Insanity Defense of Daniel McNaughtan*, New York and London: The Free Press, 1981; N. Walker, *Crime and Insanity in England, Vol. 1: The Historical Perspective*, Edinburgh: Edinburgh University Press, 1968, Ch. 5.

be argued on its own merits, however, as the Rules did not take medical opinion or categories into account, and each jury was affected by medical discourse in different ways. Furthermore, the transfer of insane convicts from prisons to asylums added to the security problems posed by a growing population of criminal lunatics, leading to calls for a separate system for dangerous lunatics, and in Ireland first then England special asylums were built for the criminally insane. The oldest secure hospital in Europe, Dublin's Dundrum Central Criminal Asylum opened in 1850 with space for 80 men and 40 women,[67] followed in 1863 by Broadmoor Criminal Lunatic Asylum in Berkshire, built to house 400 men and 100 women.[68] In Italy, Germany, France and the United States, criminal lunatics were committed to the state asylums built in increasing numbers especially after 1850.

Degeneracy, dangerousness and criminal responsibility

By the 1850s, American alienists' forays into court had become embarrassing and controversial as the monomania diagnosis was subjected to legal and public scrutiny and its weaknesses laid bare, leading to internal warfare between psychiatrists, led by John P. Gray, superintendent of the Utica State Lunatic Asylum, who equated lack of criminal responsibility with demonstrable brain lesions and intellectual impairment, and those who favoured the much broader diagnosis advocated by Ray, then superintendent of an asylum in Rhode Island.[69] Internal disagreement about the boundary between insanity and criminal responsibility also plagued German alienists, but the profession as a whole was becoming strong enough to challenge the lawyers' dominance of the decision-making process.[70] In England, where the McNaughtan Rules were silent on the question of irresistible impulses, laymen and doctors sometimes agreed that lack of sane motive was itself evidence of insanity,[71] and the association between unsoundness of mind and homicide grew closer.[72] In France, the concept of homicidal monomania had outlived its usefulness by the 1860s, as psychiatrists succeeded in establishing their profession as the nation's experts on insanity.[73]

Homicidal monomania was replaced by two new theories. Moral or instinctive insanity, which affected the emotions and instincts but not the intellect, led to the development of a strand of forensic medicine concerned with the study of perversions, mainly sexual but including disorders like kleptomania and pyromania, as exemplified by the work of the German psychiatrist Richard von Krafft-Ebing.[74] However, the links between crime, insanity and dangerousness were strongest in the idea of degeneration, which brought serious crimes within the same remit as petty offences in its understanding of insanity as an inherited physiological derangement of the nervous system brought about by moral and physical weakness.

The idea of degeneracy was first elaborated by the French alienist Bénédict-Augustin Morel (1809–73) in his *Traité des dégénérescence physique, intellectuelles et morales de l'éspèce humaine, et des causes qui produisent ces vérites maladives* (1857; *Treatise on Physical, Intellectual and Moral Degeneration in Humans and the Conditions producing these Detrimental States*). Influenced by his clinical experience as an asylum doctor, Morel devised a unique theory of hereditary degeneration in which chronic diseases, toxins and social factors were combined to explain a disparate set of mental, physical and moral illnesses which were cumulatively acquired and transmitted from generation to generation, dying out when the human host became too debilitated to reproduce. His theory was widely influential among Western psychiatrists and social thinkers until the early twentieth century, and offered a clear link between crime and insanity. It was on this basis that the Italian army doctor turned psychiatrist Cesare Lombroso (1835–1909) defined a category of 'born criminals' and founded criminal anthropology, the study of the body, mind and habits of the born criminal. His multi-causal theory of crime developed into a widespread movement involving doctors, lawyers, philosophers and sociologists, and in effect provided the foundations for the modern discipline of criminology as both his followers and his detractors investigated the influence of modern civilization on crime, and the connections between environment and criminality.[75]

As a result of a change in the biological development of the nervous centres and under the influence of climate, heredity and social factors, Lombroso thought, this class of criminals was characterized by specific bodily features and by well defined psychiatric and behavioural disorders. There were three main predisposing causes: epilepsy, which acted on the structure and function of the part of the brain that controlled movement; syphilis, which caused physical lesions observable in autopsies; and trauma, such as a head wound. In terms of their physical appearance, Lombroso labelled born criminals 'atavistic', from the Latin *atavus*, ancestor, meaning throwbacks to an earlier stage of primitive human development, atavism being an inborn tendency to revert to a lower evolutionary state. Identifying traits included a low sloping forehead, heavy lower jaw, prominent ears, abnormally long arms and insensitivity to pain or pity. He later added such social traits as the use of tattooing and criminal slang, and suggested a frequent connection with left-handedness. Criminal anthropologists rejected the phrenological map of the head and extended physical measurement to the criminal's entire body, but their emphasis on the shape of the skull and assumption that external physical features reflected internal moral states can be traced back to the earlier movement. In spite of its conjectural weakness, the strength of Lombroso's theory lay in what appeared to be its objective, quantifiable scientific underpinnings.[76]

Criminal anthropology directly challenged classical thinking, arguing that individuals committed crimes not out of free will but from biological or social determinism. Those who seemed to pose the greatest danger were the atavistic born criminals, who required removal from society no matter how small their crime. On the other hand, so-called occasional criminals, even if their crimes were serious, deserved alternatives to prison because outside environmental forces, rather than innate perversity, had tempted them to break the law. Lombroso thus shifted the focus of legal thinking once again from the crime to the criminal, a physical entity whose atavisms could be measured and counted. However, in contrast to Beccaria, he advocated judicial discretion 'to assess the degree of dangerousness posed by each defendant' as a basis for sentencing, to fit a punishment to the criminal rather than the crime. Thus, he replaced the old-fashioned philosophical approach to crime with a fashionable scientific method of study, broadly defined as positivism, and redefined dangerousness by stressing not the seriousness of the offence but the degree of criminality in the offender.[77] 'A sentence was no longer a punishment but a means of protecting society',[78] so born criminals merited perpetual imprisonment while insane criminals were to be locked up indefinitely in special asylums where they could receive psychiatric treatment.[79] The first criminal insane asylum on the Continent opened at Aversa, north of Naples, in 1876.[80]

Lombroso's ideas spread across Europe to Britain and America via two influential books, *L'uomo delinquente* (1876) and *La donna delinquente* (1893). The former was not translated into English until 1911 (*Criminal Man*), whereas *The Female Offender* appeared in English in 1895 and hence introduced British and American readers to Lombroso's work. By contrast, French readers gained early access to Lombroso via an 1887 translation of *L'uomo delinquente*, which immediately provoked controversy; its suggestion that punishing offenders was useless because they either had to be cured or removed from society was seen as practically unworkable. According to Alexandre Lacassagne, professor of forensic medicine at Lyon, it would leave societies with no option but to keep all deviants locked up in prisons or asylums. He offered an alternative suggestion which encompassed moral responsibility for the crimes that an individual committed, and it was this view that formed the foundation of the French school of criminal sociology, also positivist in its philosophy and methodology but focused on social rather than biological factors, and which became the main rival to Lombroso's Italian school. Lacassagne argued that crime was mainly the product of social causes (poverty, alcoholism, ignorance, a bad home environment and bad company), coining the famous maxim 'societies have the criminals they deserve'.[81]

Within France, however, there was controversy over the idea of free will, with lawyers arguing that it remained the fundamental source of criminality and only the threat of punishment could deter the weak-willed from offending. The opposing argument, adopted by medico-legal experts and criminologists who accepted degeneracy theory, was eventually modified to include a role for free will in hereditary determinism. By the late 1890s the French had reached a consensus that formed the basis of their national approach to criminals for the first half of the twentieth century: offenders had to be punished, because the public demanded it; but they were also treated, with an emphasis placed on helping them to re-enter society as useful and productive people.[82]

German doctors also largely rejected the notion of the born criminal, but the strength of degeneracy theory was such that many jurists and psychiatrists became convinced that habitual criminals (repeat offenders) were degenerates inherently predisposed towards crime – not insane, but not mentally healthy either. With the boundary between crime and insanity now so porous, advocates of social defence argued that individual guilt or responsibility should be irrelevant to punishment, because social defence required every criminal to be subject to whatever measures were necessary. As criminal behaviour was now a form of mental illness and future dangerousness was perceived to be as important as completed crimes, criminal justice was further medicalized, but the role of forensic psychiatry turned on its head. Formerly advocates of the accused seeking to remove them from the criminal justice system, psychiatrists now joined judges in determining the 'treatment' appropriate to each offender, replacing the prison with the asylum.[83]

The British and Americans also came to see habitual criminals as mentally weak or disabled as a consequence of environmental and biological forces, and thus less responsible and more dangerous than other criminals, but on the strength of their empirical observations of prison and asylum populations Anglo-American psychiatrists rejected the single criminal type proposed by Lombroso and maintained that some allegedly insane defendants were simply depraved and should be punished, a debate which lay at the heart of the trial of Charles Guiteau in 1881 (Case Study 4.6). The insanity defence remained

---

Case Study 4.6: Trial of Charles Guiteau for the assassination of President James Garfield (Washington DC, 1881)

On 2 July 1881 Charles Guiteau shot President Garfield in the back as he waited for a train at a Washington railway station, thereby initiating the most celebrated American insanity trial of the nineteenth century. Guiteau, a lawyer and theologian then just short of his fortieth birthday, immediately confessed, claiming the killing was done in order to unite the president's divided Republican party. After Garfield died on 19 September and Guiteau was arraigned for murder, he entered a defence of not guilty by reason of insanity. Then an unpopular defence because it was perceived as a mere dodge by the clearly guilty, the McNaughtan Rules limited the impact of any delusion that a defendant might suffer to only those that immediately affected his actions. Were Guiteau's bizarre political beliefs motive enough, or evidence of delusion and hereditary insanity? Was his careful planning, regardless of his emotional oddness, clear evidence of culpability? Psychiatrists for the prosecution argued that he understood the nature and consequences of his act and appeared to reason coherently, so was guilty by legal standards. Alienists for the defence said he was morally insane. There was little doubt that he suffered from mental illness, probably paranoid schizophrenia, in today's diagnosis: the real question was whether he was sane enough to be legally culpable. The 24 expert witnesses summoned, representing two major trends in American psychiatry, battled for supremacy: asylum psychiatrists led by John P. Gray (1825–86) claimed Guiteau was passionate and selfish but had no brain disease and so was not insane; neurologists led by Edward Spitzka (1852–1914) insisted that the assassin suffered from hereditary neurological degeneration and was not legally responsible. The public, itching for a hanging, got their wish; Guiteau was convicted, and his case has since come to occupy a prominent place in world psychiatric literature. At trial many experts endorsed contradictory views of the symptoms and aetiology of insanity, but his death marked a milestone in the American acceptance of hereditarian explanations of insanity and crime. Moral insanity died, but the professional problems inherent in the issue of legal insanity remained, and continue to plague Anglo-American forensic psychiatry.

Source: C.E. Rosenberg, *The Trial of the Assassin Guiteau: Psychiatry and Law in the Gilded Age*, Chicago: University of Chicago Press, 1968.

as controversial as ever because of the tendency of the adversarial system to pit experts against one another in court, and because psychiatrists were not always in agreement themselves about the facts of insanity – was it purely pathology of the brain or did it also involve the emotions? – they could not always persuade juries of the existence of exculpatory insanity. Diagnostic symptoms that could be examined, such as delusions and sudden personality changes, physical disease and a family history of insanity were most persuasive to juries.[84]

Conclusion

Forensic psychiatry offered a nascent discipline a way out of the asylum and into the public arena, as alienists sought to gain a place for themselves in the criminal trial process in order to strengthen national discipline-building programmes and to publicize their growing knowledge of the brain and behaviour. However, the scope of their participation was set by lawyers, judges and defendants, who needed the specialist knowledge that a professional psychiatrist could apply to ever more complicated questions of insanity and criminal responsibility.[85] In France and Germany, where the inquisitorial system had long allowed for the use of expert medical testimony, psychiatrists joined the ranks of the court-appointed experts, to provide judges with a logical and complete account of the mental state of a prisoner. In England and America, the adversarial system of justice led to clashes between experts and between doctors and lawyers over definitions of facts that were themselves often in doubt. This was also a problem in Italy, where defence psychiatrists could argue against prosecution experts until the law was changed in 1913 to allow only a single medical report by two or three experts.[86] Part of the problem was, and remains, the fact that insanity is not a medical but a legal designation, and criminal responsibility is a purely legal concept. Thus, although lawyers wanted consistency from psychiatrists, psychiatry was not always able to oblige, not least because its practitioners disputed the evolving understanding of the symptoms and aetiology of mental illness.

A further difficulty was presented by the potential for psychiatrists to usurp the judge's role, a recurring theme in the history of forensic psychiatry and a possibility that lawyers were keen to prevent. Each trial, particularly in the Anglo-American world, was thus a latent platform for debate between psychiatrists, and between psychiatry and the law. However, the problems posed by the dangerously insane forced lawyers and psychiatrists onto common ground, and by the late nineteenth century the notion of responsibility had been replaced by that of dangerousness to society, and the law and medicine were able to collaborate in removing from the judicial arena those incompetent to stand trial or to be executed.[87] This chapter has shown how the criteria used to make such judgments changed over time, as medico-legal attention, debate and eventual consensus focused in turn on the pre-modern *furiosus*, the early nineteenth-century monomaniac and the *fin-de-siècle* degenerate.

The question of mental disorder, criminal responsibility and dangerousness is one that still preoccupies jurists and forensic psychiatrists in the Western world. The American legal system, although it continues to rely on some version of the McNaughtan Rules, now takes a more conservative stance: very few defendants meet the legal standards of insanity, and when an insanity defence is successful the accused can rarely expect to be released from secure custody. In England, since the law was changed in 1991 unfitness to plead does not necessarily lead to indefinite detention and, given the alternative options available, defendants who plead insanity are relatively few in number. Those who do plead under the McNaughtan criteria tend to be suffering from physiological, for example epilepsy, rather than mental disorders, but schizophrenia diagnoses are not uncommon.[88] Nor is the insanity defence common in France, where the incidence of its use fell between the mid-1980s and 1999 to less than one per cent of all pleas, going hand in hand with a rising use of prisons to house mentally ill individuals that the cash-poor mental health system cannot accommodate in the long term.[89] The law of 1838 survived until 1990, when it was replaced by measures designed to afford additional protection to those hospitalized involuntarily on the grounds of dangerousness to themselves; but perceived weaknesses in the law's applicability in the event of dangerousness to others led to calls for city mayors to be empowered to compulsorily hospitalize people thought to pose such a risk.[90] Although most Western jurisdictions today allow for the removal of the mentally ill from the criminal process, forensic psychiatrists must be alert to the underlying tensions between patient rights, punitive values and collective security, suggesting that 'the relationship between psychiatry and criminal justice will always be, and perhaps should be, uncomfortable'.[91]

Additional reading

The references for this chapter can be found in the Bibliography, and will allow you to expand on all of the issues discussed here. If you wish to do some further reading, you may also consult the publications listed below.

Jill Newton Ainsley, '"Some mysterious agency": Women, violent crime, and the insanity acquittal in the Victorian courtroom', *Canadian Journal of History*, 2000, vol. 35, 37–55.

Vincent Barras, 'Folies criminelles au XVIIIe siècle', *Gesnerus*, 1990, vol. 47, 285–302.

Ian R. Dowbiggin, *Inheriting Madness: Professionalization and Psychiatric Knowledge in Nineteenth-Century France*, Berkeley, CA: University of California Press, 1991.

Joel Peter Eigen 'Criminal lunacy in early modern England: did gender make a difference?', *International Journal of Law and Psychiatry*, 1998, vol. 21, 409–19.

——, 'Lesion of the will: medical resolve and criminal responsibility in Victorian insanity trials', *Law and Society Review*, 1999, vol. 33, 425–59.

——, *Unconscious Crime: Mental Absence and Criminal Responsibility in Victorian London*, Baltimore, MD and London: Johns Hopkins University Press, 2003.

——, 'Delusion's odyssey: charting the course of Victorian forensic psychiatry', *International Journal of Law and Psychiatry*, 2004, vol. 27, 395–412.

Michel Foucault (ed.), *I, Pierre Rivière, having slaughtered my mother, my sister and my brother … : A Case of Parricide in the Nineteenth Century*, trans. F. Jellinek, New York: Random House, 1975.

Frank R. Freemon, 'The origin of the medical expert witness: the insanity of Edward Oxford', *Journal of Legal Medicine*, 2001, vol. 22, 349–73.

David G. Horn, *The Criminal Body: Lombroso and the Anatomy of Deviance*, New York and London: Routledge, 2003.

R.A. Houston, 'Professions and the identification of mental incapacity in eighteenth-century Scotland', *Journal of Historical Sociology*, 2001, vol. 14, 441–66.

——, 'Courts, doctors, and insanity defences in 18th and early 19th century Scotland', *International Journal of Law and Psychiatry*, 2003, vol. 26, 339–54.

Rafael Huertas and José Martínez-Pérez, 'Disease and crime in Spanish positivist psychiatry', *History of Psychiatry*, 1993, vol. 4, 459–81.

Robert M. Ireland, 'Insanity and the unwritten law', *American Journal of Legal History*, 1988, vol. 32, 157–72.

Brendan D. Kelly, 'Poverty, crime and mental illness: female forensic psychiatric committal in Ireland, 1910–48', *Social History of Medicine*, 2008, vol. 21, 311–28.

Mary Lindemann, 'Murder, melancholy and the insanity defence in eighteenth-century Hamburg', in Roberta Bivins and John V. Pickstone (eds), *Medicine, Madness and Social History: Essays in Honour of Roy Porter*, Basingstoke: Palgrave Macmillan, 2007, pp. 161–72, 269–70.

Robert Menzies, 'Contesting criminal lunacy: narratives of law and madness in West Coast Canada, 1874–1950', *History of Psychiatry*, 2001, vol. 12, 123–56.

Richard Moran, 'The punitive uses of the insanity defense: the trial for treason of Edward Oxford (1840)', *International Journal of Law and Psychiatry*, 1986, vol. 9, 171–90.

Daniel Pick, *Faces of Degeneration: A European Disorder, c.1848–c.1918*, Cambridge: Cambridge University Press, 1993.

Régine Plas, 'Hysteria, hypnosis, and moral sense in French 19th-century forensic psychiatry: the Eyraud-Bompard case', *International Journal of Law and Psychiatry*, 1998, vol. 21, 397–407.

Anthony Platt and Bernard L. Diamond, 'The origins of the "right and wrong" test of criminal responsibility and its subsequent development in the United States: an historical survey', *California Law Review*, 1966, vol. 54, 1227–60.

Pauline M. Prior, 'Murder and madness: gender and the insanity defense in nineteenth-century Ireland', *New Hibernia Review*, 2005, vol. 9, 19–36.

——, 'Roasting a man alive: the case of Mary Rielly, criminal lunatic', *Éire-Ireland*, 2006, vol. 41, 169–91.

Raymond de Saussure, 'The influence of the concept of monomania on French medico-legal psychiatry (from 1825 to 1840)', *Journal of the History of Medicine and Allied Sciences*, 1946, vol. 1, 365–97.

Svein Atle Skålevåg, 'The matter of forensic psychiatry: a historical enquiry', *Medical History*, 2006, vol. 50, 49–68.

Roger Smith, 'Expertise, procedure and the possibility of a comparative history of forensic psychiatry in the nineteenth century', *Psychological Medicine*, 1989, vol. 19, 289–300.

Janet A. Tighe, 'Francis Wharton and the nineteenth-century insanity defence: the origins of a reform tradition', *American Journal of Legal History*, 1983, vol. 27, 223–53.

——, 'The legal art of psychiatric diagnosis: searching for reliability', in Charles E. Rosenberg and Janet Golden (eds), *Framing Disease: Studies in Cultural History*, New Brunswick, NJ: Rutgers University Press, 1992, pp. 206–26.

Christina Vanja, 'Madhouses, children's wards, and clinics: the development of insane asylums in Germany', in Norbert Finzsch and Robert Jütte (eds), *Institutions of Confinement: Hospitals, Asylums, and Prisons in Western Europe and North America, 1500–1950*, Cambridge: Cambridge University Press, 1996, pp. 117–32.

Robert J. Waldinger, 'Sleep of reason: John P. Gray and the challenge of moral insanity', *Journal of the History of Medicine and Allied Sciences*, 1979, vol. 34, 163–79.

Martin Wiener, 'Judges v. jurors: courtroom tensions in murder trials and the law of criminal responsibility in nineteenth-century England', *Law and History Review*, 1999, vol. 17, 467–506.

Stephen White, 'Phrenology and the McNaughtan Rules', *Criminal Law Journal*, 1984, vol. 8, 166–83.

5 The medicalization of deviance

This chapter focuses on changing social attitudes in Western society: specifically, on how these were reflected in medico-legal thinking and practice in relation to deviant behaviour. Deviance implies a lack of compliance with social norms, by a person whose conduct and mind-set differ from accepted standards; by definition, the deviant engages in activities that society frowns upon and on which it typically imposes legal sanctions. The definition of any action as deviant is thus essentially a socio-legal matter: laws are created and abolished in relation to social trends and popular beliefs, which themselves can be influenced by medical thinking. Deviance has probably never been more sharply defined than in relation to sex and death, topics which between them encompass a vast range of human activities and which in the past formed a core of medico-legal interest. In particular, infanticide, suicide and homosexuality presented problems that society had to reconcile, a process with which forensic medicine and its practitioners were closely involved.

There can be no doubt of the historical importance of these topics, but a few statistics are in order. In late eighteenth-century Paris hundreds of people killed themselves, so that suicide was allegedly becoming so common that only the most extraordinary cases attracted much attention.[1] In England and Wales in 1856, nearly 22,000 inquests were held: of these, 476 resulted in a charge of homicide, 1,314 in a verdict of suicide, and nearly twice as many again were simply designated as 'found drowned' – frequently a euphemism for suicide.[2] Judicial statistics show that the annual number of suicides and attempted suicides kept rising during the rest of the nineteenth century, and suicide is today a leading cause of death in Western countries.[3] We cannot investigate why this is – that question exceeds the historian's expertise and belongs properly to sociology and psychology – but we do need to consider the history of social and medical attitudes to suicide in order to gain a fuller understanding of the history of forensic medicine and its importance in Western society.

Suicide was for centuries a criminal act, subject to harsh post-mortem physical and financial penalties. In contrast, for centuries infanticide was treated with remarkable lenience, being within the purview of the ecclesiastical courts, which could not impose corporal punishments, until the early modern period, when governments faced with what appeared to be a rising incidence of illegitimacy and infanticide criminalized both in an attempt to regulate female sexuality. In particular, the onus was placed on single women who gave birth in secret and whose infants subsequently died to prove they had not murdered them; those who could not provide the requisite proof were subject to capital punishment. Court cases multiplied and hundreds of convicted women perished in early modern Europe and America, but conviction rates dropped markedly during the eighteenth and nineteenth centuries even as the prevalence of violence towards infants remained disproportionately high.[4] This was largely due to changing social attitudes, in which medicine had an important role to play, especially in the use of the lung test to determine whether a child had been born alive.[5]

Finally, it was not only women's sexuality that was held up to public scrutiny; in certain circumstances men's sexual practices were subject to medico-legal investigation. In the early modern period this was largely in relation to the question of impotence, one of the only grounds available to those who wished to end a marriage. During the nineteenth century medical attention shifted to non-procreative sexualities, and studies pioneered by psychiatrists were ultimately to make sexual variance imaginable, paving the way for the broadening of twentieth-century attitudes towards sexuality.[6]

Suicide

Suicide has been a subject of academic interest for two centuries,[7] stimulated especially by the publication in 1897 of French sociologist Émile Durkheim's (1858–1917) *Suicide: A Study in Sociology*, which posited social causes for an apparently individual act. Sociologists, psychologists and psychiatrists took up the study of suicide with renewed vigour, using contemporary statistics and viewing it from the standpoint of their various disciplines, so that today there is a large body of scholarship on this important topic. Its inherent interest lies in the fact that only humans are capable of reflecting on their own existence and deciding to put an end to it, a choice to which society has never been indifferent. The ancients viewed it as a sensible or even heroic option in the face of certain defined circumstances, including incurable illness, distaste for life, political reversal of fortune, or decrepitude,[8] and the heroic martyrdom theme survived into the modern era on rare occasions, generally military or political in nature.[9] Today we consider suicide tragic and needless, but for a long time it was subject to social criticism on the grounds that it was an insult to both God and society; rejection of the gift of life and human company was a dual offence against religion and law. The religious prohibition against suicide was firmly established in Western Europe as Christianity took hold among the barbarians, and explains why, in medieval Europe, those who rejected their responsibility to God and society were considered deserving of punishment in both this world and the next.[10] Attitudes began to change towards the end of the fifteenth century, as Renaissance thinkers began to challenge the harsh penalties inflicted on suicides by approaching the issue through the notion of insanity. Indirect challenge became open defiance during the Enlightenment; the introduction of the word 'suicide', which had largely replaced the expression 'self-murder' by 1750, was a sign of change,[11] and by the end of the eighteenth century there was widespread acceptance in Britain, Europe and America of a link between suicide, melancholia and mental illness – in effect, a hybridization of suicide as both a medical and a moral problem.[12]

Until the early modern period voluntary death was seen as the result of diabolic temptation induced by despair – in which case those who succumbed to the devil could expect eternal damnation – or as mad behaviour for which the individual could not be held responsible. If deliberate self-murder was suspected, harsh punishments were inflicted on the dead body, and his or her estate was confiscated.[13] In religion, deviance was interpreted as sin, and in law as a criminal offence. The criminalization of suicide thus went hand in hand with its condemnation as a grievous sin, a breach of the religious commandment against murder, supported by communities which believed that suicides were polluting and morally dangerous: their corpses were subjected to a form of torture and execution before dishonourable burial in unconsecrated ground, just like the worst convicted criminals.[14]

Religious objections to suicide remained deep-seated during the early modern period, and physical punishments of the bodies of suicides continued; but the letter of the law was somewhat mitigated in practice, partly due to the influence of Roman law, which distinguished between culpable and excusable suicide, and partly due to long-standing popular discrimination between despair (a grave sin) and melancholy (beyond personal control and thus exculpatory).[15] In France, investigative procedures of the sixteenth century resembled criminal trials, in which rigorous standards of proof were maintained. Most jurists required a detailed report of the place where the corpse was found, a careful examination of the body by a surgeon, an investigation of the lifestyle and habits of the dead person, an inquiry into possible reasons for suicide, and someone to defend the deceased against the charge of suicide.[16] In the German-speaking lands, secular and religious authorities would relax the proscription against Christian burial depending on the suicide's mental state: mercy was extended to those who killed themselves out of mental rather than moral weakness.[17] English inquest juries, being profoundly hostile to suicide in general, were prepared to return verdicts of *felo de se*, felon of himself, or deliberate self-killing, but would sometimes use *non compos mentis* verdicts to attempt to prevent confiscation of a suicide's property.[18]

The idea that suicide might have a medical explanation grew during the seventeenth century, so that suicides could be considered more as sick people in need of treatment than demonically possessed sinners. Medical theories noted the frequent juxtaposition of melancholy and suicidal tendencies, the English physician Thomas Willis (1621–75) going furthest in positing a causal link whereby melancholy could degenerate into mania and bring on suicidal crises. Even religious beliefs could be subsumed by this new medical model: medical theorists explained religious melancholy as simply another form of disease, caused by a surplus of black bile, long associated with melancholy madness. A gap appeared between religious and secular attitudes as the power of the devil gave way to physical and psychological illness.[19] In France, the *Ordonnance criminelle* of 1670 codified contemporary procedures against suicides, which had not been nationally consistent: these were favourable to the defence but failed to specify penalties, probably because they were left to the secular authorities to determine, and were tailored to individual cases according to culpability.[20] In England, changing beliefs were reflected in inquest verdicts: less than seven per cent of inquests reported to the court of King's Bench returned *non compos mentis* verdicts in the early 1660s, but by the early eighteenth century the proportion had risen to over 40 per cent.[21] In seventeenth-century America, where the Puritan fathers had succeeded in linking melancholy to diabolical temptation, this same perception was, ironically, to erode the notion that suicide was an act freely chosen: as the idea that melancholy was a disease gained dominance during the eighteenth century, it became impossible to see it as evidence of criminal intent, whether inspired by Satan or not.[22]

The eighteenth-century impulse towards treating suicide with leniency, which resulted in its widespread decriminalization,[23] was a multi-faceted process that relied on many interacting strands of belief and practice; it was a society-wide phenomenon moulded by cultural, socio-economic, religious and political change. Paradoxically, doctors had little real role to play in this important transformation, even though the process is known as the 'medicalization' of suicide, so-called because of the shift in the perception of suicide as a sinful to an insane act, and thus of the suicidal individual from criminal to victim.[24] Although doctors contributed to the literary debate about suicide, most of which flowed from the pens of jurists, philosophers and theologians, it was not until the nineteenth century that a specifically medico-legal interest in suicide began to grow. Eighteenth-century works tended to tackle it as part of larger studies of melancholia, hypochondria and nervous maladies, perhaps most famously by the English physician George Cheyne (1671–1743), whose *The English Malady* (1733) addressed the nervous diseases supposedly rife among the elite, who seemed to be killing themselves increasingly frequently; or warned of the problems in differentiating suicide from murder. The rising number of asylums strengthened the connection between suicide and insanity in the minds of both the medical profession and the general public,[25] and it was from among the new group of alienists that explicitly medico-legal works on suicide began to appear.

In his *Traité médico-philosophique sur l'aliénation mentale ou la manie* (1801), Pinel linked suicidal tendencies to a mental defect of moral origin: sufferers were unable to view disagreeable events, be they physical or emotional, objectively and so succumbed to suicide.[26] Esquirol's 1838 classic *Des maladies mentales* devoted a large chapter to suicide, asserting its importance to clinical medicine and claiming that 'self-murder is only a phenomenon, consecutive to very different causes; ... it is, almost invariably, a symptom of mental alienation. Most of those who have failed in accomplishing their designs, remain insane for a longer or shorter period of time, or become so afterwards'. This form of insanity could be brought on by a large number of precipitating factors, including masturbation, poverty, alcohol, disease, calamity, hypochondria, monomania, passion, hatred or weariness of life and, of course, melancholy; a significant proportion of the suicidal were likely to come from families afflicted by mental alienation. Autopsy had thus far shed little light on the possible existence of organic lesions characteristic of suicide, although changes had been identified in the brain and stomach, but Esquirol was hopeful that a connection would be found.[27] He closed his chapter with a short section on what was later in the century to gain greater attention from sociologists than from medico-legal experts: the incidence of suicide, and the age, sex, methods and motives of its victims.

The well known alienist physician Forbes Winslow (1810–74), author of the first English work exclusively devoted to suicide, *The Anatomy of Suicide* (1840), aimed to establish that suicidal disposition originated in derangement of the brain and abdominal viscera, and that all suicides were committed under the influence of temporary insanity resulting from a disease of the brain, even in the absence of conclusive evidence of the nature of the organic changes that preceded and accompanied suicidal mania.[28] Since suicide was still a crime in England (it remained so until 1961), Winslow urged inquest juries to enquire carefully into the deceased's mental and physical health, as verdicts of *felo de se* were never justified. Isaac Ray devoted only two short chapters of his *Medical Jurisprudence of Insanity* (1839) to suicide, noting that it now had much less medico-legal importance as it was no longer a criminal offence in the United States, but could be an issue raised in disputes over wills.[29] He agreed with the established medical view that suicide was frequently committed under the impulse of mental derangement due to pathological or physical changes which were not as yet understood, but which were often hereditary in nature.[30] Later alienist writings, notably the encyclopaedic study of the Italian Enrico Morselli (1852–1929), *Il Suicidio: Saggio di statistica morale comparata* (1879; *Suicide: An Essay on Comparative Moral Statistics*,

---

Case Study 5.1: The suicide of Meriwether Lewis (Tennessee, 1809)

The Lewis and Clark Expedition (1804–6) to explore territory in the Great Plains and Rockies then under French sovereignty was led by Captain Meriwether Lewis (1774–1809) and Lieutenant William Clark (1770–1838), intrepid explorers who discovered a passage through the Rockies and gathered a wealth of information about western lands and peoples. Lewis was appointed governor of the Upper Louisiana

Territory in March 1808, and discovered that traversing an unmapped continent was easier than the life of a politician: he was soon in open disagreement with both the national government and his deputy, and fell into serious debt. Angry and depressed, he decided to go to Washington to confront the new president; en route, he made a will for the first time ever, and twice attempted suicide. When he arrived in Tennessee he was in such a state of intoxication and mental derangement that a local military commander insisted that he rest for two weeks. After Lewis set out again in company with three other men, he started to drink and behave oddly. On 10 October 1809 he shot himself in the forehead with one pistol and in the chest with a second; reportedly lingering some hours before death, Lewis had time to cut himself several times with a razor. In his own words, he was strong and 'hard to die'.

Americans at the time tended to attribute suicide to insanity or severe emotional distress resulting from a combination of constitutional and environmental factors. Those who knew Lewis well, including former president Thomas Jefferson, noted that he tended to become depressed whenever he followed a sedentary urban lifestyle, and the promotion to governor fit this pattern (he took up a desk job in St Louis). Others thought financial trouble caused Lewis humiliation and despair; while his deputy attributed the suicide to insanity, which itself had been the origin of his political and financial problems. The press reported his death with no hint of condemnation, connecting it to mental illness in a reflection of popular beliefs.

Although we cannot know the reasons for Lewis's suicide, a modern explanation for it shows how cultural, historical, psychological and organic factors may be linked in the causal process, and is thus revealing of current thinking on the reasons for suicide. Lewis's biography reveals patterns that are recognizable in those who attempt suicide today: repeated failure to establish lasting interpersonal relationships, as he lost his father and step-father and never married despite numerous announcements of his intention to do so, thus avoiding feared future desertion; extreme risk-taking in that he had many narrow escapes, and seemed least troubled when his life was in the greatest danger; and a compulsive desire for self-punishment given that he was an alcoholic by the age of 20 and abstained from drink only during the Expedition. His death was not merely a suicide but a sort of self-execution.

Although colonial Americans were accustomed to death, Lewis seems to have reacted to his father's decease atypically, suggesting that his suicidal urges were rooted in social, constitutional and psychological problems. The circumstances of the Revolutionary War restricted his relationship with his father and then his ability to mourn his death, as

did his mother's remarriage within six months. The historical oppor-
tunity of the Expedition provided a temporary cure for lifelong
depression and alcoholism, but with that buffer removed and personal
disappointment and financial embarrassment threatening, suicide
offered the ultimate coping mechanism.

Source: Howard I. Kushner, *Self-destruction in the Promised Land:
A Psychocultural Biology of American Suicide* (1989), New Brunswick
and London: Rutgers University Press, 1991, pp. 120–32.

1881) contended that suicide was often, though not always, the result of some
mental disease.[31]

In contrast to these views, England's leading medico-legal expert, Alfred
Swaine Taylor, argued that suicide should not be seen solely as the result of
insanity, since that implied that *all* crime was the offspring of insanity, a
viewpoint taken up later in the century by criminal anthropologists, as we saw
in Chapter 4. In his opinion, many would-be suicides were sane and deserved
punishment, and he suggested that establishing their insanity should require
stronger evidence than that admitted in murder cases. Suicide was additionally
of medico-legal importance in regard to life insurance, which became
increasingly common after mid century, since policies might be invalidated by
a deliberate, but not an insane, act of suicide.[32] However, by the end of the
nineteenth century most insurance companies had abandoned regulations
preventing payment in the event of suicide.[33]

Attempted suicide was progressively criminalized in Victorian England, as
thinking shifted away from punishing the families of suicides, as former penalties
had done, towards calling the suicidal themselves to account, and perhaps
offering them treatment in an asylum. The development of national policing
made enforcement practicable and a new area of forensic practice opened up:
prison medical officers had to provide reports on the mental health of individuals remanded for attempting suicide. It was usually policemen on the beat
and doctors who had the most contact with suicide survivors; most magistrates
took a lenient approach to them.[34] Moral and religious stigma clung to suicide
elsewhere in Europe and in America, but as it was no longer a criminal offence
medico-legal texts tended to address it largely in relation to the age-old question
of how to ensure that suicide was distinguished from accident and murder.
The sociologically inclined, like Alexandre Lacassagne, took note of rising
suicide statistics as a public health issue and urged the state to do more to
combat it,[35] while criminologists like Lombroso were interested in suicide
rates among prison inmates, as an indicator of the relationship between crime
and insanity (he considered suicide a crime of passion, when it was not
wholly due to madness) that was characteristic of his criminal anthropology.[36]

Attempts to locate the causes of suicide in the physical body continued in Europe until the twentieth century, but statistical, criminological and socio-logical enquiries began to attract more attention, culminating in Durkheim's seminal work, which emphasized the individual's emotional isolation from society.[37] During the twentieth century, research on suicide focused on social, psychological, biological, psychiatric and psychoanalytic perspectives, some or all of which may act in combination to precipitate a suicide; the study of suicide, its causes and prevention is known as suicidology, a term which came increasingly into use after World War II. The relatively new sub-field known as forensic epidemiology includes suicide, along with other unnatural deaths, within its remit to investigate the interface between forensic medicine/science and public health. Finally, the medico-legal imperative to correctly establish whether a death is suicidal remains as strong as ever, as Western nations maintain national mortality statistics which inform resource allocation and policy-making. However, neither pathology nor forensic science can necessarily prove suicide, and today suicide investigation relies as much as it always did on clues provided by the personal biography of the deceased.[38]

Infanticide

The cultural assumption that women are naturally disposed to love and nurture children is sorely tested by the crime of infanticide which, in its current legal sense, refers to the murder of an infant at the time of or soon after birth. Western notions of femininity and motherhood are at variance with the facts of the offence: the majority of perpetrators are women who, by definition, are propelled into the ranks of the deviant. This fact sets infanticide apart from other forms of homicide, for it has long been a sex-specific crime, typically perpetrated by women acting alone and in secret. Western laws, cognizant of this reality, have established prohibitions against it which have passed succes-sively through stages of leniency, extreme harshness, declining criminalization and back to relative leniency in relation to other types of killing. Just as suicide does, the offence encapsulates the transition from theological to secu-lar concerns in law and society, and thus in medical and medico-legal interest.

The word infanticide has historically been used inconsistently when refer-ring to child murder, in some cases referring to the murder of newborns, newborn child murder or in modern parlance, neonaticide; children up to the age of one year, the current definition established by English law in 1938; or even older children, now known as filicide. In the United States, Scotland, France and Germany the offence of 'infanticide' no longer exists: all homi-cides are tried as murder or manslaughter regardless of the victim's age. However other common law jurisdictions, including Ireland, Canada, Australia (three states) and New Zealand, and some European countries (Austria, Finland, Greece, Italy) have incorporated the separate offence of infanticide and legally defined it as less severe than other forms of killing. Why is this specific offence thought to be necessary, and in what circumstances did it come into being?

Infanticide was initially proscribed as sinful and unnatural by the early Christian church, and penalties against it were enacted in the Western Empire and early medieval barbarian law codes. The medieval church viewed with suspicion the apparently accidental deaths of children smothered while sleeping in the parental bed, and elevated overlaying from a venial to a mortal sin in 1237. The ecclesiastical courts had jurisdiction over infanticidal parents and took action against them, but did not regard overlaying as murder, rather as a form of negligence. If an infant's death was considered a homicide the culprit could be tried in a secular court; but many cases seem to have been viewed as accidents caused by neglect and the church courts, which could not shed blood, imposed public penances designed to enable the guilty to obtain absolution through ostracism and humiliation. If indeed infanticide by parents was widespread and under-reported in medieval Europe, it occurred most likely as a result of financial pressures on the family unit. There was little or no medical investigation of child death and no forensic procedure to follow, so it was impossible to prove premeditation, leaving few grounds on which the secular courts could prosecute.[39]

This position changed drastically during the early modern period, when rulers began to legislate against what appeared to be the predominant motive for infanticide: the need by unmarried mothers to conceal illegitimate births or dispose of illegitimate infants in order to avoid the shame and socio-economic repercussions associated with bearing a bastard. The correlation between infanticide, illegitimacy and young single women was enshrined in a series of remarkably similar capital statutes enacted all over Europe. The Carolina, promulgated in the Holy Roman Empire in 1532, defined infanticide (article 131) as the murder of a newborn by an unwed mother, or by married women or widows who had committed adultery, in order to conceal their 'sexual immorality'. Other kinds of child killing were prosecuted as murder or manslaughter under article 137. In other states, the crime was strictly limited to single women, as in the French edict of 1556, the English act of 1624, its Scottish (1690), Irish (1707), American (seventeenth century) and Canadian (eighteenth century) equivalents, and comparable laws in Sweden (1627) and elsewhere. All of these laws created a presumption of murder in cases in which an unmarried mother gave birth in secret and the baby was later found dead, even though the infant might have been stillborn or died of natural causes. Although the pervasive concern was to support a widespread social disciplining agenda by punishing sexually profligate women, these statutes were directly responsible for introducing the need for medical testimony into infanticide trials, because some judges and juries wanted proof that the child had been born alive and was then killed.[40]

The earliest works on the medico-legal aspects of infanticide appeared in the late 1600s, and autopsies on infant corpses were unknown before the mid seventeenth century.[41] To achieve convictions, legal officials relied on the external signs of childbirth displayed by a suspect woman's body: sudden reduction in size accompanied by a pale and weak appearance, the condition of the genitalia and the presence of breast milk (even though medical thinking held that childless women might lactate) were all seen as suggestive enough to justify torture, which usually led to a confession. The other principal source of proof was the child's body: if there were signs of violence upon it, it was difficult for the accused mother to credibly deny the intent to kill, despite the fact that injuries may well have been accidental. In England and colonial America, medical evidence focused on the signs of recent childbirth in the alleged mother and on the maturity and viability of the infant; if the corpse was undersized, or lacked hair or nails, midwives tended to assume that it had been stillborn. As on the Continent, signs of severe violence on the victim's body often led to conviction, and a defendant was further disadvantaged if she had a bad reputation.[42]

The introduction of the first test for live birth – one of the most important medico-legal innovations of our entire period of study – came about when key figures of the scientific revolution considered the practical utility of the long-known differences between foetal and adult lungs: the latter are paler and less dense than the former. In 1653 the English physician William Harvey (1578–1657), who had discovered the circulation of the blood (published 1628), suggested that changes in lung colour at birth, which remained even if the infant died immediately after taking its first breath, could be used to determine whether a child was born dead or alive. In 1667 Jan Swammerdam (1637–80), the Dutch naturalist, microscopist and discoverer of red blood cells, carried out a series of physiological studies of respiration which demonstrated that if an infant had breathed after birth its air-filled lungs would float in water; had the infant not breathed, the lungs would sink. This became known as 'docimasia pulmonum hydrostatica', from the Greek *dokimasia*, examination, or simply the 'hydrostatic test', 'flotation test', or 'lung test'. It was carried out by 'swimming' the lungs together and separately, or parts of them, the rationale being that lungs which had drawn a breath would contain enough air to reduce their specific gravity and therefore float. Flotation was taken as evidence that respiration had occurred and that the infant had been born alive.[43]

Karel Rayger (1641–1707), an anatomist in Bratislava, suggested that the test should be used as proof of infanticide in 1676, and five years later it was first used in a trial by the city physician of Zeitz in eastern Germany, Johannes Schreyer (1655–94), when sinking lungs helped to secure the acquittal of 15-year-old Anna Voigt.[44] The lung test entered Western medico-legal practice despite almost immediate criticism by a range of doctors in a variety of countries: lungs might float because of putrefaction or efforts at artificial respiration, or because breathing had occurred before an infant was fully born. Attempts to develop new tests based on the weight of the lungs before and after respiration were made, particularly by Wilhelm Gottfried Ploucquet (1744–1814) of Tübingen in 1781, but this and others were eventually discredited as unreliable. The determination of live birth remained a problem central to the medico-legal aspects of infanticide during the nineteenth century, when despite lingering doubts about the efficacy of the hydrostatic test, textbooks of forensic medicine were generally agreed that if it was properly done it could offer good evidence of respiration but not of live birth or separate existence from the mother.[45] The twentieth-century forensic pathologist faced precisely the same issues, as reliable signs of survival of birth become evident only after several days, but by then marked relaxation of the laws against infanticide gave mothers the benefit of the doubt.

Late eighteenth-century humanitarian sentiment combined with the fact that it was just too difficult to secure convictions against women who had been seduced and abandoned led to a growing dissatisfaction with the severity of the statutes against infanticide and so to repeal across the Western world during the course of the nineteenth century. Laws punishing the concealment of the birth of a bastard child by a fine or imprisonment were introduced (Pennsylvania 1794; England 1803; Scotland 1809; Canada 1810–36; France 1863), offering an alternative to the capital charge of killing a newborn. Proof of murder now had to be supplied in order to obtain a conviction for infanticide, making medical evidence all the more important, and courts became increasingly willing to accept pleas of insanity in mitigation; the French penal code of 1810 explicitly stated that there could be no crime if the accused mother was insane, reduced the penalty significantly if death was caused involuntarily, and furthermore required proof that the infant was viable. Judges, juries and medico-legal experts often adopted a flexible definition of insanity, recognizing that it could be a mental state experienced solely at or around the time of birth by an unmarried woman subject to fear, stress, pain, confusion and isolation as a result of male seduction. This thinking was integrated into the 1871 Imperial German Criminal Code, which defined infanticide as a crime committed against an illegitimate child by its mother at or immediately after birth, and punished it less harshly than murder or manslaughter because illegitimate births were assumed to result from male deception and the trauma of delivery was believed to diminish a mother's soundness of mind.[46]

The link between childbirth and insanity was encapsulated in the diagnosis of puerperal insanity (*psychose puerpérale*), an important step in the medicalization of infanticide. A French reform of 1824 allowed judges to impose a reduced penalty for infanticide if the accused woman's mental state had been troubled by pregnancy and childbirth, and by the mid nineteenth century alienists agreed that mental disorder could afflict women at any time from conception to weaning. It could take two forms: mania tended to be more common and to arise at the time of birth; melancholia took longer to show itself and was more difficult to treat.[47] In medico-legal practice there was an acceptance that such insanity was transitory, usually due more to a deplorable personal situation than organic disease, yet that it still negated wilful intent; the diagnosis simply supported the existing medical and social desire to treat infanticidal women with compassion. Moreover, it could be made to fit many different scenarios, from the young unmarried woman who gave birth in secret and immediately destroyed her child (Case Study 5.2) to the older married

Case Study 5.2: The murder of her newborn infant by Rose Matthews (England, 1867)

On 28 October 1867 Rose Matthews, a domestic servant aged 21, was tried at the Old Bailey for the murder of her illegitimate infant child, the sex of which was not revealed in the trial record. The evidence presented followed the established pattern for such cases. Her employer, Mary Scholefield, told the court that she had hired Rose in April and noticed within a month that she appeared to be pregnant. When asked about it, Rose had denied it, claiming that all her family had 'very peculiar figures in that way'. Early on the morning of 14 August Mrs Scholefield heard Rose wandering about the house in pain. Although she claimed she had simply over-eaten and would soon be better, the blood on her hands and clothes belied that excuse and her employer went out to look for a policeman, and then sent for a doctor.

Dr George Woolley testified that when he arrived Rose told him that she had suffered pain, diarrhoea and sickness but when he examined her it was clear that she had recently given birth. He found the baby dead in the coal cellar, and later performed an autopsy, determining that the child had been born alive and died from a large incised wound in the neck. He was closely cross-examined by Rose's (probably court-appointed) barrister about the medical evidence, and this reveals the issues that courts generally focused on in infanticide trials. Woolley said that 'the lungs were inflated', thus proving that the child was born alive, but admitted that the lungs could inflate before the child was fully separated from the mother. He did not specify how he determined live birth, though almost certainly he performed some version of the lung test; the child's size was also indicative. He further stated that although women might be delivered suddenly while standing up and the child's head consequently injured, he could not imagine that the neck wound had been made by one cut, as 'the head was nearly severed from the body' – thus strongly suggesting that the child had been deliberately murdered. Finally, he believed the prisoner to be of 'weak intellect', and in his experience 'coincident with the pains of labour there is certain mental disturbance – in the case of a person of weak intellect that mental disturbance would probably be aggravated', so opening the door to acquittal on the grounds of a mental imbalance specifically associated with childbirth.

A police officer testified to finding a knife but no baby linen, suggesting that Rose had not made preparations for the birth, and then a defence witness took the stand. John Rowland Gibson, surgeon to Newgate prison (1855–82) revealed that Rose was both deaf and of weak intellect, not capable of much reasoning or knowledge. Even more important to her case, though, was his opinion about her state of mind: 'there is a sympathetic connection between the uterine organs and the brain – during conception and child-bearing, and afterwards, when giving milk, women are more susceptible of mental disturbance than at other periods. I think there is a great tendency to mental disturbance during delivery, and in the case of a person of weak intellect I think it might be increased; there would be less power of mental control and less appreciation of facts.' But this was not to say that she was insane or did not know right from wrong. Finally, the prison chaplain – as someone who had also spent time with the prisoner – declared his confidence in Gibson's opinion. Rose Matthews was convicted not of murder but of concealing the birth of her child and sentenced to the maximum two years' imprisonment.

Her case illustrates the difficulty in proving live birth and separate existence beyond reasonable doubt, the tendency of juries to accept that even the most violent wounds might have been inflicted accidentally, and the medical belief that women were liable to temporary insanity caused by childbirth. Although very much a typical Victorian case, Rose Matthews' experience embodies many of the characteristics that have historically defined infanticide, including the refusal of pregnant young women to admit their condition, an amazing stoicism, and society's general wish to treat mothers with compassion founded on both social and medical grounds.

Source: *The Proceedings of the Old Bailey, 1674–1913*, reference number: t18671028–965, online at http://www.oldbaileyonline.org (accessed on 26 May 2010).

mother who gave birth and then, exhausted by breastfeeding a few weeks or months later (lactational insanity), killed one or more of her children, often attempting suicide at the same time.[48] Although puerperal insanity as an independent medical concept had vanished by the early twentieth century,[49] its effects on the law remained.

Consideration for the mental state of the mother at the time of delivery was used as one justification for the abolition of the death penalty for infanticide in France in 1901.[50] In the United States and Canada the death penalty still applied but acquittals, or conviction for concealment or manslaughter, were the norm.[51] In England, if the full offence could be proved a woman would be sentenced to death whether she was married or not, but no one was executed for the murder of her own infant after 1849, and acquittal or light sentences were common. However, few acquittals were on the grounds of insanity and defences tended to focus on claims of stillbirth or accident. An apparent increase in the crime during the 1860s and 1870s led to attempts to reform the law on the grounds that infanticide resulted from a mental condition induced by childbearing, but these failed for fear that it would appear to place a lesser value on infant life. An effort before World War I to abolish the pretence that a woman would be hanged for infanticide also failed, but formed the basis for the 1922 Infanticide Act.[52] This Act created a new class of homicide restricted to the killing of newly born children by their mothers, and provided a foundation for an insanity plea by applying when the mother 'had not fully recovered from the effect of giving birth to such child, and by reason thereof the balance of her mind was disturbed'. In 1938 the Act was extended to include mothers who killed infants up to the age of one year, despite a lack of 'conclusive evidence that the effects of childbirth resolved after 12 months' and the fact that psychiatrists were abandoning the concept of lactational insanity. Further, the offence really applied to two different types of murdering mothers: the killing of neonates by distressed women suffering from emotional and physical upheaval but who were not mentally ill; and the murder of older infants by women suffering some form of psychosis. The law rested on two related assumptions: first, that childbearing disturbs the balance of women's minds; second, that if a woman kills an infant it is likely to be due to the mental instability associated with childbirth.[53] Thus in the case of newborn child murder, the law found a way to adapt medical theory to fit the long-standing social consensus as to what constituted an irresistible impulse and criminal responsibility, in a marked contrast to the right/wrong test set by the McNaughton Rules.[54]

The 1938 Infanticide Act, which is still in force today, formed the basis of the Canadian law of 1948,[55] the Irish law of 1949 and the New Zealand law of 1961, as well as that of the Australian states of New South Wales, Victoria and Tasmania. It has been subject to criticism on the grounds that the psychiatric principles it rests on are unsubstantiated as no official diagnosis of postpartum psychosis exists, though there is a proven link between birth and mental disorder, and that it does not hold women properly accountable for their actions. However the 1938 Act does not presume mental illness, it allows psychiatric evidence in mitigation; it does not require proof of psychosis, merely that the balance of the mind was disturbed.[56] It seems that contrary to medico-legal tradition, 'puerperal psychotic illness is a relatively rare cause of infanticide'.[57] In essence, modern laws on infanticide reflect a policy decision to deal leniently with women who kill their infants, by sentencing them to probation or hospital instead of prison or indefinite incarceration in a forensic psychiatric facility.

Impotence

Medical expertise had a significant role to play in disputed sexual matters such as impotence, pregnancy and genital defect, which as defining characteristics of male and female, masculine and feminine – and thus of the individual's place in society – were extremely important during the medieval and early modern periods. Those who did not conform to their place in the gendered social system were exposed and ostracized, in much the same way, and for related reasons, that pregnant unmarried women were: as threats to the social order and to community values through unrestrained or unfulfilled lust. In these cases, however, it was the church courts, rather than the secular authorities, who took the medico-legal lead in investigating and revealing sex-related deviance.

Sexual defects were usually important only insofar as they related to impotence, but in the case of hermaphrodites, genital irregularity could affect a person's civil status. This was not a widespread problem, but men and women had different social and legal privileges and duties, and those who were born with genitals of both sexes risked a great deal if they were officially declared to be a sex other than the one they wished to be, as this could affect inheritance rights, the ability to marry and even how a person had to dress. By the seventeenth century the courts were deferring to medical doctors in cases of hermaphrodites and women with enlarged clitorises, who exceeded the norms of female sexual anatomy; in France, 'medical opinion could and did dramatically alter the lives of individuals, forcing them to change their gender, leave their marriages, or submit to dangerous surgery, and sometimes condemning them to punishment, exile, or imprisonment'.[58] Doctors had a

---

Case Study 5.3: The medico-legal examination of Marie le Marcis, hermaphrodite (France, 1601)

Medieval civil and canon law recognized that some individuals were born with genitals of both sexes. As there could be no legal status other than male or female, gender identity was assigned on the basis of the predominant sex and, on the assumption that a person's true nature would reveal itself at puberty, hermaphrodites were allowed to freely follow their own sexual preference. This changed during the sixteenth century, however, when legal practice in such matters began to depend more closely on medical evidence and opinion, as a consequence of the medical discovery of the clitoris and its association with what was considered deviant female sexuality: if a woman was capable of penetrating another woman, she could potentially be found guilty of the sin and crime of sodomy, which was punishable by death. At the very least, transvestism could lead to accusations of fraud.

One of the most famous cases in which these issues arose was that of Marie le Marcis, a 20-year-old chambermaid from Rouen. Raised as a girl, by the age of 15 she realized that she had a male organ which made its presence known particularly in the presence of other women, and in 1601 she abandoned female dress, changed her name to Marin, and announced her intention to marry a fellow maid, a widow with two children, named Jeane le Febvre. When they sought a dispensation to marry Marie was promptly charged with sodomy, and defended herself on the grounds that she was actually a man with a hidden penis. Visual inspection by two medical commissions failed to corroborate her claim and she was sentenced to be burned alive; Jeane was to be whipped and banished. Marie appealed to the Parlement of Rouen, and a third medical commission, composed of six physicians, two surgeons and two midwives was on the verge of confirming the original decision when one of its members, the Rouen physician Jacques Duval (1555–1615), inserted his finger into Marie's vagina and found the hidden penis. His dissenting testimony, that Marie possessed a penis that emerged only when she was aroused and that she was in fact a predominantly male hermaphrodite and thus innocent of sodomy, was enough to save her. The death sentence was commuted to a probationary period of several years, during which she was to live and dress as a woman, using neither set of genitals for sex, until she reached the age of majority (25) and it became clear which gender nature intended for her. Ten years later, Marie was living as Marin, a bearded male tailor, and Duval published an account of the case in his *Treatise on Hermaphrodites* (1612).

Sources: P. Darmon, *Trial by Impotence: Virility and Marriage in Pre-Revolutionary France* (1979), trans. P. Keegan, London: Chatto & Windus, 1985, pp. 43–46; K. Park, 'The rediscovery of the clitoris: French medicine and the tribade, 1570–1620', in D. Hillman and C. Mazzio (eds), *The Body in Parts: Fantasies of Corporeality in Early Modern Europe* (New York and London: Routledge, 1997), pp. 171–93; L. Daston and K. Park, 'The hermaphrodite and the orders of nature: sexual ambiguity in early modern France', in L. Fradenburg and C. Freccero (eds), *Premodern Sexualities*, New York and London: Routledge, 1996, pp. 117–36.

similarly persuasive effect on legal decision-making when comparable cases came to the attention of the authorities elsewhere in Europe.[59]

The most important area of the non-criminal law to rely on medico-legal opinion during the pre-modern period was the canon law of marriage, which required a couple to be physically capable of consummating their union. Once married, the only way out was via the church, which recognized inability to perform the sexual act as a reason to grant a declaration of nullity, most often on the grounds of the permanent impotence of one or the other partner. As soon as a papal decretal of the twelfth century allowed remarriage of the unaffected spouse, genital examination became an obvious method of proof and was institutionalized by Pope Innocent IV (1243–54). Inspections were made by midwives and doctors, but canonists were aware that an external view could not always resolve the issue: genital malformation was obvious enough,[60] but in its absence how could proof of inability to have sex be established, especially for men? To resolve these difficulties the highly unusual legal procedure of trial by congress was instituted,[61] quite possibly as a result of an innovation traced to the thirteenth-century English cleric Thomas of Chobham. Although canonists had already accepted that the wife should be examined by midwives, Chobham suggested that the matrons might also observe the couple together in bed over the course of many nights, advice that was taken up by the church courts within a few decades and which spread rapidly to Europe.[62]

Readers may find it surprising to learn of the ecclesiastical origins of this ultimately scandalous and ill-reputed procedure, in which a married couple had sex in the presence of medical witnesses to establish whether the husband was capable of maintaining an erection, but it clearly grew out of the evidentiary problem of establishing proof of male impotence and was thus, as were all other areas of pre-modern forensic practice, tied to the needs of the legal system. Judges and physicians, perplexed by the phenomenon of perfectly formed but impotent men, could see no other way to provide the evidence that was required to dissolve a marriage except by the testimony of eyewitnesses. From that point, the use of midwives and doctors was a short step away: the former were already mandated by canon law to examine women, and doctors soon accepted or oversaw their reports on couples' attempts at intercourse. The full-blown trial by congress, into which the practice evolved, employed medical teams in much the same way that a criminal investigation did.

Although it was known in England, Spain, Italy, Switzerland and Belgium prior to the sixteenth century (and had by then died out in England),[63] trial by congress was most closely associated with late sixteenth- and seventeenth-century France where, although it was banned in 1677, it continued during the eighteenth. Contemporaries noted that its introduction led to more and more dissolutions of marriage, though its actual incidence was probably not great. Most trials were urban rather than rural, and tended to involve people of high social status: court records indicate that 20 per cent of trials involved the nobility, who formed only three per cent of the French population. The rest concerned the liberal professions and artisan classes; peasants were excluded.[64] Perhaps five per cent of European impotence trials involved charges against women.[65]

How did it work in practice? Although people agreed to submit to it informally, it could only be legally enforced by the decision of a judge, in which case refusal implied guilt. Trials could vary in length from a few hours to several consecutive nights, and often took place on neutral territory, in a rented room or physician's home. The couple were first thoroughly examined before being left to get on with it; the matrons stayed around the bed but the male physicians and surgeons withdrew a little distance away. The number of experts varied, but there were usually three, a physician, surgeon and midwife, with more called in for the cases of wealthier aristocrats. The judge and other ecclesiastical officials were usually elsewhere in the same house. After an hour or two, or when they tired of waiting, the doctors would halt the proceedings and subject both partners to a forensic genital examination before writing the mandatory report and delivering it to the judge. Reports were nearly always unfavourable to the man unless there was clear evidence of ejaculation.[66]

Although many jurists and doctors were uneasy with the system of genital examination, and attacks on congress began in the late sixteenth century as it was both shameful and inconclusive, canon law retained a clear role for it and no one was certain what to put in its place until the Revolution legalized divorce and rejected impotence as a reason for annulment. Nineteenth-century French medico-legal experts abandoned the idea that impotence alone could nullify a marriage, though the church courts persisted; a dramatic decline in the number of trials made it possible for all cases to be submitted to Rome for approval. Forensic medical examinations continued sporadically through the first half of the twentieth century, when non-consummation of marriage was increasingly ascribed to psychological as well as physical reasons,[67] and the canonical debate about female impotence intensified with the advent of new surgical techniques like hysterectomy.[68] Today, however, impotence as an impediment to marriage is relatively unimportant in the Western world; it is more likely to be used as a defence to a charge of sexual assault.

Sexual deviance

People who have followed anomalous sexual practices – meaning any which do not fall into the ordinary procreative model stressed in Christian religious teachings – have over the centuries tended to be labelled as deviant and subjected to physical and mental repression. By far the largest group to which the label of deviance was attached were men who loved other men and sought partners of their own sex. In the past they were commonly known as sodomites, a term which by definition referred to an individual act, sodomy, not a particular group, and which included the notion of sin. Sodomitical acts could include sex between men, sex between women, sex between humans and animals, and oral or anal heterosexual sex; in essence, 'sodomy' encompassed all manner of 'unnatural' copulation, though the harshest punishments were generally reserved for male acts of anal penetration. The homosexual, by contrast, emerged during the late nineteenth century as a member of a specific social group which identified itself with same-sex love relationships and an associated lifestyle, but not necessarily with particular acts.[69] In keeping with this shift from a focus on sexual acts to the emotional life of the alleged offender, medico-legal interest in deviant sexual practices tended for a long time to centre on anal penetration; with the advent of psychiatry in the nineteenth century, medico-legal interest turned to the personality and motivations of the accused individual.

The death penalty for male same-sex practices can be traced back to the Bible, but proscription of female same-sex practices has been the preserve of secular authorities, who have not followed a uniform pattern of criminalization. Whatever the origins of the medieval sanction against what pre-modern people tended to group together under the label of 'sodomy', the crime against nature, there is no doubt that hundreds of accused men, and a much smaller number of women, were condemned to death and executed all over Europe from the late thirteenth century to the early decades of the nineteenth; the last Western execution for sodomy occurred in England in 1835.[70] On what, if any, medical evidence were these unfortunate people convicted?

For women, an enlarged clitoris could be presumptive of guilt, at least enough to justify torture, because their anatomy permitted unnatural sexual acts. Thus, in the few known examples of cases involving women accused of sodomy, medical evidence seems to have focused on that issue. When two women were tried for sodomy at Halberstadt in Saxony in 1721, the city physician, surgeon and midwife examined the main defendant, who had been living as a man for years, to find out whether she was a hermaphrodite; but her co-defendant was medically examined only after she claimed to be suffering from depression. Their convictions appear to have been due mainly to the fact that they both confessed.[71]

More evidence is available to show that medical inspection in the case of men accused of sodomy was fairly common. In 1365 a Venetian accused of having intercourse with a goat claimed in his own defence that he had been unable to sleep with a woman or to masturbate for three years due to an accident. The city authorities promptly appointed a team of two physicians and three surgeons to examine him and determine whether there was something physically wrong with him. They concluded that he was able to have an erection. Then the legal officials asked two prostitutes to test the accused, a test which he apparently failed. This established that he had a medical excuse for consorting with the goat and so, although convicted as a sodomite, he was spared the death penalty.[72] In 1467 legislation requiring surgeons to report anyone they treated for anal injuries was introduced, indicating a growing awareness of the importance of medical evidence in cases of alleged sodomy but also revealing the prevailing assumption that the passive partner was likely to be a boy or a woman, that the active partner was more culpable, yet not neglecting the utility of torture in eliciting confessions.[73] Torture and medical examination went hand in hand in other Italian jurisdictions during the Renaissance: legal records show medical involvement in sodomy cases in Florence and Lucca, where anal venereal infections were investigated along with any physical damage experienced by the passive partner.[74] A similar situation pertained in early modern Geneva, where cases could be abandoned if the medical evidence failed to support the charge of anal penetration. In cases of child molestation, prosecution relied heavily on medico-legal evidence.[75] Spanish doctors were also accustomed to performing anal examinations in sixteenth- and seventeenth-century sodomy trials conducted by both the Inquisition and the secular authorities in Spain and Mexico.[76]

Medical practitioners were however remarkably reluctant to write about this aspect of medico-legal practice, with the major exception of Paolo Zacchia, who in a very brief section of his *Quaestiones Medico-Legales* focused on the physical signs of sodomy, viewing it largely as an act of anal penetration against boys or women; women who had sex with other women were also committing sodomy. His views soon pushed the few other writings of the day into obscurity, and Zacchia became the leading seventeenth-century authority on 'the forensic implications of sodomy'. His protocol focused on anal examination by physicians and surgeons who searched for fissures, tears, haemorrhoids and loosening as signs of penetration and reported their findings to judges who would determine whether the act had occurred; the alleged perpetrator's penis also had to be examined to see whether it was capable of inflicting the injuries sustained, whilst other causes had to be ruled out.[77]

The eighteenth century marked the beginning of a turning point in medico-legal interest in deviant sexual practices. Although we know relatively little about the evidence used in court cases, medical writings on unnatural forms of lust, especially masturbation, began to approach the subject from a more holistic perspective. Rather than focusing solely on the anus, the study of same-sex practices began to consider their deleterious effects on both the body and the personality as a result of physiological weakening.[78] Scientific interest in sexuality replaced the early modern religious ascription to sin with secular notions of nature, but deviant sexuality was still seen as socially subversive.[79] When the Swiss physician Samuel Tissot (1728–97) wrote a treatise on masturbation (1760) it attracted world-wide attention because of its Enlightenment principles: the enlightened ideal of the naturally innocent child postulated bad child-rearing as a cause of self-abuse, which could then lead to a variety of wasting diseases; other forms of unacceptable sexual behaviour could lead to insanity. Tissot's model was adopted by the new medical discipline of psychiatry, while the French Revolution stimulated legal reform in areas influenced by the French: sodomy was decriminalized in France (1791), Belgium (1795), the Netherlands (1811), Bavaria (1813) and Spain (1822) on the grounds of non-interference in private affairs. Consequently, medico-legal concern shifted away from the anus of the sodomite to study his mental state; medical discourses about same-sex practices turned from the physical signs needed to secure convictions for sodomy toward the explication of what was to become the 'homosexual'.[80]

Despite the decriminalization of sodomy in some countries, penalties against same-sex behaviours were extended elsewhere (such as Austria (1852), Germany (1871) and England (1885, 1897)), and everywhere new offences against morality, such as public indecency, were introduced, along with legal ages of consent. As policing developed, medico-legal experts were increasingly confronted by sexual deviance in the courts. During the first half of the nineteenth century experts tended to believe that such offenders experienced mental and nervous disorders as a *result* of their unnatural practices and the associated social and moral failings that such activities embodied. Around mid-century, however, prompted by the encompassing rubrics of moral insanity and degeneration, psychiatrists began to suppose that (inherited) diseases of the brain and nervous system *caused* sexual deviance. Research led initially by Ambroise Tardieu in France and Johann Casper in Germany, who were among the first to report case studies of moral offenders, stimulated medical interest in the criminal responsibility of 'perverts', whose actions were redefined as biologically-based perversions rather than perversities born of vice. What is now termed 'homosexuality' was seen as a pathological condition, rather than a temporary deviation from the norm.[81]

Psychiatric interest in homosexuality was stimulated mainly by German and Austrian experiences of penalization. During the 1860s, as German uni-fication was planned and ways sought to integrate divergent criminal codes, the homosexual lawyer Karl Ulrichs (1825–95) published a series of pamph-lets on what he called 'uranism', a natural state characterized by the instinct of a woman's soul enclosed in a male body. Such inborn tendencies could not be dangerous, he argued, unsuccessfully, against the adoption by the new German Reich of the harsh Prussian penalties against same-sex practices. The words 'homosexual' and 'heterosexual' were coined in 1869 by the Hungarian journalist Karl-Maria Kertbeny (1824–82), while the psychological and neu-rological approach to homosexuality dates from the publication in 1870 of an article on 'contrary sexual feeling', later dubbed 'inversion', by the Berlin psychiatrist Carl Westphal (1833–90), which explained homosexuality as a feeling, not necessarily sexual, of being entirely alienated from one's own sex, the result of pathological under-development: that is, a person born into the wrong sexed body. In forensic medicine attention had always focused on acts, but now the interest was firmly on personalities; homosexuals became a dis-tinct group who because of heredity or childhood training chose partners of the same sex, in contrast to sodomites who were defined solely by their acts. Gradually the biological theory began to predominate over the early learning theory, laying a foundation for the development of the science of sexology.[82] In Italy, Cesare Lombroso was ahead of his time in using empirical data in support of his fairly traditional inferences about female sexuality: the Italian version of *Criminal Woman*, unlike the English abridged version, devoted sections to adultery, frigidity, lesbianism, pre-marital sex and masturbation.[83] However during the nineteenth century more innovative research was to flow from Germany, Austria and Britain than from Italy, France or elsewhere because of the criminal status of homosexuality in those countries, where its study was linked to efforts to abolish punitive laws.[84]

The most outstanding contributions to the study of non-procreative sexual practices were made by three Germans and one English physician: Richard von Krafft-Ebing (1840–1902), professor of psychiatry in Vienna; Albert Moll (1862–1939), a Berlin psychiatrist and neurologist; Magnus Hirschfeld (1868–1935), a pioneering sexologist; and Havelock Ellis (1859–1939), a sex psychologist and social reformer. Krafft-Ebing collected and catalogued information about deviant sexual practices in his famous *Psychopathia Sexualis*, first published in 1886 and in its twelfth edition by the time of his death. This classic text (it is still in print) developed a complete typology of deviant behaviours, including sadism, masochism, fetishism and contrary sexual feeling, and attributed deviations from the norm to degeneration. He thus did not hold individuals responsible for their deviant sexuality, on the grounds that heredity had overridden free will, and advocated medical treatment rather than criminal prosecution (see Case Study 5.4). Although he believed firmly

---

Case Study 5.4: The trial of Dr S and Mr G for sodomy (Germany, 1888)

Nineteenth-century German law criminalized sexual acts between men (but not women) – though only in the form of anal penetration, what Krafft-Ebing called pederasty, better known as sodomy. As medical understanding of homosexuality grew, psychiatrists who studied sexual inversion advocated a focus not only on the deed but on the perpetrator's mental condition; although a homosexual's sexual preferences may not have been to the liking of society in general, it was natural to him and punishment did no good. Men who were unfortunate enough to be charged under Germany's Paragraph 175 against sodomy sometimes turned to Krafft-Ebing for support, as in the case of two Germans whom he named only as S and G.

S, a 37-year-old married scientist and director of a city laboratory, was accused by his stepfather of having immoral relations with G, a 19-year-old butcher's son whom S and his wife had befriended. When G fell ill with gonorrhoea in February 1888 S took care of him, and in May G moved into his house. Both men later admitted that they did not really understand the strength of their feelings for each other, and gossip about them eventually led to the accusation that they had a sexual relationship. During the course of their trial, G was repeatedly examined by medical experts, who declared that his anus was pathologically changed in a manner that pointed to the probability that he was a passive sodomite, i.e. that he was accustomed to being anally penetrated. They were found guilty under Paragraph 175 of the German Criminal Code: S, as the seducer, was sentenced to eight months in prison; G, as the youthful victim, got four months.

They immediately appealed to the Supreme Court at Leipzig and collected evidence in support of their appeal: both were examined by medical experts, who declared that G's anus showed no signs of sodomy. Psychological aspects were not touched upon in the trial, but now Krafft-Ebing was asked to examine both men, who travelled to Austria to see him in December 1888. In a lengthy report, the psychiatrist concluded that S was not a homosexual and did not have sexual feelings for G, but did have a tendency to form inordinately close friendships with other men, as he had done twice before. He seems to have accepted S's claim that when he kissed or dreamed about G, there was nothing sexual in it. For his part, G did not appear to Krafft-Ebing to be a 'male courtesan', but was firmly attracted to women; he had accepted S's kisses with good grace, but initially found it unusual. G viewed S, who was a very emotional man, as a father figure. Krafft-Ebing thought S was sentimental and eccentric, but harmless.

Now his report turned to the medico-legal aspects of their case. Krafft-Ebing noted that sodomy presumed a 'congenital or acquired perversion of the sexual instinct and, at the same time, defect of moral sense that is either original or acquired'. Active or passive pederasty could be non-pathological, performed for practical reasons such as money or lack of women; or pathological, due to mental disease or the exceptional act of homosexuals more or less forced to it for some reason. It was necessary to prove that a man belonged to one of these categories to justify a conviction for sodomy. As neither S nor G fit any of these classifications, the verdict against them was, from a psychological viewpoint, legally untenable. Consequently, the defendants had a re-trial in March 1890. Evidence of S's deep friendships dovetailed with fresh medical evidence about G's alleged anal anomalies: experts called by the court conceded that these may have been due to 'digital manipulations', i.e. not a penis, whilst defence experts contested their diagnostic value. The court recognized that the offence had not been proved, and exonerated S and G.

Whether S and/or G were actually homosexual is beside the point; this case is indicative of the state of medico-legal knowledge and belief about homosexuality and homosexual practices in the late 1880s, and of legal responses to what was still a criminal offence in many Western nations. Medical science was, however slowly, beginning to view it not as a disease but as a natural state, so that the medico-legal focus slowly shifted from the homosexual's body to his mind. Krafft-Ebing was a pioneer of this changing approach, and during the 1890s he became an advocate of judicial reform and a supporter of the nascent homosexual rights movement. Paragraph 175, modelled on the Prussian successor (1794) to the Carolina's article 116, remained on the statute books from 1871 until 1994.

Source: R. von Krafft-Ebing, *Psychopathia Sexualis, with especial reference to the Antipathetic Sexual Instinct: A Medico-Forensic Study*, 12th edn, Stuttgart: Ferdinand Enke, 1903, trans. F.S. Klaf, London: Staples Press, 1965, pp. 397–405.

that only procreative sex was normal, Krafft-Ebing's theories were largely based on patient histories and so involved not only medical theory but the feelings and beliefs of those who indulged in the practices he chronicled. In contrast, Moll challenged the link between sex and procreation, arguing that people had both a sex drive and a relationship drive in his *Untersuchungen über die Libido sexualis* (1897; medical investigations on the sexual libido). In acknowledging homosexuality as the most prevalent variation of the relationship drive, Moll stimulated further research on the subject and sexology developed quickly. Hirschfeld defended the idea of a third sex as an explanation for innate homosexuality but is better known as the founder of the world's first homosexual rights organization, the Wissenschaftlich-humanitäres Komitee (Scientific Humanitarian Committee, 1897), and for replacing sexual acts with social relationships as the principal object of study. Ellis worked to emphasize the normality of practices that others considered deviant, especially homosexuality, and co-authored, with John Addington Symonds (1840–93), the first serious British study of homosexuality, *Sexual Inversion* (1897), which posited two types, congenital and acquired. Like his German contemporaries, Ellis highlighted the role of case studies and advocated liberalizing laws on same-sex relationships.[85]

Medico-legal interest in the physical effects of non-procreative sexual acts did not disappear overnight, as Case Study 5.4 shows, but it became increasingly difficult to convince a court that physical indications alone were evidence of sodomy. In 1871 the case against Ernest Boulton and Frederick Park for conspiring to commit unnatural acts collapsed, revealing a lack of medical experience and knowledge of such matters in England; later textbooks warned against relying on anal evidence and reflected the shift in interest to psychoanalytic treatments and the motives of the accused.[86] In the United States, homosexuality was viewed as a harmful aspect of modernity; initially considered a form of madness in the degenerationist mode, by the early twentieth century American physicians argued that it should be controlled in the same way as other forms of vice, by ensuring proper childhood development. It was only in the 1920s that some researchers began to accept homosexuality as a key variation of 'normal' sexuality.[87]

During the first half of the twentieth century European journals published more than twice as many articles about homosexuality than American journals did,[88] but after World War II the geographical focus of research in sexology shifted to the United States.[89] The early women's movement stimulated research on lesbianism as American doctors resisted changes in the gender hierarchy. During the 1930s a homosexual sub-culture began to develop in urban areas and the scope of obscenity laws was narrowed, leading to a surge of American medical interest in homosexuality. However, in contrast to nineteenth-century discussions about *sexual* behaviour, most of this literature focused on *gender* behaviour, and pathologized homosexuals on the grounds of deviance from the norms of masculinity and femininity.[90] The medicalization of homosexuality had negative consequences in the United States: it was seen as a potentially contagious and possibly curable illness, leading to pressure to change or psychiatric intervention, which became more common in the 1950s and 1960s, along with more extreme therapies such as aversion therapy, electroshock, castration and lobotomy. The biologist and sexologist Alfred Kinsey (1894–1956) did much to undermine the equation of homosexuality with pathology; with progressive decriminalization, the subject lost its medico-legal importance.[91] However it was many years before the legal changes that Victorian forensic experts had called for were implemented: laws prohibiting male same-sex activity were gradually dismantled in Germany from the late 1960s to 1994; homosexual acts were decriminalized in England in 1967 and in Scotland in 1980; but in the United States, despite reform of sex laws after World War II, it was not until 2003 that the Supreme Court struck down the 16 remaining state laws against 'sodomy'.

Conclusion

Forensic medicine has played an important role in developing the social understanding of behaviours which were in the past labelled as deviant and punished strictly. Medical analysis facilitated a modernization process in which scientific knowledge undercut and then replaced religious interpretations of the causes of suicide, infanticide and same-sex activities, and consequently changed investigative procedures and the legal construction of these deeply personal yet socially significant acts. Typically this was achieved by the identification of a perceived link to mental instability, through which the boundaries of legitimate illness were expanded to include deviance, a process which was most marked during the nineteenth and twentieth centuries. Medicalization should thus be viewed as a process in which new, medically informed meanings became associated with existing behaviours and beliefs. Once deviance had been redefined as a form of illness, the suicidal, infanticidal or homosexual individual could be seen in a neutral moral light, in contrast to the old emphasis on sin and criminality.

The right to care which is inherent in the notion of 'illness' has been of notable benefit to the suicidal and to infanticidal women, as suicide was decriminalized and resources allocated to its study, and women who killed their own infants were transformed from cruel wantons to seduced victims and casualties of socio-economic hardship, becoming in many twentieth-century nations legally defined as mentally altered and less culpable than other killers. The compassion which has been associated with the medicalization of behaviours previously defined as deviant has also been advantageous for those whose sexuality does not conform to heterosexual norms, as legal restrictions have been lifted or weakened. For forensic medicine, the greatest change in this regard has been the shift in focus from the bodies of the accused to their thoughts and feelings. All of these issues will retain their medico-legal importance so long as suicide rates cause social concern, arguments persist about the legal status of female child-killers who may or may not be mentally ill, and prejudice against same-sex choice continues to factor into some crimes against the person.

Additional reading

The references for this chapter can be found in the Bibliography, and will allow you to expand on all of the issues discussed here. If you wish to do some further reading, you may also consult the publications listed below.

Joseph Bajada, *Sexual Impotence: The Contribution of Paolo Zacchia (1584–1659)*, Rome: Editrice Pontificia Università Gregoriana, 1988.
Joseph Bristow, 'Remapping the sites of modern gay history: legal reform, medico-legal thought, homosexual scandal, erotic geography', *Journal of British Studies*, 2007, vol. 46, 116–42.
Peter Conrad and Joseph W. Schneider, *Deviance and Medicalization: From Badness to Sickness* (1980), revised edn, Philadelphia: Temple University Press, 1992.
Ivan Crozier, '"All the appearances were perfectly natural": the anus of the sodomite in nineteenth-century medical discourse', in Christopher E. Forth and Ivan Crozier (eds), *Body Parts: Critical Explorations in Corporeality*, Lanham, MD: Lexington Books, 2005, 65–84.
Peter Cryle, 'Female impotence in nineteenth-century France: a study in gendered sexual pathology', *French History and Civilization: Papers from the George Rudé Seminar*, 2009, vol. 3, 80–91.
Roger D. Groot, 'When suicide became felony', *Journal of Legal History*, 2000, vol. 21, 1–20.
Jörg Hutter, 'The social construction of homosexuals in the nineteenth century: the shift from the sin to the influence of medicine on criminalizing sodomy in Germany', *Journal of Homosexuality*, 1993, vol. 24, 73–93.
Mark Jackson (ed.), *Infanticide: Historical Perspectives on Child Murder and Concealment, 1550–2000*, Aldershot: Ashgate, 2002.
R.J. Kellett, 'Infanticide and child destruction – the historical, legal and pathological aspects', *Forensic Science International*, 1992, vol. 53, 1–28.
Michael MacDonald, 'The medicalization of suicide in England: laymen, physicians, and cultural change, 1500–1870', in Charles E. Rosenberg and Janet Golden (eds), *Framing Disease: Studies in Cultural History*, New Brunswick, NJ: Rutgers University Press, 1992, 85–103.
Cathy McClive, 'Masculinity on trial: penises, hermaphrodites and the uncertain male body in early modern France', *History Workshop Journal*, 2009, vol. 68, 45–68.
Angus McLaren, 'Vacher the Ripper and the construction of the nineteenth-century sadist', in John Woodward and Robert Jütte (eds), *Coping with Sickness: Medicine, Law and Human Rights – Historical Perspectives*, Sheffield: European Association for the History of Medicine and Health Publications, 2000, 55–74.
Susan K. Morrissey, *Suicide and the Body Politic in Imperial Russia*, Cambridge: Cambridge University Press, 2006.
Robert A. Nye, 'Sex difference and male homosexuality in French medical discourse, 1830–1930', *Bulletin of the History of Medicine*, 1989, vol. 63, 32–51.
Judith A. Osborne, 'The crime of infanticide: throwing out the baby with the bathwater', *Canadian Journal of Family Law*, 1987, vol. 6, 47–59.

George Painter, 'The sensibilities of our forefathers: the history of sodomy laws in the United States' (1991–2005), online at Sodomy Laws, http://www.glapn.org/sodomylaws/ sensibilities/introduction.htm (26 May 2010).

Elizabeth Reis, 'Impossible hermaphrodites: intersex in America, 1620–1960', *Journal of American History*, 2005, vol. 92, 411–41.

Vernon A. Rosario (ed.), *Science and Homosexualities*, London and New York: Routledge, 1997.

Robert Roth, 'Juges et médecins face à l'infanticide à Genève au XIXe siècle', *Gesnerus*, 1977, vol. 34, 113–28.

Jens Rydström, *Sinners and Citizens: Bestiality and Homosexuality in Sweden, 1880–1950*, Chicago and London: University of Chicago Press, 2003.

Eltjo Schrage, 'Suicide in canon law', *Journal of Legal History*, 2000, vol. 21, 57–62.

Roger Smith, 'Defining murder and madness: an introduction to medicolegal belief in the case of Mary Ann Brough, 1854', in Robert A. Jones and Henrika Kuklick (eds), *Knowledge and Society: Studies in the Sociology of Culture Past and Present*, Vol. 4, Greenwich, CT and London: JAI Press Inc., 1983, 173–225.

Lieven Vandekerckhove, 'On the origins of the punishment of suicidal behaviour in Old-European law – historical versus sociological explanation', *European Journal of Crime, Criminal Law and Criminal Justice*, 1999, vol. 7, 314–30.

Mary Nagle Wessling, 'Infanticide trials and forensic medicine: Württemberg 1757–93', in Michael Clark and Catherine Crawford (eds), *Legal Medicine in History*, Cambridge: Cambridge University Press, 1994, 117–44.

Melanie Williams, 'Medico-legal stories of female insanity: three nullity suits', *Feminist Legal Studies*, 1998, vol. 6, 3–31.

6 Twentieth-century developments in forensic medicine and science

Previous chapters have demonstrated the pace at which forensic medicine developed during the eighteenth and nineteenth centuries: professional ambitions and intellectual advancements, especially in toxicology and psychiatry, led to the emergence of the modern expert witness, an individual who was increasingly likely to be employed by one of the growing number of universities, asylums, hospitals, laboratories and, on the Continent, medico-legal institutions that sprang up during the period. However, at the *fin-de-siècle* the discipline's sphere of activity was by no means limited to bodies living or dead: organic stains of blood, semen, meconium and breast milk; prints and marks on fabrics and other surfaces; and fibres and hair all lay within the purview of forensic medicine.[1] The inevitable consequence of advancing knowledge was increased specialization within forensic medicine and a growing demarcation between forensic medicine and forensic science – processes that characterized the twentieth-century history of the discipline. By 1950 it was clear that forensic medicine had become an umbrella term, as medico-legal practitioners differentiated themselves according to professional expertise: pathologists, psychiatrists and toxicologists were joined by serologists as specialists who recognized that no single individual could hope to attain the breadth of experience that nineteenth-century experts had had, making collaboration a progressively more common feature of working practice. Furthermore, as the scientific investigation of all types of crimes grew in importance, the field of forensic science expanded to include chemistry, physics, biology, botany, zoology, entomology, anthropology, geology and, most recently and dramatically, genetics.[2] Applied social science also established its value to the criminal justice system, most notably through forensic psychology and behavioural analysis.[3]

The spectacular growth of forensic medicine and science in the twentieth century makes any attempt to provide a comprehensive overview of the key developments impractical. Instead, this chapter will consider some of the most innovative and significant medical, scientific and institutional advances made during the century, many of which will be familiar to readers accustomed to the modern media fascination with all things forensic: the diagnosis of physical and sexual abuse in children; the laboratory based organization of forensic medicine and science; establishing identity and time since death; blood typing and DNA analysis; and offender profiling. Although these areas of forensic significance are associated with late twentieth-century advancements, with the exception of DNA analysis each had an earlier history. Thus, this chapter explores both the foundations and the content of modern forensic practice, highlighting the challenges that have been and will remain integral to the field.

The diagnosis of physical and sexual abuse in children

While it is largely correct to view child abuse as a social problem that was officially 'discovered' by the American paediatrician C. Henry Kempe (1922–84) in the early 1960s with the aid of X-ray diagnosis, forensic practitioners had been aware of the physical and sexual abuse of children for centuries. However, the low status accorded to children, lack of diagnostic certainty, and social and gender bias delayed medical and public acceptance of what is now a major area of societal concern, so much so that in the case of Anglo-American child sexual abuse it is more accurate to speak of its 'rediscovery' in the 1970s.[4] Child sexual abuse was acknowledged by early and mid nineteenth-century medico-legal practitioners in Britain and the United States, but tended to disappear from public view during later decades as medical professionals struggled with the implications of finding venereal disease to be widespread in young girls. In light of diagnostic difficulties, doctors relied on the character and history of the patient and her family, and so often ignored the possibility of sexual abuse, particularly incest in middle-class families, while working class girls were assumed to be suffering from nothing more sinister than bad hygiene.[5] In Europe, Richard von Krafft-Ebing and his medico-legal colleagues were aware of a rising number of sexual crimes against children throughout France, Germany and Britain,[6] though the criminal statistics seem to have reflected increased prosecution rather than increasing incidence, and certainly underestimated the extent of the problem.[7] Moreover, while the Victorians were clearly conscious of the non-sexual abuse of children, they framed arguments against it in terms of 'cruelty to children', as just one aspect of family violence that might inspire criminal tendencies in juveniles.[8] Thus, although detailed information about child abuse existed at the dawn of the twentieth century, the way it was interpreted and acted upon in most western nations was repeatedly and severely compromised until after World War II.

Unlike infanticide, we do not have very much information about what early modern doctors thought about child abuse, but by the seventeenth century it was well enough known for the greatest forensic practitioner of the day to use the example of a child in a discourse about head injuries published in the 1651 edition of his *Quaestiones Medico-Legales*. However, it is unlikely that Paolo Zacchia considered the terrible damage that some children sustained to be symptomatic of a form of adult deviance worthy of criminalization, though he did accept that death could result from the blows inflicted by parents and other authority figures.[9] Other doctors also referred to what seems to have been the physical abuse of children. In 1682 the Genevan physician and pathologist Théophile Bonet (1620–89) published *A Guide to the Practical Physician* (English translation 1684), which included a section on children. He noted that some mothers could not or would not care for their babies because they were 'diseased and sometimes also of bad manners', and also that head contusions in young babies 'may be the nurse's fault in letting the child fall and dashing it against a thing'. Bonet observed that under the age of seven injuries occurred in which the skin might not be damaged, but referred to fractures in children only in passing.[10] Jean Devaux included a report on a case of child rape resulting in venereal disease in his *L'art de faire les raports en chirurgie* (1703),[11] and physicians, surgeons and midwives treated numerous child victims of rape during the eighteenth century, testifying at any ensuing trials.

Undoubtedly medical practitioners also treated the victims of parental physical abuse, but in an age when parents and guardians had absolute authority over children it is little surprise that doctors focused their attentions on the symptoms rather than the causes. No clear diagnosis of the problem really emerged until the nineteenth century. In 1835 a book on child rearing written by a female British aristocrat plainly set out circumstances typical of what is now recognized as child abuse: 'Blows on the head from harsh instruction have been suspected to produce water on the brain, and the mode in which some people gratify their anger towards children by shaking them violently might also lead to serious consequences'.[12]

The key nineteenth-century medico-legal expert on this subject was Ambroise Tardieu, the most famous doctor to comment in print on the prevalence of abuse by parents.[13] In an 1859 monograph on sexual offences, the third edition of his *Étude médico-légale sur les attentats aux moeurs*, he noted that sexual crimes against children under 16 had more than tripled between 1826 and 1850; of 400 cases in which he had been consulted, over three-quarters of female victims were children, and a handful of boys had been molested by women.[14] In 1860 Tardieu published a forensic study of child cruelty, describing in detail a series of 32 abused children, 18 of whom had died. Of all the children 24 had been harmed by their parents and 53 per cent were under the age of five. Tardieu recognized burns, blows, suffocation, extreme deprivation and isolation as examples of possible abuse, and noted that abused children might exhibit recognizable injuries and behaviours, such as frozen watchfulness. He thought it unlikely that parents who abused their children were insane, and although most claimed that the injuries were accidental, this was easily refuted; the bruises and marks on the child victims of abuse differed in location and number from those caused by true accidents, and were often accompanied by the identifiable imprints of restraints or the objects used in beatings.[15]

Although France was ahead of other Western nations in acknowledging the existence of physical and sexual child abuse, and in deciding to do something about it,[16] Tardieu was unsuccessful in his attempt to draw immediate attention to the plight of children within their own families, because of the widespread

Victorian notion that parents had absolute rights over their offspring. Subsequently, some French, German and Austrian medico-legal experts cast doubt on the clinical signs of abuse that he described, and warned that children were prone to invent tales of rape and maltreatment,[17] but attitudes did slowly begin to change. French societies concerned with child welfare began to appear in the 1860s, sparking a rise in prosecutions of nonsexual crimes against children,[18] and there was a marked increase in the reporting of incest in France, which was probably related to fears about degeneration.[19] Governments began to legislate for the safety of children outside the home, enacting laws against child labour and cruelty in France, Britain and America and raising the age of consent, but medico-legal approaches thereafter tended to diverge. Sexual abuse was considered separately from child-beating, and although swift action was taken against abuse that occurred at the hands of strangers, doctors were unwilling to admit that incest and mistreatment by parents and relatives were commonplace. Krafft-Ebing coined the term 'erotic paedophilia' to describe the four child-loving men he had encountered,[20] but the explicit recognition of child abuse as a form of deviance remained elusive as long as doctors continued to assume that such acts were restricted to the working classes and people of moral and/or mental weakness, who had succumbed to the effects of poverty, alcohol or both.[21]

Although venereal disease in girls had long been seen by British and American courts as probative evidence in cases of alleged child rape, medical doubts were raised as early as the late eighteenth century in relation to the nature and cause of gonorrhoea, a disease which was eventually determined to be of bacterial origin. Defendants were however frequently convicted if the victim displayed evidence of genital trauma, infection and semen stains, and if the accused was also infected.[22] In 1879 the German bacteriologist Albert Neisser (1855–1916) identified the bacterium *Neisseria gonorrhoeae* as the cause of gonorrhea, but it remained difficult to diagnose until 1884 when Hans Christian Gram (1853–1938), a Danish bacteriologist, published a technique that utilized a system of coloured stains and visual identification under a microscope. Ironically, the discovery of this test for gonorrhoea led medical practitioners to recoil from its use as a diagnostic of sexual abuse in girls. The disease was found to be so prevalent among middle class girls who had not complained of sexual assault that medical and legal evidence showing that children were being sexually assaulted at home was ignored, in favour of assumptions that abuse was something that happened mainly outside the family and the girls that it happened to were in some way delinquent. A new disease aetiology was constructed, one which broke the link between gonorrhoea in children and sexual assault and instead posited a link between infected family members and poor hygiene, via everyday contact with linens, toilet seats, towels, bathwater and other objects which obviated the medico-legal implications of the diagnosis.[23] At a stroke this took the medical gaze off incest as a crime that occurred within 'respectable' families, by providing an alternative diagnosis: yet successful prosecutions remained possible (Case Study 6.1).

Case Study 6.1: The rape of Melba McAfee (California, 1926)

In November 1926 11-year-old Melba McAfee testified against her father Robert at his trial for incest. She recounted how, on an outing in early April, he had stopped at the side of the road, ordered her to sit down and spread her legs, and proceeded to force his penis into her vagina, aided by the contents of a jar of Vaseline. After telling her that he had taken her 'maiden's head', he did it again, despite the fact that she was bleeding heavily. He threatened to kill her if she told anyone, and two months later he assaulted her again. This time her stepmother saw the blood on Melba's underclothes, and the girl told her what had happened, but no action was taken until more than a week later, after Melba had been sent to live with her mother. Her daughter's sickness, pain and constant crying alerted Nancy McAfee that something was wrong, and finally Melba confided in her. She was immediately taken to the police who, when they learned she had a vaginal discharge, sent her to a doctor. Using a microscope, Dr Thomas Sidney Whitelock examined a smear and diagnosed Melba with gonorrhoea. At the trial he stated that it could only be acquired from someone who already had it, via sexual contact. The defence alleged that McAfee could not have infected his daughter because although he had been infected seven years ago he did not now have any symptoms. Then they turned the tables on the victim, claiming that she must have been having sex with boys her own age and had then made false claims of rape at the instigation of her jealous mother. This tactic did not work, however: McAfee was convicted.

The attack made on Melba McAfee's honesty and innocence was typical of the defence strategy in cases of incest and child sexual assault, but because evidence corroborating the sexual trauma she had suffered was clear, there was no point in suggesting that she had been infected by a toilet seat or any other non-sexual mode of transmission. Instead they focused on when the infection had been transmitted, suggesting it had preceded the date of the alleged assault by her father. In the first half of the twentieth century it was common for defence counsel to allege that children suffering from venereal disease were morally damaged goods; this was the alternative to accepting that father–daughter incest was as rampant as the statistics on gonorrhoea in pubescent girls suggested. Such a view could not have achieved widespread currency were it not for the pervasive acceptance that incest occurred only among immigrant, non-white and poor people.

Source: L. Sacco, *Unspeakable: Father–Daughter Incest in American History*, Baltimore, MD: Johns Hopkins University Press, 2009, pp. 182–88.

Medico-legal interest in child-beating during the late nineteenth century was if anything under-developed relative to child sexual abuse. In Britain, the first medical reporting of what is now called child abuse appeared in a paper read by Dr Samuel West in 1888, in which he described several young children from the same family who had developed painful swellings over the limb bones; he concluded that the cause was rickets, having also considered scurvy and syphilis but not violence.[24] In the United States and Britain physicians treated the physical injuries of maltreated children, and national societies for the prevention of cruelty to children prosecuted parents of all classes for assault and neglect, though the signs of child abuse were not seen as unique indicators of a particular form of deviance; no clear diagnostic label existed. In France, where a complete review of child physical abuse published in 1929 reported cases severe enough for criminal charges over a period of 22 years, the subject had been otherwise neglected since Tardieu.[25] Change came in the middle third of the twentieth century, when a series of British, French but mostly American clinicians published studies of hospitalized children with very similar fractures, subdural haematomas (a haemorrhage between the brain membranes usually caused by trauma), retinal haemorrhages and bony lesions indicative of multiple trauma to the same area of the body. The use of X-rays marked a turning point and established the radiological features now commonly associated with physical child abuse. In 1946 the paediatrician John Caffey (1895–1978) linked fractures to haematomas for the first time, in 1953 a landmark article by Frederic N. Silverman (1914–2006), a founder of paediatric radiology, defined *inflicted* trauma as the cause of the bony lesions, and in 1955 paediatrician P.V. Woolley and radiologist W.A. Evans 'blasted the medical profession … for its reluctance to concede that the multiple injuries to children were committed willfully'.[26]

By the late 1950s more and more physicians had begun to accept that the damage they saw in some children was due to deliberate physical abuse, but the key turning point was the public lecture given by C. Henry Kempe in 1961 and subsequently published in the *Journal of the American Medical Association* in 1962. This paper referred to 'battered child syndrome', the first British paper to do the same was published the following year, and the universal recognition of battered children as a significant medico-legal problem followed swiftly, stimulating intervention in the form of laws, regulations and guidelines for reporting.[27] The first International Congress on Child Abuse and Neglect was held in Geneva in 1976, and has been held every other year since then. In 1977 the International Society for the Prevention of Child Abuse and Neglect was established, and the first issue of *Child Abuse and Neglect* was published under Kempe's editorship.[28] By affixing a label to behaviour that previously had no name, the medical profession succeeded in defining the perpetrators as a deviant group.[29]

The rubric 'child abuse' was widened to include sexual abuse following the rediscovery of incest in the 1970s, when doctors once again noticed a high prevalence of gonorrhoea in girls. Following the revelations of child physical abuse, there was more willingness to investigate the involvement of family members, and this was reinforced in 1977 when Kempe delivered an influential speech which identified sexual abuse as another hidden paediatric problem. The notion of non-sexual transmission of venereal disease came into question, but many family physicians remained so resistant to the idea that incest was widespread that in 1991 the American Academy of Paediatrics reminded paediatricians to keep an open mind to the possibility, and in 1997 paediatric residencies added a mandatory component on child abuse. The feminist movement of the 1970s and 1980s played an important role in identifying incest as a key feature of domestic violence, one which was not limited to marginalized sections of society; their work was bolstered by the emergence of published survivor narratives. Yet, at the end of the century, child sexual abuse remained subject to under-reporting and the assumption that it occurred mainly at the hands of strangers,[30] a conjecture reinforced by eager media reporting of the relatively rare cases of children abducted or assaulted by complete strangers, and the pervasive fear of predatory paedophiles.

The medico-legal aspects of child physical and sexual abuse are better understood today, and Western society is more fully informed than at any time in the past. Warning signs are well documented and diagnostic techniques have been improved and expanded, especially by the introduction of DNA analysis and the so-called rape kit used during the medical examination of victims. Moreover, the public is alert to the possibility that parents abuse their children. As recent failures in Britain, Austria and elsewhere attest,[31] however, the ability to accurately identify abusive family situations is linked both to personal and professional experience and to attitudes to children, parents and family violence.

The organization of forensic medicine and science in the twentieth century

In Chapter 3 we noted the importance of forensic pathology in the twentieth century, and the different medico-legal systems established in Britain, Europe and the United States. Since the early nineteenth century major European cities have had modern morgues and trained pathologists based in university or hospital departments of forensic medicine. In many countries, medico-legal specialists are trained both in pathology and clinical forensic medicine involving wounds and injuries to the living. In the United Kingdom, the work of the forensic pathologist is based almost exclusively on autopsies.[32] In England, the system of retaining a forensic pathologist remained informal until the 1950s, when a register of Home Office approved pathologists who have the skill and experience to conduct a medico-legal autopsy was instituted. There are currently 38 Home Office pathologists,[33] and university based or NHS consultant pathologists also do some medico-legal work. The police can request a specific expert, but the final decision rests with the coroner. In Scotland, the Scottish Executive directly funds forensic pathology departments within the major universities. In the United States, the spread of the medical examiner system contributed to the close integration of forensic pathology and police investigative procedures. By the end of the twentieth century almost half the American population was served by the ME system and in 22 states there were no coroners at all, though locally elected coroners still exist in the west and south, and the expansion of the ME system slowed after 1990.[34] States which use the coroner system either have medical examiners on staff or make arrangements with local police and hospitals to secure the relevant pathological expertise.

At the beginning of the twentieth century the locus of medico-legal knowledge and research lay largely in university departments and medical examiners' offices, but the use of scientific methods to study crime was gaining momentum, going hand in hand with the rise of criminology, the theories of Lombroso and the identification techniques pioneered by Bertillon, whose Department of Judicial Identity was created in Paris in 1888. While the Paris police worked closely with the Medico-Legal Institute (founded in 1868) and the Toxicology Laboratory, and the police in other regions could draw upon university and hospital based medico-legal expertise, it was not until 1912 that the first police laboratory was set up in Lyon by Edmond Locard, a former assistant to Alexandre Lacassagne, the first professor of forensic medicine at Lyon and a pioneer in the use of scientific methods in forensic medicine. Locard, who was qualified in medicine and law and had spent some time working with Bertillon, resigned his post at the University of Lyon in 1910 to set up a police laboratory known from 1912 as the Police Scientific Laboratory of Lyon, which later became the technical police laboratory for the prefecture of the Rhône.[35] Today there are five scientific police laboratories in France, at Paris, Lille, Lyon, Marseille and Toulouse, operating under the aegis of the National Police.[36]

Locard justifiably gained a reputation as the first true forensic scientist, and is probably most closely associated with the principle identified by his name: the Locard exchange principle, which holds that 'every contact leaves a trace'. It is the foundation for the use of what is called trace evidence, which depends on comparing traces of materials found on a suspect with materials from the scene of a crime. However, Locard never claimed that every contact leaves a trace; rather, he recognized that when a perpetrator committed a violent crime some trace of their presence would remain, and that such traces could be identified by using a microscope.[37] The principle was seen to be startlingly successful in 1912, when bank clerk Emile Gourbin was suspected of strangling his girlfriend, Marie Latelle, but had set up a solid alibi. Locard took samples from the victim's neck and matched them to skin scraped from beneath the suspect's fingernails. An even stronger indicator of Gourbin's guilt emerged when the skin flakes were found to be coated with a fine pink powder that matched the chemical composition of the victim's custom-made face powder. When confronted with the evidence, Gourbin made a full confession.[38] By the end of the twentieth century, however, trace evidence had become much less central to forensic science, due to its labour intensiveness and the more clear-cut results offered by DNA.[39]

Locard established not only a guiding principle for forensic science, but also an institutional format that was followed all over the West. Since the early twentieth century forensic science has been located in laboratories divided into different scientific sections. Some are associated with the local medico-legal institute, but it is far more common for them to be attached to government chemical or toxicological laboratories, or to be under the exclusive direction of the police, which is the most typical situation in the United States. The first university department of forensic science was established at the University of Lausanne in Switzerland by Rudolphe Reiss (1876–1929), who had worked with Bertillon and as a result established his own photography course in 1902, which by 1909 had developed into a programme of study in forensic science. By the 1930s his department had evolved into the Lausanne Institute of Police Science, and had become one of several police science laboratories across Europe.[40] In 2007 there were an unknown number of European forensic science laboratories, of which 53 were members of the European Network of Forensic Science Institutes.[41]

European developments did not go unnoticed in early twentieth-century England, which lacked a comparable institutional basis for forensic science; when needed, the police could turn on an ad hoc basis to the public analysts, the Laboratory of the Government Chemist (1842) and the National Physical Laboratory (1900). English medico-legal practitioners recognized that there was a problem and encouraged the Home Office to establish a central medico-legal institute in association with the University of London. However, this was conceived more in terms of forensic medicine and pathology than forensic science, and the Home Office preferred instead to create a network of regional forensic laboratories that would be geared towards solving a rising tide of property crimes. This was part of a drive to modernize police methods, including the use of forensic science, and in 1935 the Metropolitan Police opened their Forensic Laboratory at Hendon; in 1974 it moved to Lambeth. The newly formed Home Office Forensic Science Service established five laboratories around the country, the first opening at Nottingham in 1936. The network still exists today: in 1996 the Metropolitan Police Laboratory merged with the Forensic Science Service to create a national organization.

Thus, in Britain and Europe forensic science is generally located in a system of national laboratories and services, sometimes in association with universities. Initially this was the model followed in the United States: in 1923 the first forensic science laboratory was established at Los Angeles under the chief of police August Vollmer (1876–1955), with strong links to the University of California at Berkeley; in 1930 the Scientific Detection Crime Laboratory at Northwestern University opened under the directorship of Calvin Goddard (1891–1955), formerly of the Bureau of Forensic Ballistics in New York (founded in 1915), as a direct result of his work during the investigation of the 1928 St Valentine's Day Massacre in Chicago. The police and university academics collaborated in Indiana during the 1940s to develop methods of breath-alcohol testing, and the collaboration continued during the career of Robert Borkenstein (1912–2002), who worked for both the state police and Indiana University. But generally the main pattern of provision has been through the 'own service' path: state police created their own laboratories.[42] In 1932 the Bureau of Investigation, soon to become the Federal Bureau of Investigation, set up its Technical Laboratory, which now as the FBI Laboratory provides forensic services and training to federal, state and local law enforcement agencies. FBI Director J. Edgar Hoover modelled the Technical Laboratory on the first North American facility of its kind, Montreal's Laboratoire de Recherches Médico-légales, founded in 1914 by Dr Wilfrid Derome (1877–1931) along the lines suggested by Locard, to support police investigations through scientific means.[43]

Regardless of their institutional affiliation, forensic laboratories today share common features. They are likely to be arranged by discipline, with forensic pathology remaining quite separate from the various sub-specialities of forensic science. Because the information needed to solve crimes can come from many different areas of forensic practice, the work increasingly requires contributions from a team of investigators. The nineteenth-century model of the lone expert has vanished. However, although medico-legal practice in the twentieth century became far more complex and multi-disciplinary than it had been, one characteristic did not change: the importance of the human body as a source of evidence. The next section examines the twentieth-century relationship between medicine, science and crime – themes pursued throughout this book – through the history of the development of some of the key modern areas of forensic practice. The focus will lie on techniques closely related to the body, to the evidence that can be gained from bodies, and on 'offender profiling', which uses information drawn from forensic psychology to interpret the links between offences and an offender's way of thinking. In some areas, most notably DNA analysis, cutting-edge academic research migrated to forensic practice; in others, for example estimation of time of death, research was driven by the needs of the criminal justice system. Thus the questions that have always concerned forensic medicine – what happened to the victim, how and when did it happen, and who did it – are now answered using a combination of medical and scientific knowledge.

Establishing identity and time since death

The foundations of modern forensic science were laid in the nineteenth century, a fact that becomes evident when we consider a series of techniques which are more closely associated with the present day. In the early 1830s Mathieu Orfila noted that maggots play an important role in decomposition, while Alexandre Lacassagne was the first to show a correlation between markings on a bullet and the rifling inside the barrel of the weapon that fired it.[44] Dental evidence was crucial to the conviction of Harvard professor John

Webster for the murder of Dr George Parkman in 1849, a case notable also for the early use of forensic anthropology to identify the remains of the victim.[45] The first test for blood, the Teichmann test for haemoglobin, was developed in 1853 and used until the late twentieth century,[46] and in 1868 the professor of forensic medicine at Glasgow, Harry Rainy (1792–1876), suggested that the cooling of dead bodies could be used to determine time since death.[47] Cesare Lombroso's concept of the criminaloid, a type of occasional offender, can be interpreted as a crude form of profiling in its matching of criminal tendencies to occupational temptations,[48] and medico-legal interest in the serial sex killer was stimulated by the cases of Jack the Ripper (1888) and Joseph Vacher (1869–98).[49] Finally, the team work that is now the watchword of complicated murder investigations was evident at the beginning of the twentieth century, for example in the Crippen case of 1910.[50]

The rest of this chapter will examine the subsequent development of these forensic specialties, focusing on identification and estimation of time since death. Entomology typically aids in estimating time of death using the history of fly larval development. Anthropology uses the physical characteristics of bones to identify the species, gender, race, stature and age of remains, and may shed light on the manner and cause of death, or even individual identity. Odontology, the study of teeth, is of increasing importance as a means of international identification, as more and more dental records are kept throughout the world. Serology, the study of body tissues including blood, semen and saliva provides another identification technique. Ballistics uses marks on bullets and weapons to discern links between crimes, suspects and victims; ballistics specialists may need to liaise with pathologists because there is a relationship between wounds and the bullets that cause them. Psychology, the branch of science mainly responsible for criminal profiling, aids in the understanding of repeat offending. DNA typing has the shortest history, dating only from the 1980s, but has provided the greatest advance in the identification of the origin of biological materials.[51]

There are a number of changes that take place in a body after death that can be helpful in estimating the time at which someone died. The normal human body temperature is 37°C. As soon as someone dies, their temperature starts to fall, so the temperature of a body will give some indication of how long it has been dead. A number of different factors will affect how quickly the body temperature drops. A body cools more slowly inside a building than if it is left outside, so external temperature and weather conditions have to be taken into consideration. A naked body will cool much faster than a clothed one, and a body wrapped in blankets will cool even more slowly. By the end of the nineteenth century estimates based on rectal temperature were relatively common, but it remained difficult to deal with complex environmental conditions. The problem was not seriously addressed by forensic pathologists until 1955, when G.S.W. de Saram (1896–1963) and two of his colleagues at the University of Ceylon developed a formula which could take external factors into account.[52] Research since then has tended to focus on body and ambient temperature measurements, computerized calculations and muscle contractions. The most reliable body temperatures are those taken in the brain, and it is now known that a typical body loses temperature at a rate of 0.8°C during the first eight hours, then 0.6°C an hour until the body temperature reaches equilibrium with the surrounding environment; but temperature-based estimates of time since death remain approximations.[53]

Pathologists can also use rigor mortis to estimate time of death. At death, the heart stops pumping blood around the body and the brain stops functioning within minutes. However some tissues, especially muscle, effectively stay alive for a few minutes longer. When they finally die, the muscle fibres no longer slide smoothly past each other, but lock solid. This produces a stiffening effect known as rigor mortis, which was first studied in detail by the Belgian-French doctor Pierre Nysten (1771–1818) in 1811 and mentioned in textbooks of legal medicine by the 1880s. On average it starts about two to four hours after death, takes between six and eight hours to take full effect, moving downward from head to toe, and has completely passed within three to four days. The time it takes to begin is related to the levels of a muscle enzyme called adenosine triphosphate, ATP. If there is a lot of it rigor mortis takes longer to start. Normal quantities in the muscles are related to individual genetics and physical fitness, but it is used up by exercise in a phenomenon known as cadaveric spasm, which explains why rigor starts very quickly in cases of drowning – victims use up all their ATP in struggling to stay afloat. In 1977 the importance of temperature to the development and breaking of rigor was established, but rigor mortis remains one of the least certain indicators of time since death.[54]

A third type of change that takes place in the body after death can be used to establish when someone died. Once the heart stops beating, the blood slowly drains by gravity to the lowest parts of the body. The top regions become very pale, while the lower regions are dark red. These colour changes, known as hypostasis, lividity or livor mortis, begin within a couple of hours of death and become permanent within 12 hours; contact areas with firm surfaces remain pale. Once it is fixed, lividity can indicate whether a body has been moved: for example, if a corpse is found face downwards, but lividity is visible on the back, it was probably moved sometime after death, perhaps in an attempt to hide it. An imprint of the surface on which the victim expired may also be revealed; hypostasis can however sometimes flow from one part of the body to another. The colour too can be indicative, for example the cherry pink of carbon monoxide or cyanide poisoning, or the presence of pressure whitening around the nose and mouth in cases of suffocation. It is important to distinguish livor mortis from ante-mortem bruising. Research published between 1905 and 1964 showed how variable the timings associated with post-mortem blood pooling can be, and generally the subject is less well researched than rigor mortis, with which it is on a par in regard to reliability of time-since-death estimates.[55]

Finally, the body begins to decay, following a predictable pattern. Within two to three days of death, a greenish colour begins to appear around the chest and abdomen due to bacterial action, which spreads over a period of weeks. Further discoloration, bloating and a distinctive smell of decomposition develop; after three weeks the whole body will be substantially disfigured and the hair will slip from the scalp; after four weeks 'there is slimy liquefaction of the whole body'. The rate at which these changes occur varies depending on external conditions like temperature, weather, levels of oxygen in the air and animal predation. If conditions are damp, body fats are transformed into adipocere, taking four to five months around the head and five to six months around the trunk. In the Crippen case, the presence of adipocere helped to establish that the victim had been interred for several months when discovered.[56]

The processes of decomposition have been known for centuries, but little or no research had been carried out on the extended post-mortem interval before 1981 when Bill Bass (b. 1928) began what was to become a world-renowned study. Bass, an anthropology professor at the University of Knoxville in Tennessee since 1971, and also the state forensic anthropologist, was called to a supposed crime scene on 29 December 1977: an old grave had been disturbed and a headless body discovered. The flesh was still pink and the body was in a sitting position atop the coffin, which had been buried in 1864. The assumption was that this was a recent murder victim who had been buried in the grave of Civil War veteran Colonel William Shy, who had been killed in battle. Knowing what he did about Civil War graves, Bass did not believe that any part of its original occupant would remain. Then, the missing skull was found on 3 January, revealing the cause of death to be a massive gunshot wound to the head. It was only when he took a close look at the teeth that Bass began to realize whose skull this was. There was no sign that the 'murder victim' had ever visited a dentist, and to the great embarrassment of Bass and the police, the body was revealed to be none other than Col. Shy. 'Instead of a recent murder victim crammed partway into a coffin, the body was an old soldier pulled mostly *out* of the coffin, losing his head and some appendages' along the way. Shy was reburied and Bass set out to rectify his critical error. How could he have misjudged the time of death by 113 years? It was partly because the body had been embalmed, partly due to the airtight cast-iron coffin, but it was mostly because so little was known about post-mortem processes.[57]

In May 1981 Bass founded the Anthropology Research Facility, better known as the Body Farm, at the University of Knoxville, an outdoor research 'laboratory' dedicated to enhancing the understanding of what happens when human bodies decay in a range of different conditions. The bodies are donated by people who wish to further scientific knowledge, and at the Body Farm's secluded site, about 30 bodies are under observation at any one time. Some are buried, some are not, some are rolled up in carpet, stuffed in dustbin bags or car boots, some are in damp areas, yet others are exposed to the full effects of the weather. By monitoring the rate of change until nothing remains but bone, the research team has compiled useful information that will aid forensic investigations all over the world. By 1999 the Body Farm's time-since-death database, the first and only one of its kind charting the processes and timetable of decomposition, held results gleaned from over 300 corpses.[58]

One of the most important factors in the decomposition process involves insect activity on and in the body, providing further valuable data about time of death. When a person dies and the body is exposed to the elements, insects find it quickly, within minutes of death, and colonize it. Flies and other insects lay eggs in the natural openings of the body, like the eyes, nose and mouth, but also in wounds, and different insects do this at different times. Other insects such as beetles and wasps will attack and feed off the insects and their eggs. Depending on temperature and other environmental factors, this parade of visitors takes place at surprisingly consistent time intervals. By inspecting the corpse, forensic entomologists can give a good estimate of the time since death. They know the detailed lifecycle of blowflies and other bugs likely to seek out corpses, and how this varies with different conditions and temperature: Bill Bass, for example, has noted that blowflies will not fly if the temperature drops below 52°F. This information can be used to help estimate how long a body has been in the place it was found. Additionally, there is information available by studying the insects themselves. If a person has been poisoned, the flies will ingest some of the poison; toxicologists can then analyze the bugs, extract the poison and identify it.[59]

French and German medico-legal experts had noticed that buried bodies are inhabited by a variety of insects before the nineteenth century, but the first case report was published in 1855 by M. Bergeret, a hospital physician at Arbois in eastern France near Besançon. In 1850 he was asked to examine a mummified child's corpse found in a flat, to determine the time interval between birth and death. Pathology could estimate the child's age, but to work out how long the body had been there, Bergeret used blowfly pupae and larval moths to conclude that the child had died in 1848. The death could therefore be traced to the tenant who had lived in the house at that time.[60] Forensic entomological studies on human corpses were subsequently carried out by French, German, American and Canadian doctors and scientists, the most important work being that of Jean Pierre Mégnin (1828–1905), a French doctor and veterinarian whose *La Faune des cadavres* (1894) described eight stages of insect infestation in exposed bodies (two for buried corpses), allowing estimation of time since death.[61] Research during the first half of the twentieth century was marked by systematic studies of insect ecosystems, particularly after the 1920s, when numerous books and articles on insect biology relative to human cadavers were published, often referring to specific criminal cases but remaining largely descriptive.[62] The earliest British case in which insect evidence was used successfully in a murder investigation occurred in 1935, when in a trial notable for its many forensic innovations, entomology was used to support other evidence pointing to Buck Ruxton's guilt (Case Study 6.2).

Case Study 6.2: The identification of Isabella Ruxton and Mary Rogerson, murdered by Dr Buck Ruxton (Scotland, 1935)

On 29 September 1935 police at Moffat, a town 50 miles south of Edinburgh, received reports of human remains lying below a bridge. The gruesome finds were retrieved and inventoried: despite extensive dismemberment, it was immediately evident that the body parts belonged to two people. Amongst the bundles in which the bodies were wrapped pieces of newspaper were found dated on or before 15 September; some were identified as part of an issue local to Morecambe and Lancaster, 100 miles south in England. Body parts continued to be found until early November, but the police already had a good idea of who they belonged to. Two women had disappeared in Lancaster on 14 September: 34-year-old Isabella Kerr, the common-law wife of Buck Ruxton, an Indian-born doctor aged 37; and her nursemaid, Mary Rogerson (19). On 13 October Ruxton was charged with Rogerson's murder, and on 5 November with the murder of his wife. In order to positively identify the victims, the police relied on the forensic evidence provided by a team of Scottish experts.

All distinguishing features had been removed or mutilated: Mrs Ruxton had prominent teeth and Mary Rogerson had a squint, but many teeth and the eyes had been removed. Head 1 seemed to be that of a young woman, but Head 2 appeared to be male. Local doctors conducted the initial examination, but on 1 October John Glaister, professor of forensic medicine at the University of Glasgow and W. Gilbert Millar, lecturer in pathology at the University of Edinburgh acting for the professor of forensic medicine, Sydney Smith, were called in. They soon realized that careful reconstruction and detailed examination would be required and transferred the remains to Edinburgh, where responsibility for different aspects of the work was divided between several specialists. Millar and Glaister took on the pathology and medico-legal aspects of the case, and tested the bloodstains found in Ruxton's house. The anatomical investigation to ascertain age, sex, height and features that might aid identification was done by James Couper Brash, professor of anatomy at Edinburgh, assisted by a radiographer. Dental examination of the skulls was carried out by Arthur Hutchinson, dean of the dental school at Edinburgh. Towards the end of the investigation, Smith worked on the medico-legal implications of the evidence: the dismemberment would have taken about eight hours and revealed that the culprit had trained in anatomy; Body 2 died from asphyxia; the hand of Body 1 appeared to be that of someone who did manual labour. Dr Alexander Mearns of Glasgow's Institute of Hygiene identified the species of maggot that infested the corpses and estimated the time since the bodies were dumped as 12 to 14 days before they were examined on 1 October.

Body 1 was clearly that of a woman; its age and stature, confirmed by evidence from the teeth, bones and numerous anatomical features, as well as fingerprints, identified it as Rogerson. When Head 2 was definitively matched to Body 2, which was also female, the experts had a problem, as its age appeared to be over 40, and its stature was difficult to determine exactly. Most of the identifying features had been removed, but although Body 2 was more mutilated than Body 1 the mutilations drew attention to the characteristics they were designed to conceal. The remaining features, including the left foot, which fitted a shoe, and the breasts, were consistent with Mrs Ruxton. To positively identify her, X-rays of the skulls were superimposed on life-size photographs of the victims, the first time such a comparison had been made in a criminal case. Although the match was surprisingly good for Head 2, Brash could not state with absolute certainty that it was Mrs Ruxton. On the whole, however, the balance of evidence suggested that Body 2 was hers.

Buck Ruxton was tried for the murder of his wife at Manchester assizes in March 1936; he was convicted on the eleventh day. He was not tried for the murder of the maid, but evidence concerning her was admitted to prove the killing and identification of Isabella. His appeal failed when the lord chief justice stated that the identification evidence was overwhelming, as was the evidence that Ruxton had committed the crime, proved by circumstantial and blood evidence, among other things. Ruxton confessed before his execution: he strangled his wife in a fit of jealous rage, then killed Rogerson (probably by cutting her throat) when she discovered the crime.

This extraordinary case is notable primarily because of the novel and extensive methods of anatomical reconstruction that the scope and character of the mutilations inflicted on the two victims necessitated. Collaborative work between different branches of forensic medicine and other specialized fields was essential, and the comparison of skulls and portraits together with the life-size enlargements were among a number of completely new techniques developed in order to solve this case. Others included testing whether casts of the feet fit the shoes of the missing women; experimental post-mortem tooth extraction to trace the formation of blood clots; and the identification of fly maggots – the first use of forensic entomology in a British police investigation.

Source: J. Glaister and J.C. Brash, *Medico-Legal Aspects of the Ruxton Case*, Edinburgh: E. & S. Livingstone, 1937.

Post-war research focused more closely on developing scientific under-standing of the relationship between insect evidence and factors, such as temperature and access to the body, which influence the determination of time since death. In 1952 Hubert Caspers of the Zoological Institute in Hamburg introduced the use of caddis-fly casings as a source of forensic information. The body of a woman clad only in red socks had been found in 1948, with a fly casing partly made out of red fibres attached to one sock. Since the body was wrapped in a sack, it appeared that the fly had begun making the casing before landing on the sock, and had then finished the casing after the body was put in the sack. Since the attachment process was known to last several days, Caspers deduced that the body had been stored elsewhere before it was dumped. Between the 1960s and mid 1980s forensic entomology was most closely associated with medical doctor Marcel Leclercq (1924–2008) in Belgium and biology professor Pekka Nuorteva (b. 1926) in Finland, and as soon as the Body Farm opened in 1981 Bill Rodriguez, then one of Bill Bass's graduate students, began a series of pioneering experi-ments on blowfly activity. Since then the field has progressed rapidly due to improved technical facilities, better experimental design and interdisciplinary cooperation.[63] It is only relatively recently that forensic entomology has gained a distinctive institutional identity. The French Gendarmerie established a forensic entomology department within its Criminal Research Institute in 1992, and the first autonomous unit of forensic entomology in Germany was created in 2000 within the department of legal medicine at Frankfurt. The FBI and several crime labs in the United States now have forensic entomolo-gists on staff, and leading authorities run seminars and workshops to train law enforcement professionals to recognize and preserve insect evidence. The European Association for Forensic Entomology was founded in 2002 to pro-mote the discipline, and its first meeting in 2003 attracted delegates from 18 countries including Australia, Canada and the United States.[64]

Blood typing and DNA analysis

We have seen that victims' bodies are important objects of medico-legal study in relation to time and cause of death, but bodies also offer another kind of evidence, related to the identity of the victim and perhaps even that of a killer or rapist. Forensic serology, the study of body fluids such as blood, saliva, semen, sweat, urine and tears, was the mainstay of forensic examination in the twentieth century, until in the 1980s DNA analysis was introduced and rapidly became the key way to link a crime to the criminal. Both these branches of forensic science share a core aim: the identification and classifi-cation of biological evidence, the most important of which is blood.

Fresh blood is easily identifiable due to its colour, consistency and odour; but dried and decomposed blood becomes brown and is difficult to differ-entiate from other brownish materials. The importance of this problem was recognized in the nineteenth century, and in 1853 the anatomist Ludwig

Teichmann (1823–95) of Göttingen developed a test that converted hae-moglobin into microscopically distinctive crystals when blood was heated in the presence of chloride, iodide and bromide in acetic acid. This was the first specific test for blood, on which many future modifications were based, including the more robust and reliable test introduced by Masaeo Takayama in 1912, in which blood mixed with pyridine produces feathery pink crystals.[65]

The first screening test for blood was described by Christian Schönbein (1799–1868), a German chemist at the University of Basel better known for his discovery of ozone and guncotton. In 1863 he advocated the use of hydrogen peroxide to determine whether a stain might be blood, as it decomposed violently in the presence of haemoglobin. This reaction is cata-lyzed by an enzyme which is found in many substances, so is not specific to blood. Since then, screening tests have relied on colour-change reactions involving peroxide and a colourless compound that changes when catalyzed by haemoglobin. The earliest of these was benzidine (1904), the use of which was phased out in the 1970s after it was found to be carcinogenic. The Kastle-Meyer phenolphthalein test (1901) is still used today and produces a characteristic pink colour. Luminol was recognized as a good indicator in 1937 but did not become a routine form of testing until later in the century. Instead of a colour-change reaction, the test produces luminescence: the area has to be dark so the light can be seen, but the reaction is sensitive and does not interfere with subsequent blood analysis.[66]

Blood stains could not be accurately attributed to a specific species until 1901, when two immunologists made important discoveries. The Austrian Karl Landsteiner (1868–1943) identified ABO blood groups and the German Paul Uhlenhuth (1870–1957) was able to differentiate the blood stains of one mammal from another, including humans. It was some years before blood groups could be used to examine stains, but Uhlenhuth's test was used in a forensic case the very year of its discovery. In 1901 two little boys, brothers Hermann and Peter Stubbe, were dismembered and their body parts scattered across woodland on the island of Rügen off the north-east coast of Germany. Ludwig Tessnow, a carpenter from the nearby village of Baabe who had been seen talking to the boys on the day they disappeared, was questioned and a search of his house yielded boots and clothes marked with dark brown stains. He explained that they were wood dye, but was brought before a magistrate, Johann Schmidt, who recalled a similar case that had occurred three years earlier when two little girls had been found murdered and mutilated near Osnabrück in north-west Germany. The same carpenter, Tessnow, had been seen in the woods where their bodies were found and questioned about dark brown stains on his clothes. They looked like blood but Tessnow had said they were wood dye; since they resembled the stains produced by the dye he used, the police had released him. Armed with this information, Schmidt and local prosecutor Ernst Hubschmann continued to investigate Tessnow, and discovered that three weeks before the Stubbe brothers were discovered on 2 July, a farmer had seen a man running from a field where seven sheep were found mutilated and dismembered. The farmer picked Tessnow from an identity parade, but he denied any wrong-doing and there was no direct evidence apart from the stains on his clothing. As luck would have it, Hubschmann had heard of Uhlenhuth's work and sent him Tessnow's clothes. On 8 August Uhlenhuth submitted a report: many of the stains were human blood, others were sheep's blood. Tessnow, the 'monster of Rügen', was executed at Greifswald prison in 1904 at the age of 32.[67]

The precipitin test, as it is called, relies on the fact that invertebrates produce antibodies to repel foreign substances, as a consequence of which the blood serum of one species will react with that of another to form a cloudy precipitate (precipitin). When an extract of a suspected bloodstain is mixed with an anti-serum produced by a specific species, the reaction, or lack of reaction, indicates what species the blood could, or could not, have come from. Uhlenhuth developed the concept of an anti-serum on the strength of the earlier research of Jules Bordet (1870–1961), a Belgian immunologist who showed that vaccination produced specific antibodies which would later react with the foreign substance. The substances responsible for the production of antibodies are called antigens, and Landsteiner found that the presence or absence of two of these antigens, which he called A and B, in human blood formed four distinct groups – the ABO blood group system. Within a few years scientists recognized that blood group is inherited, so paving the way for its use in establishing paternity; the German courts admitted such evidence for the first time in 1930. In 1916 Leone Lattes (1887–1954) of the Institute of Forensic Medicine in Turin developed a method of identifying the blood group of dried samples of blood; by 1923 he had refined his technique so that it could be performed on small stains, and in 1931 the Austrian Franz Holzer (1903–74) improved the typing of smaller and older stains. In the United States, Alexander Weiner (1907–76) of the New York City medical examiner's office brought blood typing into routine forensic practice, and was the first to use body fluids other than blood for typing. In March 1943 a murder suspect confessed when confronted with his own sweat-stained clothes, which Weiner had matched to his blood group. This was possible because in 1925 serologists had discovered that 80 per cent of the population belong to a group called 'secretors': their body fluids carry a water-soluble form of the substances that determine their blood group. It is this trait that makes saliva such a good source of forensic evidence.[68]

Further improvements in typing procedures were made after the war, notably by an employee of the Forensic Science Service in England, Stuart Kind (1925–2003), whose absorption technique for isolating samples was adopted by the Metropolitan Police Laboratory, which became a world leader in blood typing. Electrophoresis, the motion of dispersed particles in a gel under the influence of an electric field, was the other key post-war development: it became the basis for increasingly sophisticated methods of separating forensic samples from other materials they were mixed with, and allowed the discovery of further genetic markers in blood serum. These serum proteins enabled greater discrimination between individuals subject to ABO typing, but although several hundred systems were known, only a handful were routinely used in forensic practice. Efforts to refine these techniques were ongoing during the 1980s when a new discovery rendered serology all but redundant.[69]

Forensic biologists knew that the key to identifying specific individuals lay in genes rather than blood groups, because the former are unique to the individual; DNA was discovered in 1953, and geneticists had been working to develop techniques to isolate its variable regions from those shared by all humans. In the early 1980s Alec Jeffreys (b. 1950) discovered a method for identifying individuals, and was working on applying it to paternity testing when he was contacted by police investigating two murders; the importance of his discovery to forensic science quickly became apparent (Case Study 6.3).

Case Study 6.3: The introduction of DNA fingerprinting into forensic science – the identification of Colin Pitchfork (England, 1987)

In November 1983 15-year-old Lynda Mann was raped and strangled in Narborough, a village in Leicestershire. A semen sample was taken from her body, but at that time scientists could only distinguish the attacker's blood group: he was a Group A secretor, one of only 10 per cent of English adult males in this group. Despite the best efforts of the police, including blood testing 150 potential suspects, no one was charged. Three years later another 15-year-old girl, Dawn Ashworth, was found murdered in the same manner, in the same area. All the evidence suggested this was the work of the same man: the semen samples showed that the blood groups matched.

The police had a suspect – a local youth who confessed to Dawn's murder but denied having anything to do with Lynda's death, but the officers in charge of the case were convinced that if he had committed one crime, he must have committed the other too. They contacted Dr Alec Jeffreys at the University of Leicester, because in 1985 he had published work showing how new DNA analysis techniques – now known as DNA or genetic fingerprinting – could be used to help solve crimes, by uniquely identifying individuals on the basis of the genetic 'profile' obtained from bodily fluids. When Jeffreys ran a comparison between the semen collected from the bodies of both victims, and the blood of the suspect, he found that the same man had certainly carried out both murders, but was not the man who had confessed. The police then decided to set up a mass screening of all the adult males in the three villages in the area where the girls had lived and died. This was carried out by the Forensic Science Service: 5,000 men gave samples, and DNA profiling was carried out on those who had the same blood group as the killer. None of the DNA matched the killer and the case was left hanging, until a local woman overheard a colleague boasting that he had given his DNA sample under a false name. He had done a favour for a friend and claimed to be Colin Pitchfork when he gave his saliva sample. The woman went to the police, the real Colin Pitchfork, a baker aged 26, was arrested in September 1987, and his DNA was tested. The results showed that it was his semen that had been recovered from the victims, he confessed, and in January 1988 he was jailed for life for the two murders.

Subsequent experience has shown that DNA evidence can be crucial in prompting a suspect to confess, and in solving 'cold' cases.

Sources: J. Wambaugh, *The Blooding*, London: Bantam Books, 1989; J. Ward, *Crimebusting: Breakthroughs in Forensic Science*, London: Blandford Press, 1998, pp. 176–87.

Other convictions based largely on DNA evidence quickly followed, the examination of stains being one goal of forensic research, the development of more rapid and sensitive analyses another. 'The forensic community quickly embraced DNA typing, but it was not a smooth transition': it was clear that strict procedural and quality protocols had to be agreed or the admissibility of DNA profiles in court could be challenged, as occurred in the 1989 trial of Joseph Castro in New York. Although guilty of a double murder to which he later confessed, Castro was acquitted because DNA evidence was disallowed on procedural grounds. To further complicate matters, commercial laboratories entered the field, providing testing kits that made the analytical process simpler but which dictated how testing would be carried out; this brought private industry into the ongoing relationship between science, medicine and the law. To get the most out of each test, that is to allow matches to be found between unsolved cases and named individuals, national databases to store the data had to be created, the first in the world being that launched by the UK's Forensic Science Service in April 1995. In the United States the CODIS database (Combined DNA Index System) pilot project (1990) became fully operational in 1998, and both have proved their effectiveness many times over as more and more reference samples taken from people convicted of certain offences are added. Civil liberties issues are of course a concern, as those arrested but not convicted argue against inclusion and those convicted worry that the data might be used for health or other screening. Australia and European countries have their own DNA databases, their forensic value lying in their demonstrated ability to convict the guilty and exonerate the innocent.[70] DNA analysis now has the sort of public awareness that most scientists can only dream about, and perhaps the only other forensic technique that can match it in terms of public expectation is offender profiling.

Offender profiling

Offender profiling refers to the use of information about a crime, a crime scene and a victim, together with available information on convicted offenders, to infer the likely characteristics of an unknown offender. It is used in cases where the police have few clues, most frequently the investigation of serial rape, murder and, to a lesser extent, arson. In response to the perceived rise in serial homicide, the psychological profiling of killers has seen an upsurge of awareness not only among the general public but also within law enforcement agencies, but it is because profiling is most useful in cases of attacks by strangers that it garners so much media attention. Its importance lies in the fact that these serious offences involve direct contact between a perpetrator and victim and are thus, from a psychological point of view, most likely to reveal aspects of the offender's personality and motivation.[71]

Profiling has a short history in comparison to other forensic techniques. During the hunt for Jack the Ripper, police surgeon Thomas Bond (1841–1901) made a number of deductions about the killer, based mainly on the wounds inflicted on the victims: all the attacks had been carried out by the same person, who had no anatomical knowledge but took some care over his personal appearance. A profile of Adolf Hitler was compiled during World War II, which successfully predicted that he would commit suicide rather than flee.[72] However it was not until the 1950s, and the work of the American psychiatrist James A. Brussel (1905–82), that psychological detection really began. Then in private practice in New York and serving as the state's assistant commissioner of mental hygiene, he received a visit from the police that prompted him to reverse the psychiatrist's usual method. Psychiatrists study people and make intelligent predictions about what they may do in the future, particularly how they would respond to certain situations, but Brussel studied an individual's responses and actions to make deductions about the sort of person they were. His earliest and most famous success with this method was his role in the 1957 identification of New York's Mad Bomber, George Metesky, who planted 32 homemade bombs in a 16-year crusade against his former employer, the Consolidated Edison power company. Amazingly, no one had been killed, but apart from a series of notes, sometimes handwritten but often assembled from words cut from newspapers and magazines, the police had no leads. Finally they called in Brussel, who had a reputation as a forensic psychiatrist. He read the case file and constructed a remarkably detailed psychological profile, then suggested that the police release it to the media, to entice the bomber to reveal himself, and it worked: Metesky telephoned Brussel. Meanwhile, the profile gave the police enough information to lead them to former employees of the power company, and after searching staff records they found the man who matched the profile. Metesky was tried and found guilty but insane, and confined in Matteawan State Hospital for the criminally insane until 1973. He died in 1994, aged 90.[73] Brussel assisted the New York police from 1956 until 1972.

Subsequently, police forces sought the views of psychiatrists and psychologists on an occasional basis, but formal interest in applying profiling techniques to solving crimes dates to the early 1970s and is especially associated with the FBI. Special Agent Howard Teten began teaching applied criminology, including profiling techniques, in 1970, having been influenced by Brussel, among others, and in 1972 the FBI set up the Behavioral Science Unit under the leadership of Jack Kirsch. In 1985 the FBI's National Center for the Analysis of Violent Crime was created during an expansion of the BSU, and profiling units can now be found in law enforcement agencies around the world, including Australia, Canada, Britain, the Netherlands and South Africa. In 1999 the Academy of Behavioral Profiling was founded, the first international, independent, multidisciplinary professional organization of its kind working to develop standards of practice and ethical guidelines.[74]

Profiles are built by analyzing elements such as victim traits, witness reports and modus operandi, to produce a list of identifying features including gender, age group, marital status, sexual preference, occupation and criminal record, which can provide leads and help to focus investigations. Based on the assumption that the behaviour shown at a crime scene will reflect basic consistencies in an offender's personality, choices and actions, the goal is to narrow the range of likely suspects as far as possible. However, profiling is not a substitute for careful policing: serial killers Peter Sutcliffe, Ted Bundy and Gary Ridgeway were all good matches to the profiles created for them, but were not investigated closely for several years. This revealed a fundamental reality: reliance on coordinated analysis of available information is particularly important in cases that are not confined to a small area. To solve this problem, the FBI introduced VICAP, the Violent Criminal Apprehension Program, in 1985, to serve as a central information hub for national crime reports. The United Kingdom equivalent, HOLMES, the Home Office Large Major Enquiry System, was available nationally by 1988.[75]

Approaches to profiling have largely been dominated by the methods used by the FBI, who have focused on creating descriptive classifications, some of which are based on statements made by convicted criminals. Criticism has thus pointed out that the FBI's system lacks a foundation in sufficiently rigorous empirical research and has not been reliably verified; that while the construction of typologies suggests that offenders' motivations are consistent, research indicates that this is not the case; and that there has been a lack of comparison studies to determine what the levels of certain behaviours are in the general population.[76] Even the degree to which the FBI actually rely on psychology has been questioned, a key critic in this regard being David Canter (b. 1944), a psychologist and pioneering profiler now at the University of Huddersfield.

During the 1980s Canter used statistical analysis of witness statements to aid the police during the hunt for the rapist and murderer John Duffy, dubbed the Railway Rapist, the first English criminal identified by psychological profiling and subsequently convicted (1988). Canter considers his profiling work to be a branch of applied psychology, bases it on accepted models and methods, and argues that perpetrator–victim interactions are governed by the same behaviour that influences the offender's other social relations. By examining offender behaviour, Canter and his colleagues identified five characteristics that can help in rape investigations, of which the first two have been found to be the most useful: residential location; criminal biography; social characteristics; personal characteristics; and occupational or educational history. Drawing on environmental psychology, Canter has also found that mental maps influence offenders' choice of target-area: they operate in locations related to their place of residence, in which they believe they will not arouse suspicion. This aspect of profiling allows the technique to be applied to criminals such as burglars. However, despite the foundation in a scientific method, profiles created in this way are still only probabilities: they rely on statistical analysis and are therefore limited by the accuracy of the available data.[77]

There is no international agreement on approaches to profiling, though most countries have adopted some form of the FBI's methods. Profilers in the Netherlands open their work to more scientific scrutiny than the FBI does, using it to steer investigations and combine detective experience with behavioural psychological knowledge. Psychiatric insights into offending tend to draw inferences about a single offender, linked to their developmental experiences and/or current mental state. Understanding a perpetrator's mental world can help the police target particular individuals or predict whether they will offend again. A clinical psychological approach can offer insights into motivation. Since human behaviour is complex, it is unlikely that there is only one 'right' approach to profiling, and the ultimate assessment of reliability should rest on empirical testing. Criminal profiling is not yet a science nor still an art; there is still room to develop its potential if scientific theory and policing practice are increasingly brought together.[78]

Conclusion

Although they are now quite different disciplines, contemporary forensic medicine and forensic science share a concern with the human body and mind reminiscent of that of earlier times. Their institutional organization, personnel, methods and techniques have changed significantly over the past century but, just as in the medieval, early modern and Victorian periods, forensic practitioners seek information about time, manner and cause of death or injury and try to deduce information about offenders' state of mind. Individual expert witnesses may become figures of controversy, but expert witnesses in general are recognized as critical elements in the modern medico-legal process and, as in the past, medico-scientific debate tends to lead eventually to consensus. Earlier chapters have shown how this happened during the nineteenth century as regards the importance of toxicology and psychiatry to the courts, with DNA testing providing a modern, much faster, counterpart; the process is still ongoing with respect to offender profiling. In many respects, modern forensic practice is distinguished from its forebears largely by the speed at which developments occur, as a consequence of the worldwide expansion and progress of medicine and science.

What then is the current status of forensic medicine in the West? The key development of the twentieth century was its separation from forensic science, so that now forensic medicine means 'pathology', while forensic science encompasses dozens of specialist subjects, many based specifically in institutes and police laboratories of forensic science, others remaining within universities until called upon by the police. As in the past, the needs of the state are a constant feature in medico-legal developments. On the Continent, the entire system of death investigation is geared primarily to suspected crimes and thus the police or judiciary make the decisions about which cases should be subject to medico-legal investigation. By contrast, in Britain and the United States the coroner and medical examiner systems cast much wider nets, because their remit is to investigate cases of sudden or unnatural death, not just suspicious deaths.[79] In other words, variations in political, legal and educational structures still influence medico-legal practice.

In terms of educational provision, forensic medicine is well represented in European and Scottish medical schools, increasingly so in the United States since the 1970s, but almost not at all in England, where its status as a medical specialty was hit hard by its exclusion from the NHS and the consequent lack of specific career paths, combined with government preference to support forensic science. It remains to be seen whether the upsurge of public interest in what is now called 'forensics' will be translated into tangible increases in funding for or teaching of forensic medicine, but it is already clear that security needs will be a driving force in advancements in forensic science. With crime rates a significant area of public concern and the increasing sophistication of criminals and terrorists, we can be certain that forensic medicine and science will continue to play a key role in serving the needs of the law.

Additional reading

The references for this chapter can be found in the Bibliography, and will allow you to expand on all of the issues discussed here. If you wish to do some further reading, you may also consult the publications listed below.

Jacques Côté, *Wilfrid Derome: expert en homicides*, Montréal: Boréal, 2003.
Arthur Daemmrich, 'The evidence does not speak for itself: expert witnesses and the organization of DNA-typing companies', *Social Studies of Science*, 1998, vol. 28, 741–72.
Zakaria Erzinçlioğlu, *Maggots, Murder and Men: Memories and Reflections of a Forensic Entomologist*, Colchester: Harley Books, 2000.

Colin Evans, *The Father of Forensics: The Groundbreaking Cases of Sir Bernard Spilsbury, and the Beginnings of Modern CSI*, New York: Berkley Books, 2006.

Estelle B. Freedman, '"Uncontrolled desires": the response to the sexual psychopath, 1920–60', *Journal of American History*, 1987, vol. 74, 83–106.

Patrizia Guarnieri, '"Dangerous girls", family secrets, and incest law in Italy, 1861–1930', *International Journal of Law and Psychiatry*, 1998, vol. 21, 369–83.

Saul Halfon, 'Collecting, testing and convincing: forensic DNA experts in the courts', *Social Studies of Science*, 1998, vol. 28, 801–28.

Dan Healey, *Bolshevik Sexual Forensics: Diagnosing Disorder in the Clinic and Courtroom, 1917–1939*, DeKalb, IL: Northern Illinois University Press, 2009.

Michael Lynch and Sheila Jasanoff, 'Contested identities: science, law and forensic practice', *Social Studies of Science*, 1998, vol. 28, 675–86.

Kenneth M. Pinnow, 'Cutting and counting: forensic medicine as a science of society in Bolshevik Russia, 1920–29', in David L. Hoffmann and Yanni Kotsonis (eds), *Russian Modernity: Politics, Knowledge, Practices*, Basingstoke: Macmillan, 2000, 115–37.

Sir Sydney Smith, *Mostly Murder*, London: Harrap, 1959.

Frank Smyth, *Cause of Death: The Story of Forensic Science*, London: Orbis Publishing, 1980.

P.H.A. Willcox, *The Detective-Physician: The Life and Work of Sir William Willcox*, London: William Heinemann Medical Books, 1970.

Notes

Introduction

1 Y.V. O'Neill and G.L. Chan, 'A Chinese coroner's manual and the evolution of anatomy', *Journal of the History of Medicine and Allied Sciences*, 1976, vol. 31, 3–16; Sung Tz'u, *The Washing Away of Wrongs: Forensic Medicine in Thirteenth-Century China*, trans. B.E. McKnight, Ann Arbor: Center for Chinese Studies, University of Michigan, 1981; D. Bodde, 'Forensic medicine in pre-Imperial China', *Journal of the American Oriental Society*, 1982, vol. 102, 1–15; L. Gwei-Djen and J. Needham, 'A history of forensic medicine in China', *Medical History*, 1988, vol. 32, 357–400; D. Asen, 'Vital spots, mortal wounds, and forensic practice: finding cause of death in nineteenth-century China', *East Asian Science, Technology and Society*, 2009, vol. 3, 453–74.
2 W.J. Curran, 'Titles in the medicolegal field: a proposal for reform', *American Journal of Law and Medicine*, 1975, vol. 1, p. 2; E.H. Ackerknecht, 'Early history of legal medicine', in C.R. Burns (ed.), *Legacies in Law and Medicine*, New York: Science History Publications, 1977, pp. 253–56.
3 Curran, 'Titles in the medicolegal field', pp. 2–3.
4 Ibid., p. 3; W. Keil, A. Berzlanovich and B. Madea, 'Textbooks on legal medicine in the German-speaking countries', *Forensic Science International*, 2004, vol. 144, 289–302.
5 Curran, 'Titles in the medicolegal field', pp. 3–4; A. Lacassagne, *Précis de médecine judiciaire* (1886), Chestnut Hill, MA: Elibron Classics, 2006, p. 28: 'the art of providing medical knowledge in the service of the administration of justice'.
6 Curran, 'Titles in the medicolegal field', pp. 4–6.
7 Ibid., p. 6; B. White, 'Training medical policemen: forensic medicine and public health in nineteenth-century Scotland', in M. Clark and C. Crawford (eds), *Legal Medicine in History*, Cambridge: Cambridge University Press, 1994, 145–63.
8 M. Clark and C. Crawford, 'Introduction', in Clark and Crawford (eds), *Legal Medicine in History*, p. 2.
9 Readers interested in learning more about these issues may consult in the first instance the following: K. Jones, 'The Windham Case: the enquiry held in London in 1861 into the state of mind of William Frederick Windham, heir to the Felbrigg Estate', *British Journal of Psychiatry*, 1971, vol. 119, 425–33; J. Basten, 'The court expert in civil trials – a comparative appraisal', *Modern Law Review*, 1977, vol. 40, 174–91; M. Jackson, '"It begins with the goose and ends with the goose": medical, legal and lay understandings of imbecility in Ingram *v.* Wyatt, 1824–32', *Social History of Medicine*, 1998, vol. 11, 361–80; D. Mendelson, 'The expert deposes, but the court disposes: the concept of malingering and the function of a medical expert witness in the forensic process', *International Journal of Law and Psychiatry*, 1995, vol. 18, 425–36; D. Mendelson, 'English medical experts

and the claims for shock occasioned by railway collisions in the 1860s: issues of law, ethics, and medicine', *International Journal of Law and Psychiatry*, 2002, vol. 25, 303–29; J.C. Mohr, 'The origins of forensic psychiatry in the United States and the great nineteenth-century crisis over the adjudication of wills', *Journal of the American Academy of Psychiatry and the Law*, 1997, vol. 25, 273–84; J. Sim, *Medical Power in Prisons: The Prison Medical Service in England 1774–1989*, Milton Keynes: Open University Press, 1990; E. Hasson, 'Capability to marry: law, medicine and conceptions of insanity', *Social History of Medicine*, 2010, vol. 23, 1–20.

10 J. Duffin, *History of Medicine: A Scandalously Short Introduction*, Basingstoke: Macmillan, 2000, pp. 64–66; L.S. King and M.C. Meehan, 'A history of the autopsy', *American Journal of Pathology*, 1973, vol. 73, 514–44.

11 R. Porter, *The Greatest Benefit to Mankind: A Medical History of Humanity from Antiquity to the Present*, London: HarperCollins, 1997, pp. 255–99.

12 Duffin, *History of Medicine*, pp. 119–20.

13 Ibid., p. 119.

14 M.I. Roemer, 'Government's role in American medicine – a brief historical survey', in Burns (ed.), *Legacies in Law and Medicine*, p. 191.

15 Duffin, *History of Medicine*, pp. 212, 224.

16 A.W. Russell (ed.), *The Town and State Physician in Europe from the Middle Ages to the Enlightenment*, Wolfenbüttel: Herzog August Bibliothek, 1981.

17 W.F. Bynum, E.J. Browne and R. Porter (eds), *Macmillan Dictionary of the History of Science*, London: The Macmillan Press, 1983, pp. 325–26 (entry on 'physic').

18 T.N. Bonner, *Becoming a Physician: Medical Education in Britain, France, Germany, and the United States, 1750–1945* (1995), Baltimore and London: Johns Hopkins University Press, 2000. On military medical schools and the 'rapprochement' of medicine and surgery, see pp. 54–58.

19 Burns (ed.), *Legacies in Law and Medicine*; Clark and Crawford (eds), *Legal Medicine in History*.

20 E. Fischer-Homberger, *Medizin vor Gericht: Gerichtsmedizin von der Renaissance bis zur Aufklärung*, Bern: Verlag Hans Huber, 1983; J. Shatzmiller, *Médecine et Justice en Provence Médiévale: Documents de Manosque, 1262–1348*, Aix-en-Provence: Université de Provence, 1989; A. Pastore, *Il medico in tribunale: La perizia medica nella procedura penale d'antico regime (secoli XVI-XVIII)*, Bellinzona: Edizioni Casagrande, 1998; F. Chauvaud, *Les experts du crime: la médecine légale en France au XIXe siècle*, Paris: Aubier, 2000; M. Renneville, *Crime et folie: deux siècles d'enquêtes médicales et judiciaires*, Paris: Fayard, 2003; A. Pastore and G. Rossi (eds), *Paolo Zacchia: alle origini della medicina legale 1584–1659*, Milan: FrancoAngeli, 2008.

21 P. Cassar, *Landmarks in the Development of Forensic Medicine in the Maltese Islands*, Valetta: International Academy of Legal Medicine and Social Medicine, 1974; R. Smith, *Trial by Medicine: Insanity and Responsibility in Victorian Trials*, Edinburgh: Edinburgh University Press, 1981; T.R. Forbes, *Surgeons at the Bailey: English Forensic Medicine to 1878*, New Haven, CT and London: Yale University Press, 1985; M.A. Crowther and B. White, *On Soul and Conscience. The Medical Expert and Crime: 150 Years of Forensic Medicine in Glasgow*, Aberdeen: Aberdeen University Press, 1988; J.C. Mohr, *Doctors and the Law: Medical Jurisprudence in Nineteenth-Century America*, Baltimore, MD and London: Johns Hopkins University Press, 1993; J.P. Eigen, *Witnessing Insanity: Madness and Mad-Doctors in the English Court*, New Haven, CT and London: Yale University Press, 1995; J.R. Bertomeu-Sánchez and A. Nieto-Galan (eds), *Chemistry, Medicine, and Crime: Mateu J.B. Orfila (1787–1853) and His Times*, Sagamore Beach, MA: Science History Publications, 2006. This last uses Orfila as a point of departure for an international perspective, but each chapter focuses

largely on developments in only one nation. I. Goold and C. Kelly (eds), *Lawyers' Medicine: The Legislature, the Courts and Medical Practice, 1760–2000*, Oxford and Portland, OR: Hart Publishing, 2009, considers the influence that medical practitioners have had on the development of the law.

1 The legal inheritance

1 C. Crawford, 'Legalizing medicine: early modern legal systems and the growth of medico-legal knowledge', in M. Clark and C. Crawford (eds), *Legal Medicine in History*, Cambridge: Cambridge University Press, 1994, p. 89.

2 D.M. Dwyer, 'Expert evidence in the English civil courts, 1550–1800', *Journal of Legal History*, 2007, vol. 28, 93–118; V. McMahon, 'Reading the body: dissection and the "murder" of Sarah Stout, Hertfordshire, 1699', *Social History of Medicine*, 2006, vol. 19, 19–35. D. Harley, 'Political post-mortems and morbid anatomy in seventeenth-century England', *Social History of Medicine*, 1994, vol. 7, 1–28 suggests that physicians abandoned autopsy to the surgeons at the end of that century, a supposition that my own work on eighteenth-century England and Wales supports.

3 The French and Italians produced medico-legal treatises from the late sixteenth century, and the Germans from the early eighteenth century: E.H. Ackerknecht, 'Early history of legal medicine', in C.R. Burns (ed.), *Legacies in Law and Medicine*, New York: Science History Publications, 1977, pp. 252–60.

4 H.J. Berman, *Law and Revolution I: The Formation of the Western Legal Tradition*, Cambridge, MA and London: Harvard University Press, 1983; R.C. van Caenegem, *Legal History: A European Perspective*, London and Rio Grande: The Hambledon Press, 1991, Ch. 4, 'Methods of proof in Western medieval law', pp. 71–113.

5 The term 'barbarian' is used to denote a member of one of the large number of tribes that migrated into western Europe from eastern Germany and areas east of the Black Sea during the fourth and fifth centuries. Only some of these tribes had a lasting influence on the legal systems that developed after the fall of the Roman Empire, particularly the Visigoths of Spain, the Burgundians, the Franks and the Anglo-Saxons.

6 P.S. Barnwell, 'Emperors, jurists and kings: law and custom in the late Roman and early medieval west', *Past and Present*, 2000, vol. 168, p. 11.

7 van Caenegem, *Legal History*, Ch. 5, 'Law in the medieval world', p. 117.

8 Barnwell, 'Emperors, jurists and kings', p. 15. Roman customary law was strongest in the provinces, where men educated in the written law were – particularly in rural areas – few and far between.

9 H. Janin, *Medieval Justice: Cases and Laws in France, England, and Germany, 500–1500*, Jefferson, NC and London: McFarland, 2004, p. 11.

10 Barnwell, 'Emperors, jurists and kings', pp. 15–18.

11 D.W. Amundsen and G.B. Ferngren, 'The forensic role of physicians in Roman law', *Bulletin of the History of Medicine*, 1979, vol. 53, p. 52.

12 J.F. Winkler, 'Roman law in Anglo-Saxon England', *Journal of Legal History*, 1992, vol. 13, 101–27; L. Waelkens, 'Traces Romano-canoniques dans les preuves "Germaniques"', *Legal History Review*, 2007, vol. 75, 321–31.

13 G. Halsall, 'Violence and society in the early medieval west: an introductory survey', in G. Halsall (ed.), *Violence and Society in the Early Medieval West*, Woodbridge: The Boydell Press, 1998, p. 15.

14 Barnwell, 'Emperors, jurists and kings', p. 17; S. Rubin, 'The bot, or composition in Anglo-Saxon law: a reassessment', *Journal of Legal History*, 1996, vol. 17, 144–54; M. Elsakkers, 'Inflicting serious bodily harm: the Visigothic *Antiquae* on violence and abortion', *Legal History Review*, 2003, vol. 71, p. 61 which notes that the fines varied according to the status of those concerned.

15 R.P. Brittain, 'Origins of legal medicine: Leges Barbarorum', *Medico-Legal Journal*, 1966, vol. 34, pp. 21–22.
16 Rubin, 'The bot, or composition in Anglo-Saxon law: a reassessment', p. 151.
17 van Caenegem, *Legal History*, p. 74. Preparations for performing ordeals were often made in church.
18 See for example R. Bartlett, *Trial by Fire and Water: the Medieval Judicial Ordeal*, Oxford: Oxford University Press, 1986, pp. 153–66, and the riposte by R.C. van Caenegem, 'Reflexions on rational and irrational modes of proof in medieval Europe', *Legal History Review*, 1990, vol. 58, 263–79.
19 van Caenegem, 'Reflexions on rational and irrational modes of proof in medieval Europe', p. 270.
20 Janin, *Medieval Justice*, p. 13; van Caenegem, *Legal History*, p. 73; Bartlett, *Trial by Fire and Water*, p. 2.
21 R.H. Helmholtz, 'Crime, compurgation and the courts of the medieval church', *Law and History Review*, 1983, vol. 1, p. 13.
22 Ibid.
23 For a discussion of the circumstances in which ordeals were used in England, see Bartlett, *Trial by Fire and Water*, Ch. 3.
24 Janin, *Medieval Justice*, p. 14.
25 Ibid., pp. 14–16. For a description of the religious formulas used for conducting ordeals see the Internet Medieval Sourcebook, http://www.fordham.edu/halsall/sbook.html (accessed on 2 June 2010).
26 Janin, *Medieval Justice*, p. 16.
27 M.H. Kerr, R.D. Forsyth and M.J. Plyley, 'Cold water and hot iron: trial by ordeal in England', *Journal of Interdisciplinary History*, 1992, vol. 22, 573–95.
28 van Caenegem, 'Reflexions on rational and irrational modes of proof in medieval Europe', p. 264.
29 Bartlett, *Trial by Fire and Water*, Ch. 5; van Caenegem, *Legal History*, pp. 83–89.
30 Helmholz, 'Crime, compurgation', p. 26; van Caenegem, *Legal History*, pp. 93–94; J.H. Baker, *An Introduction to English Legal History*, 4th edn, London: Butterworths, 2002, p. 74.
31 In England, where trial by battle was introduced by the Normans after 1066, its use in civil cases was never common. See M.J. Russell, 'Trial by battle and the writ of right', *Journal of Legal History*, 1980, vol. 1, 111–34.
32 Janin, *Medieval Justice*, p. 17.
33 M.J. Russell, 'Trial by battle and the appeals of felony', *Journal of Legal History*, 1980, vol. 1, p. 145. For details of English procedure, see M.J. Russell, 'Trial by battle procedure in writs of right and criminal appeals', *Legal History Review*, 1983, vol. 51, 123–34.
34 Russell, 'Trial by battle and the appeals of felony', pp. 149–53.
35 E. Jager, *The Last Duel: A True Story of Crime, Scandal, and Trial by Combat in Medieval France*, New York: Broadway Books, 2004.
36 Sir J. Hall (ed.), *Trial of Abraham Thornton*, Glasgow: William Hodge, 1926, pp. 33–35.
37 'Abraham Thornton', *The Newgate Calendar*, http://exclassics.com/newgate/ng574.htm (accessed 9 June 2009).
38 Ibid.
39 59 Geo III c. 46 (1819).
40 Janin, *Medieval Justice*, pp. 26–30.
41 Ibid., p. 32.
42 Ibid., pp. 31–34; van Caenegem, *Legal History*, pp. 128–31.
43 A. Esmein, *A History of Continental Criminal Procedure with special reference to France*, trans. J. Simpson (1913), Union, NJ: Lawbook Exchange, 2000, pp. 288–95; van Caenegem, *Legal History*, pp. 131–32.

44 H.J. Berman, *Law and Revolution II: The Impact of the Protestant Reformations on the Western Legal Tradition*, Cambridge, MA and London: Belknap Press, 2003, p. 4.

45 J.H. Langbein, *Torture and the Law of Proof: Europe and England in the Ancien Régime* (1976), Chicago: University of Chicago Press, 2006, pp. 5–8; R.M. Fraher, 'Conviction according to conscience: the medieval jurists' debate concerning judicial discretion and the law of proof', *Law and History Review*, 1989, vol. 7, 23–88; M. Damaška, 'The death of legal torture', *Yale Law Journal*, 1978, vol. 87, 860–84.

46 Janin, *Medieval Justice*, pp. 64–68.

47 Ibid., p. 74; van Caenegem, *Legal History*, pp. 95–98.

48 Baker, *An Introduction to English Legal History*, pp. 72–76.

49 J.D.J. Havard, *The Detection of Secret Homicide: A Study of the Medico-legal System of Investigation of Sudden and Unexplained Deaths*, London: Macmillan, 1960, pp. 11–27.

50 Crawford, 'Legalizing medicine', p. 95.

51 At Charlemagne's death the Carolingian empire encompassed the modern countries of France, Germany, Belgium, the Netherlands, Austria, Switzerland and northern Italy.

52 Janin, *Medieval Justice*, pp. 148–53.

53 Berman, *Law and Revolution II*, pp. 131–37.

54 Esmein, *A History of Continental Criminal Procedure with special reference to France*, pp. 39–40.

55 van Caenegem, *Legal History*, pp. 97–98.

56 J.H. Langbein, *Prosecuting Crime in the Renaissance: England, Germany, France* (1974), Clark, NJ: Lawbook Exchange, 2005, pp. 177–78, 217.

57 C. Emsley, *Crime and Society in England 1750–1900*, 3rd edn, Harlow: Pearson Education, 2005, Ch. 8.

58 The proceedings held at the Old Bailey, the central court for the City of London and county of Middlesex, were a notable exception, as written trial reports first appeared in 1674. See http://www.oldbaileyonline.org (accessed on 24 May 2010).

59 Langbein, *Prosecuting Crime in the Renaissance*, p. 131.

60 Ibid.

61 Berman, *Law and Revolution II*, pp. 133–36; Langbein, *Prosecuting Crime in the Renaissance*, pp. 148–52; Esmein, *A History of Continental Criminal Procedure with special reference to France*, pp. 107–14; van Caenegem, *Legal History*, pp. 99–102.

62 J. Pardo-Tomás and À. Martínez-Vidal, 'Victims and experts: medical practitioners and the Spanish Inquisition', in J. Woodward and R. Jütte (eds), *Coping with Sickness: Medicine, Law and Human Rights – Historical Perspectives*, Sheffield: European Association for the History of Medicine and Health Publications, 2000, p. 15; Langbein, *Torture and the Law of Proof*, p. 14.

63 Langbein, *Prosecuting Crime in the Renaissance*, p. 223.

64 Ibid., p. 307.

65 Crawford, 'Legalizing medicine', p. 103; Ackerknecht, 'Early history of legal medicine', pp. 253, 266–71; Esmein, *A History of Continental Criminal Procedure with special reference to France*, p. 257; H. Skoda, 'Violent discipline or disciplining violence? Experience and reception of domestic violence in late thirteenth- and early fourteenth-century Paris and Picardy', *Cultural and Social History*, 2009, vol. 6, p. 18.

66 Esmein, *A History of Continental Criminal Procedure with special reference to France*, p. 506; R.M. Andrews, *Law, Magistracy, and Crime in Old Regime Paris, 1735–1789, Vol. 1, The System of Criminal Justice*, Cambridge: Cambridge University Press, 1994, p. 425.

67 van Caenegem, *Legal History*, Ch. 6, 'Reflexions on the place of the low countries in European legal history', p. 158.

68   P. Spierenburg, 'Faces of violence: homicide trends and cultural meanings: Amsterdam, 1431–1816', *Journal of Social History*, 1994, vol. 27, 701–16.
69   Berman, *Law and Revolution II*, pp.141–43; Crawford, 'Legalizing medicine', pp. 101–5; Langbein, *Prosecuting Crime in the Renaissance*, pp. 198–202; S. De Renzi, 'Witnesses of the body: medico-legal cases in seventeenth-century Rome', *Studies in History and Philosophy of Science*, 2002, vol. 33, 219–42.
70   M. Jackson, 'Suspicious infant deaths: the statute of 1624 and medical evidence at coroners' inquests', in Clark and Crawford (eds), *Legal Medicine in History*, pp. 64–86.
71   Crawford, 'Legalizing medicine', p. 109.

2 Medico-legal practice before the modern period

  1   The literature on this subject is vast, and focuses mainly on the Anglo-American and French contexts. See for example C.A.G. Jones, *Expert Witnesses: Science, Medicine, and the Practice of Law*, Oxford: Clarendon Press, 1994; T. Golan, *Laws of Men and Laws of Nature: The History of Scientific Expert Testimony in England and America*, Cambridge, MA and London: Harvard University Press, 2004; F. Chauvaud and L. Dumoulin, *Experts et expertise judiciaire: France, XIXe et XXe siècles*, Rennes: Presses Universitaires de Rennes, 2003.
  2   C. Rabier (ed.), *Fields of Expertise: A Comparative History of Expert Procedures in Paris and London, 1600 to Present*, Newcastle: Cambridge Scholars Publishing, 2007.
  3   V. Nutton, 'Continuity or rediscovery? The city physician in classical antiquity and mediaeval Italy', in A.W. Russell (ed.), *The Town and State Physician in Europe from the Middle Ages to the Enlightenment*, Wolfenbüttel: Herzog August Bibliothek, 1981, pp. 11–17.
  4   D.W. Amundsen and G.B. Ferngren, 'The physician as an expert witness in Athenian law', *Bulletin of the History of Medicine*, 1977, vol. 51, p. 204.
  5   Ibid., pp. 204–13.
  6   R.P. Brittain, 'Origins of legal medicine: Roman law: Lex Duodecim Tabularum', *Medico-Legal Journal*, 1967, vol. 35, p. 71.
  7   F. Collard, *Pouvoir et Poison: histoire d'un crime politique de l'Antiquité à nos jours*, Paris: Éditions du Seuil, 2007, pp. 55–57.
  8   D.W. Amundsen and G.B. Ferngren, 'The forensic role of physicians in Roman law', *Bulletin of the History of Medicine*, 1979, vol. 53, pp. 40–44.
  9   Ibid., pp. 46–52.
 10   On Roman civic doctors see Nutton, 'Continuity or rediscovery?', pp. 17–21.
 11   Ibid., pp. 21–23; D.W. Amundsen and G.B. Ferngren, 'The forensic role of physicians in Ptolemaic and Roman Egypt', *Bulletin of the History of Medicine*, 1978, vol. 52, pp. 338–44.
 12   Amundsen and Ferngren, 'The forensic role of physicians in Ptolemaic and Roman Egypt', pp. 339–42, 351–53.
 13   D.W. Amundsen, 'Visigothic medical legislation', *Bulletin of the History of Medicine*, 1971, vol. 45, pp. 553–65.
 14   For the effects on learned medicine of the fall of the Roman Empire, see R. Porter, *The Greatest Benefit to Mankind: A Medical History of Humanity from Antiquity to the Present*, London: Harper Collins, 1997, pp. 83–92.
 15   R.P. Brittain, 'Origins of legal medicine: Leges Barbarorum', *Medico-Legal Journal*, 1966, vol. 34, p. 21; E.H. Ackerknecht, 'Early history of legal medicine', in C.R. Burns (ed.), *Legacies in Law and Medicine*, New York: Science History Publications, 1977, p. 250.
 16   Brittain, 'Origins of legal medicine', p. 21.

17 S.P. Scott (trans.), *The Visigothic Code: Forum Judicum*, Boston: Boston Book Company, 1910, book 6, title 4, p. 209; online, http://libro.uca.edu/vcode/visigoths. htm (accessed 28 June 2009).

18 'The Salic Law, Title XVII, Concerning Wounds', in E.F. Henderson (trans. and ed.), *Select Historical Documents of the Middle Ages*, London: G. Bell and Sons, 1910, pp. 176–89; online at Medieval Sourcebook, http://www.fordham.edu/halall/ source/salic-law.html and at The Avalon Project, http://avalon.law.yale.edu/medieval/ salic.asp (accessed 28 June 2009).

19 Ibid.

20 Scott, *The Visigothic Code*, p. 208.

21 For a wider discussion of what practices like cruentation reveal about northern European beliefs about the dead body, the very different Italian beliefs, and what these meant for attitudes towards opening the body, see K. Park, 'The life of the corpse: division and dissection in late medieval Europe', *Journal of the History of Medicine and Allied Sciences*, 1995, vol. 50, 111–32.

22 R.P. Brittain, 'Cruentation in legal medicine and in literature', *Medical History*, 1965, vol. 9, pp. 82–83; P. Volk and H.J. Warlo, 'The role of medical experts in court proceedings in the medieval town', in H. Karplus (ed.), *International Symposium on Society, Medicine and Law: Jerusalem, March 1972*, Amsterdam: Elsevier, 1973, pp. 107–8.

23 E. Cohen, *The Crossroads of Justice: Law and Culture in Late Medieval France*, Leiden: E.J. Brill, 1993, pp. 139–40.

24 Brittain, 'Cruentation in legal medicine and in literature', pp. 83–87.

25 National Library of Wales, Great Sessions 4/380/6 (Breconshire), Gwenllian David, 25 March 1753.

26 Brittain, 'Cruentation in legal medicine and in literature', p. 86.

27 For a detailed description of how the Carolingian legal system worked, but which neglects discussion of the role of medical witnesses, see A. Barbero, *Charlemagne: Father of a Continent*, trans. A. Cameron, Berkeley, CA: University of California Press, 2004, pp. 196–212.

28 R.P. Brittain, 'The history of legal medicine: Charlemagne', *Medico-Legal Journal*, 1966, vol. 34, p. 122; C. Desmaze, *Histoire de la médecine légale en France*, Paris: G. Charpentier, 1880, p. xii.

29 P.W. Edbury (ed.), *John of Ibelin: Le Livre des Assises*, Leiden and Boston, MA: Brill, 2003, pp. 473–74; P.D. Mitchell, *Medicine in the Crusades: Warfare, Wounds and the Medieval Surgeon*, Cambridge: Cambridge University Press, 2004, pp. 15–16, 222. My thanks to Professor Edbury for his clarification of the Old French text.

30 R.P. Brittain, 'The history of legal medicine: the Assizes of Jerusalem', *Medico-Legal Journal*, 1966, vol. 34, pp. 72–73.

31 R.P. Brittain, 'Origins of legal medicine: the origin of legal medicine in France', *Medico-Legal Journal*, 1966, vol. 34, pp. 168–69.

32 For the shift in the notion of expertise from practical experience to intellectual understanding, see Chapter 3.

33 J. Shatzmiller, *Médecine et Justice en Provence Médiévale: Documents de Manosque, 1262–1348*, Aix-en-Provence: Université de Provence, 1989, p. 21; 'at the demand of the court or of interested persons'.

34 Ibid., pp. 32–43.

35 Y.V. O'Neill, 'Innocent III and the evolution of anatomy', *Medical History*, 1976, vol. 20, pp. 430–31.

36 R.P. Brittain, 'Origins of legal medicine: the origin of legal medicine in Italy', *Medico-Legal Journal*, 1965, vol. 33, p. 170; G. Tourdes and E. Metzquer, *Traité de médecine légale: théorique et pratique*, Paris: Asselin et Houzeau, 1896, p. 18.

37 A. Simili, 'The beginnings of forensic medicine in Bologna', in Karplus (ed.), *International Symposium*, pp. 91–100; Brittain, 'Legal medicine in Italy', pp. 168–69; Shatzmiller, *Médecine et Justice*, pp. 33–34. Nutton, 'Continuity or rediscovery?', pp. 26–27 points out that Hugo had been under contract as Bologna's city doctor since 1214, while Mitchell, *Medicine in the Crusades* p. 26, notes that the already elderly Hugo went on crusade to Egypt 1218–21.

38 K. Park, *Secrets of Women: Gender, Generation, and the Origins of Human Dissection*, New York: Zone Books, 2006, pp. 52–53, 123.

39 J. Shatzmiller, 'The jurisprudence of the dead body: medical practition (sic) at the service of civic and legal authorities', *Micrologus*, 1999, vol. 7, pp. 226–30.

40 G. Ruggiero, 'The cooperation of physicians and the state in the control of violence in Renaissance Venice', *Journal of the History of Medicine and Allied Sciences*, 1978, vol. 33, pp. 158, 160–64.

41 Park, *Secrets of Women*, p. 37; K. Park, 'The criminal and the saintly body: autopsy and dissection in Renaissance Italy', *Renaissance Quarterly*, 1994, vol. 47, pp. 8–11.

42 Ackerknecht, 'Early history of legal medicine', p. 251: Padua (1316), Genoa (fourteenth century), Mirandola (1386), Bassano (1389), Florence (1415), Verona (1450), Brescia (1470), Milan (1480), Ferrara (1506) and Urbino (1556).

43 Park, *Secrets of Women*, pp. 20, 113, 312n108; 'The criminal and saintly body', pp. 10–11; 'The life of the corpse', pp. 114–15.

44 E.H. Ackerknecht, 'Early history of legal medicine', p. 251; Brittain, 'Legal medicine in Italy', p. 171; Desmaze, *Histoire de la médecine légale en France*, p. xv.

45 R. van Dülmen, *Theatre of Horror: Crime and Punishment in Early Modern Germany*, trans. E. Neu, Cambridge: Polity Press, 1990, pp. 19, 20, 21; A. Pastore, *Il medico in tribunale: La perizia medica nella procedura penale d'antico regime (secoli XVI–XVIII)*, Bellinzona: Edizioni Casagrande, 1998, pp. 37–42.

46 J. Pardo-Tomás and À. Martínez-Vidal, 'Victims and experts: medical practitioners and the Spanish Inquisition', in J. Woodward and R. Jütte (eds), *Coping with Sickness: Medicine, Law and Human Rights – Historical Perspectives*, Sheffield: European Association for the History of Medicine and Health Publications, 2000, pp. 16–17.

47 Brittain, 'Legal medicine in Italy', p. 171.

48 Ackerknecht, 'Early history of legal medicine', pp. 251, 267.

49 See Desmaze, *Histoire de la médecine légale en France*, pp. 11–20 and Brittain, 'Origins of legal medicine in France', pp. 169–72, though they give no examples for the fifteenth century.

50 Desmaze, *Histoire de la médecine légale en France*, p. 31 states that the office was suppressed in 1577, but it must have been revived soon after as C. McClive, 'Blood and expertise: the trials of the female medical expert in the ancien-régime courtroom', *Bulletin of the History of Medicine*, 2008, vol. 82, p. 92 shows that the Parlement of Paris issued rulings confirming the sworn-surgeons' monopoly in 1597, 1675 and 1722.

51 Ackerknecht, 'Early history of legal medicine', p. 253.

52 Desmaze, *Histoire de la médecine légale en France*, pp. 42–44.

53 R.P. Brittain, 'Origins of legal medicine: The origin of legal medicine in France: Henri IV and Louis XIV', *Medico-Legal Journal*, 1967, vol. 35, p. 25; Desmaze, *Histoire de la médecine légale en France*, p. 10.

54 Brittain, 'Henri IV and Louis XIV', pp. 25–26.

55 J.H. Langbein, *Prosecuting Crime in the Renaissance: England, Germany, France* (1974), Clark, NJ: Lawbook Exchange, 2005, p. 141.

56 For a discussion of Charlemagne's influence on Europe's socio-political development see Barbero, *Charlemagne*, pp. 102–15.

57 For more on the legal history of the German Empire before the Carolina see Langbein, *Prosecuting Crime in the Renaissance*, pp. 141–52.

58 M. Stürzbecher, 'The physici in German-speaking countries from the Middle Ages to the Enlightenment', in Russell (ed.), *The Town and State Physician in Europe from the Middle Ages to the Enlightenment*, p. 124.

59 Volk and Warlo, 'The role of medical experts in court proceedings in the medieval town', pp. 101–4, 111, 112.

60 For details of the Bamberg Capital Court Statute and its importance as a model for legislation in other German principalities, see H.J. Berman, *Law and Revolution I: The Formation of the Western Legal Tradition*, Cambridge, MA and London: Harvard University Press, 1983, pp. 137–46 and Langbein, *Prosecuting Crime in the Renaissance*, pp. 163–66.

61 Volk and Warlo, 'The role of medical experts in court proceedings in the medieval town', pp. 104–6, 109–11.

62 Langbein, *Prosecuting Crime in the Renaissance*, pp. 198–202; C. Crawford, 'Legalizing medicine: early modern legal systems and the growth of medico-legal knowledge', in M. Clark and C. Crawford (eds), *Legal Medicine in History*, Cambridge: Cambridge University Press, 1994, p. 104.

63 R.P. Brittain, 'Origins of legal medicine: Constitutio Criminalis Carolina', *Medico-Legal Journal*, 1965, vol. 33, p. 126.

64 For the gradual process by which the duties of the medieval coroner were established and distinguished from those of other officials, see R.F. Hunnisett, 'The origins of the office of coroner', *Transactions of the Royal Historical Society*, 5th series, 1958, vol. 8, 85–104.

65 T.R. Forbes, 'Crowner's quest', *Transactions of the American Philosophical Society*, 1978, vol. 68, pp. 5–8; A.K. Mant, 'Milestones in the development of the British medicolegal system', *Medicine, Science and the Law*, 1977, vol. 17, pp. 155–58.

66 See for example R.F. Hunnisett (ed.), *Calendar of Nottinghamshire Coroners' Inquests 1485–1558*, Nottingham: Thoroton Society, 1969; T.R. Forbes, 'London coroner's inquests for 1590', *Journal of the History of Medicine and Allied Sciences*, 1973, vol. 28, 376–86.

67 See Chapter 1 n.2 and also J.D.J. Havard, *The Detection of Secret Homicide: A Study of the Medico-legal System of Investigation of Sudden and Unexplained Deaths*, London: Macmillan, 1960, pp. 1–36; M. MacDonald and T.R. Murphy, *Sleepless Souls: Suicide in Early Modern England*, Oxford: Clarendon Press, 1990, pp. 225–26; R.F. Hunnisett (ed.), *East Sussex Coroners' Records 1688–1838*, Lewes: Sussex Record Society, 2005; P.J. Fisher, 'The politics of sudden death: the office and role of the coroner in England and Wales, 1726–1888', PhD thesis, University of Leicester, 2007, pp. 184–92.

68 K. Watson, *Poisoned Lives: English Poisoners and their Victims*, London: Hambledon and London, 2004, p. 155; Havard, *The Detection of Secret Homicide*, p. 36.

69 Watson, *Poisoned Lives*, pp. 156–60; Havard, *The Detection of Secret Homicide*, pp. 37–66; R.F. Hunnisett (ed.), *Wiltshire Coroners' Bills 1752–1796*, Devizes: Wiltshire Record Society, 1981, pp. xlviii–l. Hunnisett thought that the Wiltshire coroners might be unique, but in 1796 the Flintshire coroner Robert Davies was a surgeon (National Library of Wales, Crime and Punishment Database, http://www.llgc.org.uk/sesiwn_fawr/index_s.htm, accessed on 1 June 2010) and it seems likely that there were others.

70 For the generally good reputation enjoyed by early modern European midwives, see D. Harley, 'Historians as demonologists: the myth of the midwife-witch', *Social History of Medicine*, 1990, vol. 3, 1–26.

71 M.H. Green, 'Gendering the history of women's healthcare', *Gender & History*, 2008, vol. 20, 488–96; M.H. Green, *Making Women's Medicine Masculine: The Rise of Male Authority in Pre-Modern Gynaecology*, Oxford: Oxford University Press, 2008, pp. viii–xiv.

72　Pastore, *Il medico in tribunale*, pp. 140–44; McClive, 'Blood and expertise', pp. 92–93; Lisa Forman Cody, *Birthing the Nation: Sex, Science, and the Conception of Eighteenth-Century Britons*, Oxford: Oxford University Press, 2005, pp. 271–75.

73　Green, 'Gendering the history of women's healthcare', pp. 492, 498.

74　E.H. Ackerknecht, 'Midwives as experts in court', *Bulletin of the New York Academy of Medicine*, 1976, vol. 52, 1224–28; T.G. Benedek, 'The changing relationship between midwives and physicians during the Renaissance', *Bulletin of the History of Medicine*, 1977, vol. 51, 550–64; H. Marland (ed.), *The Art of Midwifery: Early Modern Midwives in Europe*, London and New York: Routledge, 1993.

75　Amundsen and Ferngren, 'The forensic role of physicians in Roman law', p. 47; Benedek, 'The changing relationship between midwives and physicians during the Renaissance', p. 552; J.C. Oldham, 'On pleading the belly: a history of the jury of matrons', *Criminal Justice History*, 1985, vol. 6, p. 2.

76　Ackerknecht, 'Midwives as experts in court', p. 1225.

77　Ibid., pp. 1225–26; Oldham, 'On pleading the belly', pp. 19–21; Pastore, *Il medico in tribunale*, pp. 129–48.

78　Ackerknecht, 'Midwives as experts in court', pp. 1226–28; Marland (ed.), *The Art of Midwifery*, see under 'court appearances and investigations'.

79　J.C. Oldham, 'The origins of the special jury', *University of Chicago Law Review*, 1983, vol. 50, 137–221.

80　Oldham, 'On pleading the belly', pp. 30–31.

3 Experts and expertise

1　K.D. Watson, 'Medical and chemical expertise in English trials for criminal poisoning, 1750–1914', *Medical History*, 2006, vol. 50, p. 375. I wish to thank the editors for permission to quote extensively from this article.

2　I. Burney, *Poison, Detection, and the Victorian Imagination*, Manchester and New York: Manchester University Press, 2006, p. 6.

3　T. Ward, 'English law's epistemology of expert testimony', *Journal of Law and Society*, 2006, vol. 33, p. 572. This is the current common law test of admissibility of expert evidence valid in England, the United States and other common law jurisdictions such as Canada and Australia, but it closely mirrors the French understanding of what an expert witness does; see C. Restier-Melleray, 'Experts et expertise scientifique: le cas de la France', *Revue française de science politique*, 1990, vol. 40, pp. 549–53.

4　E.H. Ash, *Power, Knowledge and Expertise in Elizabethan England*, Baltimore, MD and London: Johns Hopkins University Press, 2004, pp. 213–16; C. Rabier, 'Introduction: expertise in historical perspectives', in C. Rabier (ed.), *Fields of Expertise: A Comparative History of Expert Procedures in Paris and London, 1600 to Present*, Newcastle: Cambridge Scholars Publishing, 2007, pp. 1–2.

5　Ash, *Power, Knowledge and Expertise in Elizabethan England*, p. 10.

6　Rabier, 'Introduction', pp. 2–15.

7　T. Robisheaux, 'Witchcraft and forensic medicine in seventeenth-century Germany', in S. Clark (ed.), *Languages of Witchcraft: Narrative, Ideology and Meaning in Early Modern Culture*, Basingstoke: Macmillan, 2001, 197–215; S. De Renzi, 'Witnesses of the body: medico-legal cases in seventeenth-century Rome', *Studies in History and Philosophy of Science*, 2002, vol. 33, 219–42.

8　Y. Mausen, 'Ex scientia et arte sua testificatur: A propos de la spécificité du statut de l'expert dans la procédure judiciaire médiévale', *Rechtsgeschichte*, 2007, vol. 10, 127–35; O. Cavallar, 'Agli albori della medicina legale: I trattati "De percussionibus" e "De vulneribus"', *Ius Commune: Zeitschrift für Europäische*

Rechtsgeschichte, 1999, vol. 26, 27–89; O. Cavallar, 'La "benefundata sapientia" dei periti: Feritori, feriti e medici nei commentari e consulti di Baldo degli Ubaldi', *Ius Commune: Zeitschrift für Europäische Rechtsgeschichte*, 2000, vol. 27, 215–81.

9 J. Shatzmiller, *Médecine et Justice en Provence Médiévale: Documents de Manosque, 1262–1348*, Aix-en-Provence: Université de Provence, 1989; A. Pastore, *Il medico in tribunale: La perizia medica nella procedura penale di antico regime (secoli XVI–XVIII)*, Bellinzona: Casagrande, 1998; S. De Renzi, 'Medical expertise, bodies, and the law in early modern courts', *Isis*, 2007, vol. 98, p. 318 (quote).

10 Mausen, 'Ex scientia et arte sua testificatur', p. 135.

11 De Renzi, 'Witnesses of the body', pp. 222–27.

12 M. Redmayne, *Expert Evidence and Criminal Justice*, Oxford: Oxford University Press, 2001, p. 124; D.J. Gee and J.K. Mason, *The Courts and the Doctor*, Oxford: Oxford University Press, 1990, p. 26.

13 C. Hamlin, 'Scientific method and expert witnessing: Victorian perspectives on a modern problem', *Social Studies of Science*, 1986, vol. 16, 485–513; T. Golan, 'The history of scientific expert testimony in the English courtroom', *Science in Context*, 1999, vol. 12, 7–32; T. Golan, *Laws of Men and Laws of Nature: The History of Scientific Expert Testimony in England and America*, Cambridge, MA and London: Harvard University Press, 2004; M. Essig, 'Poison murder and expert testimony: doubting the physician in late nineteenth-century America', *Yale Journal of Law and the Humanities*, 2002, vol. 14, 177–210.

14 I.R. Freckelton, *The Trial of the Expert: A Study of Expert Evidence and Forensic Experts*, Melbourne and Oxford: Oxford University Press, 1987; C.A.G. Jones, *Expert Witnesses: Science, Medicine, and the Practice of Law*, Oxford: Clarendon Press, 1994; Redmayne, *Expert Evidence and Criminal Justice*.

15 Ward, 'English law's epistemology of expert testimony'; J.H. Langbein, *The Origins of Adversary Criminal Trial*, Oxford: Oxford University Press, 2003; S. Landsman, 'Of witches, madmen, and products liability: a historical survey of the use of expert testimony', *Behavioral Sciences and the Law*, 1995, vol. 13, 131–57; S. Landsman, 'One hundred years of rectitude: medical witnesses at the Old Bailey, 1717–1817', *Law and History Review*, 1998, vol. 16, 445–94.

16 I.A. Burney, *Bodies of Evidence: Medicine and the Politics of the English Inquest, 1830–1926*, Baltimore, MD and London: Johns Hopkins University Press, 2000; J.C. Mohr, *Doctors and the Law: Medical Jurisprudence in Nineteenth-Century America*, Baltimore, MD and London: Johns Hopkins University Press, 1993; T.R. Forbes, *Surgeons at the Bailey: English Forensic Medicine to 1878*, New Haven, CT and London: Yale University Press, 1985; R. Smith and B. Wynne (eds), *Expert Evidence: Interpreting Science in the Law*, London: Routledge, 1989; C.J. Crawford, 'The emergence of English forensic medicine: medical evidence in common-law courts, 1730–1830', DPhil thesis, Oxford University, 1987; M. Clark and C. Crawford (eds), *Legal Medicine in History*, Cambridge: Cambridge University Press, 1994.

17 See for example Restier-Melleray, 'Experts et expertise scientifique'; F. Chauvaud, *Les experts du crime: la médecine légale en France au XIXe siècle*, Paris: Aubier, 2000; F. Chauvaud and L. Dumoulin, *Experts et expertise judiciaire: France, XIXe et XXe siècles*, Rennes: Presses Universitaires de Rennes, 2003; Rabier (ed.), *Fields of Expertise*.

18 E.J. Engstrom, V. Hess and U. Thoms (eds), *Figurationen des Experten: Ambivalenzen der Wissenschaftlichen Expertise im ausgehenden 18. und fruhen 19. Jahrhundert*, Frankfurt: Peter Lang, 2005.

19 This paragraph and the one following are taken from Watson, 'Medical and chemical expertise in English trials for criminal poisoning, 1750–1914', pp. 376–78.

20 Landsman, 'One hundred years of rectitude', pp. 446–47; Golan, *Laws of Men and Laws of Nature*, pp. 18–22; D.M. Dwyer, 'Expert evidence in the English civil courts, 1550–1800', *Journal of Legal History*, 2007, vol. 28, 93–118.

21   Langbein, *The Origins of Adversary Criminal Trial*, pp. 67–105.
22   Ibid., pp. 8–9; Redmayne, *Expert Evidence and Criminal Justice*, pp. 198–220; Gee and Mason, *The Courts and the Doctor*, pp. 143–46.
23   Golan, *Laws of Men and Laws of Nature*, pp. 22–51, especially pp. 44–45.
24   Ibid., pp. 52–54; Sir G. Gilbert, *The Law of Evidence, considerably enlarged by Capel Lofft*, 4 vols, London: A. Strahan and W. Woodfall, 1791, Vol. 1, pp. 298–302.
25   Golan, 'The history of scientific expert testimony in the English courtroom', pp. 14–15, 26; Jones, *Expert Witnesses*, pp. 57–60; Landsman, 'Of witches, madmen, and products liability', pp. 144–50.
26   See for example J.Z. Fullmer, 'Technology, chemistry, and the law in early 19th-century England', *Technology and Culture*, 1980, vol. 21, 1–28; M.A. Crowther and B.M. White, 'Medicine, property and the law in Britain 1800–1914', *Historical Journal*, 1988, vol. 31, 853–70; Mohr, *Doctors and the Law*, pp. 94–108, 207–8, 254; K.D. Watson, 'The chemist as expert: the consulting career of Sir William Ramsay', *Ambix*, 1995, vol. 42, 143–59; Golan, *Laws of Men and Laws of Nature*, pp. 54–106.
27   Dwyer, 'Expert evidence in the English civil courts, 1550–1800', pp. 111–12.
28   Gilbert, *Law of Evidence*, Vol. 1, p. 301.
29   Dwyer, 'Expert evidence in the English civil courts, 1550–1800', p. 96.
30   Chauvaud, *Les experts du crime*, pp. 9–16 (quote on p. 10). The definition is taken from the Larousse dictionary of 1870: 'the activities undertaken by people who have special knowledge of an art, science or trade, with a view to resolving a question put to them by the judge. Experts are those charged with carrying out this activity, and the act of stating it is called the report'.
31   Rabier, 'Introduction', p. 2.
32   R. Porter, *The Greatest Benefit to Mankind: A Medical History of Humanity from Antiquity to the Present*, London: Harper Collins, 1997, p. 287.
33   L. Brockliss and C. Jones, *The Medical World of Early Modern France*, Oxford: Oxford University Press, 1997, p. 9.
34   Ibid., pp. 818–34.
35   Chauvaud, *Les experts du crime*, p. 244n3: the chairs were created by a law of 14 frimaire an III, 4 December 1794.
36   For more on the importance of the Morgue see C. Desmaze, *Histoire de la médecine légale en France*, Paris: G. Charpentier, 1880, pp. 287–90, and V.R. Schwartz, *Spectacular Realities: Early Mass Culture in Fin-de-Siècle Paris*, Berkeley, CA and London: University of California Press, 1998, Ch. 2.
37   S.E. Chaillé, 'Origins and progress of medical jurisprudence, 1776–1876' (1876), *Journal of Criminal Law and Criminology*, 1949, vol. 40, p. 399; A. Lacassagne, *Précis de médecine judiciaire* (1886), Chestnut Hill, MA: Elibron Classics, 2006, pp. 18, 30–32 (19 ventôse an XI).
38   Benjamin F. Martin, *Crime and Criminal Justice Under the Third Republic: The Shame of Marianne*, Baton Rouge, LA and London: Louisiana State University Press, 1990, pp. 42–48.
39   Ibid., p. 79; Simon A. Cole, *Suspect Identities: A History of Fingerprinting and Criminal Identification*, Cambridge, MA and London: Harvard University Press, 2001, pp. 32–59.
40   Chauvaud, *Les experts du crime*, pp. 47–48.
41   R. Harris, *Murders and Madness: Medicine, Law, and Society in the Fin de Siècle*, Oxford: Clarendon Press, 1989, pp. 138–46; Chauvaud, *Les experts du crime*, pp. 53–70. Autopsy fees in Paris compared favourably with those in England circa 1913, when 25F was worth approximately one guinea.
42   Chauvaud, *Les experts du crime*, pp. 43–46; Chauvaud and Dumoulin, *Experts et expertise judiciaire*, pp. 101–14.

43 E. Baccino, A. Dorandeu, E. Margueritte, P. Fornes and A. Soussy, 'Medicolegal activity in France: who really are the médecins légistes', *Journal of Clinical Forensic Medicine*, 1999, vol. 6, 208.

44 Redmayne, *Expert Evidence and Criminal Justice*, pp. 206–11.

45 Porter, *The Greatest Benefit to Mankind*, pp. 287–88.

46 Chaillé, 'Origins and progress of medical jurisprudence, 1776–1876', p. 399; J. Nemec, *Highlights in Medicolegal Relations*, Bethesda: National Library of Medicine, 1968, p. 21, online at http://www.nlm.nih.gov/hmd/pdf/highlights.pdf (accessed on 25 May 2010); E.H. Ackerknecht, 'Early history of legal medicine', in C.R. Burns (ed.), *Legacies in Law and Medicine*, New York: Science History Publications, 1977, p. 259.

47 Ackerknecht, 'Early history of legal medicine', p. 258.

48 Ibid., p. 259.

49 W. Keil, A. Berzlanovich and B. Madea, 'Textbooks on legal medicine in the German-speaking countries', *Forensic Science International*, 2004, vol. 144, pp. 289–94.

50 W. Krauland, 'The history of the German Society of Forensic Medicine', *Forensic Science International*, 2004, vol. 144, p. 101. For details of nineteenth-century German periodical literature on forensic medicine, see H-J. Wagner, 'On the prehistory of the German Society of Legal Medicine', *Forensic Science International*, 2004, vol. 144, pp. 90–93.

51 R. Virchow, *Post-Mortem Examinations: With Especial Reference to Medico-Legal Practice*, trans. T.P. Smith, 3rd American edn, Philadelphia: P. Blakiston, 1896, pp. 11, 139–43. Virchow clearly distinguished those who performed medico-legal autopsies from routine anatomization: 'the expert may allow himself to make alterations [to the plan of examination]' (p. 15); 'In puzzling cases (which, I admit, do occur to the expert, and even to the anatomist) … ' (p. 25).

52 Krauland, 'The history of the German Society of Forensic Medicine', pp. 99–100; F. Fischer, M. Graw and W. Eisenmenger, 'Legal medicine in the Federal Republic of Germany and after reunification', *Forensic Science International*, 2004, vol. 144, 137–41. Most institute medical staff are accredited *Gerichtsärzte*.

53 T.N. Burg, 'Forensic medicine in the nineteenth-century Habsburg monarchy', Center for Austrian Studies, University of Minnesota, June 1996, online at http://cas.umn.edu/assets/pdf/wp962.pdf (accessed on 25 May 2010).

54 Ibid.

55 G. Bauer, 'Austrian forensic medicine', *Forensic Science International*, 2004, vol. 144, 143–49.

56 Ibid.

57 Porter, *The Greatest Benefit to Mankind*, pp. 289–90.

58 Ibid., pp. 290–93; A. Digby, *Making a Medical Living: Doctors and Patients in the English Market for Medicine, 1720–1911*, Cambridge: Cambridge University Press, 1994, pp. 233–40.

59 On the origins and socio-medical importance of the Anatomy Act, see R. Richardson, *Death, Dissection and the Destitute*, 2nd edn with a new afterword, London: Phoenix Press, 2001.

60 C. Crawford, 'A scientific profession: medical reform and forensic medicine in British periodicals of the early nineteenth century', in R. French and A. Wear (eds), *British Medicine in an Age of Reform*, London and New York: Routledge, 1991, 203–30.

61 M.A. Crowther and B. White, *On Soul and Conscience. The Medical Expert and Crime: 150 Years of Forensic Medicine in Glasgow*, Aberdeen: Aberdeen University Press, 1988, p. 7.

62 N.G. Coley, 'Alfred Swaine Taylor, MD, FRS (1806–80): forensic toxicologist', *Medical History*, 1991, vol. 35, 409–27; Watson, 'Medical and chemical expertise in English trials for criminal poisoning, 1750–1914'.

63 Chaillé, 'Origins and progress of medical jurisprudence, 1776–1876', p. 400.
64 R.D. Summers, 'History of the police surgeon', *The Practitioner*, 1978, vol. 221, 383–87; Gee and Mason, *The Courts and the Doctor*, p. 26.
65 In 1924 the fee for attending an inquest and performing an autopsy was two guineas, and the same fee was payable to the county analyst for attending and carrying out a toxicological analysis: see Oxfordshire Record Office, COR VII/10. In 1989 the fee for carrying out a post-mortem examination for an inquest was £46.50; by 2006 the fee had risen to £87.70 and the first ever audit of autopsies in England, Wales and Northern Ireland found that a quarter were of a poor or unacceptable standard: see Gee and Mason, *The Courts and the Doctor*, p. 204 and BBC News 19 Oct 2006, 'Autopsy quality concerns raised', http://news.bbc.co. uk/1/hi/health/6061552.stm (accessed on 25 May 2010).
66 Burney, *Bodies of Evidence*.
67 N. Ambage and M. Clark, 'Unbuilt Bloomsbury: medico-legal institutes and forensic science laboratories in England between the wars', in Clark and Crawford (eds), *Legal Medicine in History*, 293–313.
68 A.K. Mant (ed.), *Taylor's Principles and Practice of Medical Jurisprudence*, 13th edn, London: Churchill Livingstone, 1984, pp. 5–10.
69 See note 65 and BBC News 18 Aug 2009, 'Major hospital halts post-mortems', http://news.bbc.co.uk/1/hi/wales/wales_politics/8206981.stm (accessed on 1 June 2010).
70 M.H. Kaufman, 'Origin and history of the Regius Chair of Medical Jurisprudence and Medical Police established in the University of Edinburgh in 1807', *Journal of Forensic and Legal Medicine*, 2007, vol. 14, 121–30.
71 Crowther and White, *On Soul and Conscience*.
72 Ibid., p. 3.
73 Ambage and Clark, 'Unbuilt Bloomsbury'.
74 E.A. Cawthon, *Medicine on Trial: A Sourcebook with Cases, Law, and Documents*, Indianapolis, IN: Hackett Publishing, 2004, p. 59.
75 J. Johnson, 'Coroners, corruption and the politics of death: forensic pathology in the United States', in Clark and Crawford (eds), *Legal Medicine in History*, pp. 269–70.
76 Chaillé, 'Origins and progress of medical jurisprudence, 1776–1876', pp. 410–11; Cyril H. Wecht, 'The history of legal medicine', *Journal of the American Academy of Psychiatry and the Law*, 2005, vol. 33, pp. 247–48.
77 J.A. Tighe, 'The New York Medico-Legal Society: legitimating the union of law and psychiatry (1867–1918)', *International Journal of Law and Psychiatry*, 1986, vol. 9, 231–43.
78 Essig, 'Poison murder and expert testimony', pp. 192–208; J.C. Mohr, 'The trial of John Hendrickson, Jr: medical jurisprudence at mid-century', *New York History*, 1989, vol. 70, pp. 23–26.
79 Mohr, *Doctors and the Law*, pp. 237–49.
80 Cawthon, *Medicine on Trial*, pp. 23–38.
81 Wecht, 'The history of legal medicine', pp. 249–50.
82 J. Johnson-McGrath, 'Speaking for the dead: forensic pathologists and criminal justice in the United States', *Science, Technology & Human Values*, 1995, vol. 20, p. 455; Johnson, 'Coroners, corruption and the politics of death', pp. 281–82.
83 Cawthon, *Medicine on Trial*, pp. 17–38.
84 Landsman, 'Of witches, madmen, and products liability', pp. 155–57; Ward, 'English law's epistemology of expert testimony'.
85 K.D. Watson and P. Wexler, 'History of toxicology', in P. Wexler (ed.), *Information Resources in Toxicology*, 4th edn, San Diego, CA and Oxford: Academic Press, 2009, pp. 13, 15.

86 J. Thorwald, *Proof of Poison*, trans. R. and C. Winston, London: Thames and Hudson, 1966, pp. 19, 21. For examples of seventeenth-century French practice, see Desmaze, *Histoire de la médecine légale en France*, pp. 76–97.
87 Desmaze, *Histoire de la médecine légale en France*, p. 21.
88 W. Roughead (ed.), *Trial of Mary Blandy* (1914), Charleston, SC: BiblioBazaar, 2006, pp. 98–107.
89 Gee and Mason, *The Courts and the Doctor*, p. 23.
90 R.F. Bud and G.K. Roberts, *Science Versus Practice: Chemistry in Victorian Britain*, Manchester: Manchester University Press, 1984, pp. 47–69; F.L. Holmes, *Eighteenth-Century Chemistry as an Investigative Enterprise*, Berkeley, CA: Office for History of Science and Technology, University of California, 1989, pp. 85–102.
91 Watson, 'Medical and chemical expertise in English trials for criminal poisoning, 1750–1914', pp. 381–82.
92 M.J.B. Orfila, *Traité des poisons tirés des règnes minéral, végétal et animal, ou toxicologie générale, considérée sous les rapports de la physiologie, de la pathologie et de la médecine légale*, 2 vols, Paris: Crochard, 1814–15.
93 R. Christison, *A Treatise on Poisons, in Relation to Medical Jurisprudence, Physiology, and the Practice of Physic*, Edinburgh: Adam Black, 1829.
94 Watson and Wexler, 'History of toxicology', p. 16; Mohr, *Doctors and the Law*, pp. 24–28, 69–71.
95 M. Ortolani, 'L'empoisonnement à Nice sous la Restauration: enquête judiciaire et expertise toxicologique', *Legal History Review*, 2008, vol. 76, pp. 117–31; J.R. Bertomeu-Sánchez and A. Nieto-Galan (eds), *Chemistry, Medicine and Crime: Mateu J.B. Orfila (1787–1853) and His Times*, Sagamore Beach, MA: Science History Publications, 2006, see especially the chapters by Bertomeu-Sánchez, Burney, Crowther, Tomic and Watson.
96 Lacassagne, *Précis de médecine judiciaire*, pp. 387–92; M.I. Septon, 'Les femmes et le poison: l'empoisonnement devant les jurisdictions criminelles en Belgique au XIXe siècle, 1795–1914', PhD thesis, Marquette University, 1996, Ch. 2 part 2, p. 248; K. Watson, *Poisoned Lives: English Poisoners and their Victims*, London: Hambledon and London, 2004, pp. 42–45.
97 On nineteenth-century medical education in cross-national comparison, see T.N. Bonner, *Becoming a Physician: Medical Education in Britain, France, Germany, and the United States, 1750–1945* (1995), Baltimore, MD and London: Johns Hopkins University Press, 2000; Watson, 'Medical and chemical expertise in English trials for criminal poisoning, 1750–1914', pp. 383–88.
98 Essig, 'Poison murder and expert testimony', pp. 181–82.
99 Ibid., p. 182.
100 These included the trials of Dr Couty de la Pommerais (digitalis, France, 1864); Dr George Henry Lamson (aconitine, England, 1882); Carlyle Harris (morphine, New York, 1892); Dr Hawley Harvey Crippen (hyoscine, England, 1910). The tendency for doctors to choose these drugs is unmistakeable (Harris was a medical student).
101 Home Office Analysts 1872–1954:

Name	Junior	Senior	Hospital	Death
Sir Thomas Stevenson	1872–81	1881–1908	Guy's	1908
Dr Charles M. Tidy	1882–92		The London	1892
Dr Arthur P. Luff	1892–1908		St Mary's	1938
Mr John Webster	1900–15	1915–27	St Mary's	1927
Sir William H. Willcox	1904–08	1908–19	St Mary's	1941
Dr Gerald Roche Lynch	1920–27	1927–54	St Mary's	1957

4 Criminal responsibility and the insanity defence

1 D.N. Robinson, *Wild Beasts and Idle Humours: The Insanity Defense from Anti-quity to the Present*, Cambridge, MA and London: Harvard University Press, 1996, pp. 29–31.
2 *The Digest of Justinian*, Vol.1, trans. C.H. Monro, Cambridge: Cambridge University Press, 1904, pp. 59–60.
3 V. Barras and J. Bernheim, 'The history of law and psychiatry in Europe', in R. Bluglass and P. Bowden (eds), *Principles and Practice of Forensic Psychiatry*, Edinburgh: Churchill Livingstone, 1990, pp. 103–4.
4 Robinson, *Wild Beasts and Idle Humours*, p. 32.
5 Ibid., pp. 33–44.
6 S.P. Scott (trans.), *The Visigothic Code: Forum Judicum*, Boston: Boston Book Company, 1910, p. xxxiv; online, http://libro.uca.edu/vcode/visigoths.htm (accessed 28 June 2009).
7 Robinson, *Wild Beasts and Idle Humours*, pp. 53–71.
8 H.C. Erik Midelfort, *A History of Madness in Sixteenth-Century Germany*, Stanford, CA: Stanford University Press, 1999, pp. 189–91.
9 Barras and Bernheim, 'The history of law and psychiatry in Europe', p. 104; D. Forshaw and H. Rollin, 'The history of forensic psychiatry in England', in Bluglass and Bowden (eds), *Principles and Practice of Forensic Psychiatry*, p. 79.
10 Robinson, *Wild Beasts and Idle Humours*, p. 71; G. Magherini and V. Biotti, 'Madness in Florence in the 14th–18th centuries: judicial inquiry and medical diagnosis, care, and custody', *International Journal of Law and Psychiatry*, 1998, vol. 21, 355–68; G. Ruggiero, 'Excusable murder: insanity and reason in early Renaissance Venice', *Journal of Social History*, 1982, vol. 16, 109–19 points out that the Venetians assessed criminal responsibility, including that of the insane, in terms of reason: the less reason involved in a crime, the less serious the crime was considered (p. 115).
11 N.D. Hurnard, *The King's Pardon for Homicide before AD 1307*, Oxford: Clarendon Press, 1969, pp. 159–70.
12 A. Esmein, *A History of Continental Criminal Procedure with special reference to France*, trans. J. Simpson (1913), Union, NJ: Lawbook Exchange, 2000, p. 155.
13 J. Shatzmiller, *Médecine et Justice en Provence Médiévale: Documents de Manosque, 1262–1348*, Aix-en-Provence: Université de Provence, 1989, pp. 29, 119.
14 Midelfort, *A History of Madness in Sixteenth-Century Germany*, p. 191.
15 Ibid., pp. 193–94.
16 Ibid., p. 196.
17 For details of Weyer's biography and other writings see G. Mora (ed.), *Witches, Devils, and Doctors in the Renaissance: Johann Weyer, De praestigiis daemonum*, Binghamton, NY: Center for Medieval and Early Renaissance Studies, State University of New York at Binghamton, 1991, pp. xxvii–xlv.
18 Midelfort, *A History of Madness in Sixteenth-Century Germany*, pp. 198–201.
19 The Latin term for witch is *lamia*; the plural is *lamiae*.
20 Mora, *Witches, Devils, and Doctors in the Renaissance*, p. 567 (Ch. 27 in Weyer's book).
21 For a discussion of the medieval and early modern intellectual foundations of the European witch-hunt, see B.P. Levack, *The Witch-hunt in Early Modern Europe*, 3rd edn, Harlow: Pearson Education Limited, 2006, pp. 30–73.
22 Mora, *Witches, Devils, and Doctors in the Renaissance*, p. lxii.
23 Ibid., pp. lxv–lxix.
24 Midelfort, *A History of Madness in Sixteenth-Century Germany*, pp. 204–6.
25 Ibid., pp. 213–27; Mora, *Witches, Devils, and Doctors in the Renaissance*, pp. lxix–lxxi.
26 Midelfort, *A History of Madness in Sixteenth-Century Germany*, pp. 217–23.

27   Barras and Bernheim, 'The history of law and psychiatry in Europe', p. 105.
28   Ibid., pp. 105–6.
29   Midelfort, *A History of Madness in Sixteenth-Century Germany*, p. 219.
30   H. Steinberg, A. Schmidt-Recla and S. Schmideler, 'Forensic psychiatry in nineteenth-century Saxony: the case of Woyzeck', *Harvard Review of Psychiatry*, 2007, vol. 15, p. 175.
31   Midelfort, *A History of Madness in Sixteenth-Century Germany*, pp. 223–26.
32   N. Walker, *Crime and Insanity in England, Vol. 1: The Historical Perspective*, Edinburgh: Edinburgh University Press, 1968, pp. 27–29
33   O. Williams, 'Exorcising madness in late Elizabethan England: *The Seduction of Arthington* and the criminal culpability of demoniacs', *Journal of British Studies*, 2008, vol. 47, 30–52.
34   Robinson, *Wild Beasts and Idle Humours*, pp. 115–16.
35   Ibid., pp. 116–17.
36   G. Geis and I. Bunn, *A Trial of Witches: A Seventeenth-century Witchcraft Prosecution*, London: Routledge, 1997, pp. 148–55.
37   Forshaw and Rollin, 'The history of forensic psychiatry in England', p. 82.
38   Sir M. Hale, *The History of the Pleas of the Crown*, Vol. 1, 1st American edn, Philadelphia: Robert H. Small, 1847, pp. 31–32.
39   M.J. Wiener, *Men of Blood: Violence, Manliness, and Criminal Justice in Victorian England*, Cambridge: Cambridge University Press, 2004, pp. 255–79.
40   Walker, *Crime and Insanity in England, Vol. 1*, pp. 36–41; Hale, *The History of the Pleas of the Crown*, Vol. 1, pp. 29–36.
41   C. Beccaria, *On Crimes and Punishments* (1764), trans. D. Young, Indianapolis, IN: Hackett Publishing, 1986, pp. xi–xv.
42   J.A. Sharpe, *Judicial Punishment in England*, London: Faber and Faber, 1990.
43   Barras and Bernheim, 'The history of law and psychiatry in Europe', pp. 106–7.
44   J.P. Eigen, *Witnessing Insanity: Madness and Mad-doctors in the English Court*, New Haven, CT and London: Yale University Press, 1995, pp. 18–30, 182–89.
45   D. Rabin, *Identity, Crime and Legal Responsibility in Eighteenth-Century England* Basingstoke: Palgrave Macmillan, 2004.
46   D. Kaufmann, 'Boundary disputes: criminal justice and psychiatry in Germany, 1760–1850', *Journal of Historical Sociology*, 1993, vol. 6, 276–87.
47   Barras and Bernheim, 'The history of law and psychiatry in Europe', p. 106.
48   R. Porter, *The Greatest Benefit to Mankind: A Medical History of Humanity from Antiquity to the Present*, London: Harper Collins, 1997, p. 494; see Ch. 16 for the history of psychiatry.
49   Ibid., p. 495; Barras and Bernheim, 'The history of law and psychiatry in Europe', p. 107.
50   J.M. Quen, 'The history of law and psychiatry in America', in Bluglass and Bowden (eds), *Principles and Practice of Forensic Psychiatry*, p. 111; J. Colaizzi, *Homicidal Insanity, 1800–1985*, Tuscaloosa, AL and London: University of Alabama Press, 1989, pp. 8, 24–25; N. Rafter, 'The unrepentant horse-slasher: moral insanity and the origins of criminological thought', *Criminology*, 2004, vol. 42, 979–1008.
51   Steinberg et al, 'Forensic psychiatry in nineteenth-century Saxony', pp. 174–75.
52   J. Goldstein, *Console and Classify: The French Psychiatric Profession in the Nineteenth Century*, Cambridge: Cambridge University Press, 1987, rev. ed. 2001, pp. 173–78; J-E. Esquirol, 'Note sur la monomanie-homicide', in J-C. Hoffbauer, *Médecine légale relative aux aliénés et aux sourds-muets*, trans. A-M. Chambeyron, Paris: J-B. Baillière, 1827, pp. 309–59.
53   Forshaw and Rollin, 'The history of forensic psychiatry in England', p. 83.
54   L. Guignard, 'Aliénation mentale, irresponsabilité pénale et dangerosité sociale face à la justice du XIXe siècle: étude d'un cas de fureur', *Crime, History & Societies*, 2006, vol. 10, 83–100.

55   C. Desmaze, *Histoire de la médecine légale en France*, Paris: G. Charpentier, 1880, pp. 141–45.
56   Steinberg et al, 'Forensic psychiatry in nineteenth-century Saxony', pp. 173, 177.
57   Colaizzi, *Homicidal Insanity*, pp. 20–29; M. Foucault, 'About the concept of the dangerous individual in nineteenth-century legal psychiatry', *International Journal of Law and Psychiatry*, 1987, vol. 1, pp. 3–11.
58   Foucault, 'About the concept of the dangerous individual in nineteenth-century legal psychiatry', pp. 3–6; J. Goldstein, 'Professional knowledge and professional self-interest: the rise and fall of monomania in 19th-century France', *International Journal of Law and Psychiatry*, 1998, vol. 21, pp. 389–91.
59   Barras and Bernheim, 'The history of law and psychiatry in Europe', p. 108.
60   Ibid.; see also Desmaze, *Histoire de la médecine légale en France*, pp. 146–55.
61   Goldstein, *Console and Classify*, pp. 276–92.
62   Desmaze, *Histoire de la médecine légale en France*, pp. 167–77.
63   Colaizzi, *Homicidal Insanity*, pp. 27–30; J.C. Mohr, *Doctors and the Law: Medical Jurisprudence in Nineteenth-Century America*, Baltimore, MD and London: Johns Hopkins University Press, 1993, pp. 144–46.
64   Porter, *Greatest Benefit to Mankind*, pp. 499–500; N. Rafter, 'The murderous Dutch fiddler: criminology, history and the problem of phrenology', *Theoretical Criminology*, 2005, vol. 9, pp. 70–72.
65   Colaizzi, *Homicidal Insanity*, pp. 30–39; Rafter, 'The murderous Dutch fiddler', pp. 75–81.
66   Tragically, Parkman achieved lasting fame not as a psychiatrist but as the murder victim of Harvard professor John Webster in 1849, a case which was itself of forensic significance: see *The Trial of Professor John White Webster*, with an introduction by G. Dilnot, London: Geoffrey Bles, 1928.
67   P. Prior, *Madness and Murder: Gender, Crime and Mental Disorder in Nineteenth-Century Ireland*, Dublin: Irish Academic Press, 2008, pp. 24–33.
68   R. Partridge, *Broadmoor: A History of Criminal Lunacy and its Problems*, London: Chato and Windus, 1953.
69   Mohr, *Doctors and the Law*, pp. 148–53; Quen, 'The history of law and psychiatry in America', p. 114.
70   Steinberg et al, 'Forensic psychiatry in nineteenth-century Saxony', p. 173; Kaufmann, 'Boundary disputes'.
71   R. Smith, *Trial by Medicine: Insanity and Responsibility in Victorian Trials*, Edinburgh: Edinburgh University Press, 1981, pp. 103–23.
72   M.J. Wiener, *Reconstructing the Criminal: Culture, Law, and Policy in England, 1830–1914*, Cambridge: Cambridge University Press, 1990, pp. 269–79.
73   Goldstein, *Console and Classify*, pp. 189–96.
74   R. von Krafft-Ebing, *Psychopathia Sexualis, with especial reference to the Antipathetic Sexual Instinct: A Medico-Forensic Study*, 12th edn, Stuttgart: Ferdinand Enke, 1903, trans. F.S. Klaf, London: Staples Press, 1965 (238 case studies). The first edition (1886) included 45 case studies.
75   Barras and Bernheim, 'The history of law and psychiatry in Europe', p. 109.
76   Ibid., pp. 108–9; G. Wright, *Between the Guillotine and Liberty: Two Centuries of the Crime Problem in France*, Oxford: Oxford University Press, 1983, pp. 117–20; P. Guarnieri, 'Alienists on trial: conflict and convergence between psychiatry and law (1876–1913)', *History of Science*, 1991, vol. 29, pp. 400–402; C. Lombroso, *Criminal Man*, translated with a new introduction by M. Gibson and N.H. Rafter, Durham, NC and London: Duke University Press, 2006, pp. 7–26.
77   Lombroso, *Criminal Man*, pp. 13–15; Foucault, 'About the concept of the dangerous individual in nineteenth-century legal psychiatry', pp. 13–14.
78   Barras and Bernheim, 'The history of law and psychiatry in Europe', p. 109.
79   Lombroso, *Criminal Man*, p. 14.

80 *Museo Criminologico*, 'The establishment of criminal asylums', http://www.museocriminologico.it/manicomi_uk.htm (accessed 1 August 2009).
81 Wright, *Between the Guillotine and Liberty*, pp. 119–22.
82 Ibid., pp. 123–28.
83 R.F. Wetzell, 'The medicalization of criminal law reform in Imperial Germany', in N. Finzsch and R. Jütte (eds), *Institutions of Confinement: Hospitals, Asylums, and Prisons in Western Europe and North America, 1500–1950*, Cambridge: Cambridge University Press, 1996, pp. 275–83; R. Schulte, *The Village in Court: Arson, Infanticide, and Poaching in the Court Records of Upper Bavaria, 1848–1910*, Cambridge: Cambridge University Press, 1994, pp. 58–68.
84 Smith, *Trial by Medicine*; Mohr, *Doctors and the Law*, pp. 164–79.
85 Mohr, *Doctors and the Law*; Goldstein, *Console and Classify*; Smith, *Trial by Medicine*; Guarnieri, 'Alienists on trial'; Eigen, *Witnessing Insanity*; Kaufmann, 'Boundary disputes'.
86 Guarnieri, 'Alienists on trial', p. 404.
87 R. Harris, *Murders and Madness: Medicine, Law, and Society in the Fin de Siècle*, Oxford: Clarendon Press, 1989, pp. 147–54; Wiener, *Men of Blood*, pp. 279–88. T. Ward, 'Law, common sense and the authority of science: expert witnesses and criminal insanity in England, ca. 1840–1940', *Social and Legal Studies*, 1997, vol. 6, pp. 348, 356 points out that the McNaughtan Rules were interpreted more liberally over time, as shown by the proportion of murder defendants found insane: 14.6 per cent in 1861–70, 34.3 per cent in 1900–10 and 59.9 per cent in 1929–38, reflecting the impact of degeneracy theory as well as common-sense understandings of insanity.
88 N. Walker, 'McNaughtan's innings: a century and a half not out', *Journal of Forensic Psychiatry and Psychology*, 1993, vol. 4, 207–13; J. McEwan, *The Verdict of the Court: Passing Judgment in Law and Psychology*, Oxford: Hart Publishing, 2003, pp. 71–83; C.P. Ewing, *Insanity: Murder, Madness, and the Law*, Oxford: Oxford University Press, 2008.
89 M. Renneville, *Crime et folie: deux siècles d'enquêtes médicales et judiciaires*, Paris: Fayard, 2003, Ch. 15.
90 V. Savoja, P.F. Godet and J. Dubuis, 'Compulsory treatments in France', *International Journal of Mental Health*, 2008–9, vol. 37, 17–32.
91 T. Harding, 'A comparative survey of medico-legal systems', in J. Gunn and P.J. Taylor (eds), *Forensic Psychiatry: Clinical, Legal and Ethical Issues*, Oxford: Butterworth-Heinemann, 1993, p. 124.

5 The medicalization of deviance

 1 J. Merrick, 'Patterns and prosecutions of suicide in eighteenth-century Paris', *Historical Reflections*, 1989, vol. 16, 1–53.
 2 W.A. Guy, *Principles of Forensic Medicine*, 2nd edn, London: Henry Renshaw, 1861, p. xviii. Coroners held a total of 21,801 inquests in 1856 and recorded 2,681 deaths by drowning, exclusive of deaths at sea, a fair proportion of which were probably suicides.
 3 M. Williams, *Suicide and Attempted Suicide* (1997), London: Penguin, 2001, pp. 18–44.
 4 L. Rose, *Massacre of the Innocents: Infanticide in Great Britain 1800–1939*, London: Routledge & Kegan Paul, 1986, p. 8 shows that in England 1863–87 the under-ones formed 61 per cent of all homicide victims but constituted only 2.5–3 per cent of the population. A. Tardieu, *Étude médico-légal sur l'infanticide*, Paris: J-B. Baillière et Fils, 1868, pp. 6–7 noted that infanticide was frequent in France, Germany and Britain, and that the numbers could not be attributed simply to better detection but must be related to adverse administrative measures imposed

on unmarried mothers (the 1834 New Poor Law in England, and the gradual suppression after 1833 of the French hospital *tours* which allowed for large-scale infant abandonment). O. Ulbricht, 'Infanticide in eighteenth-century Germany', in R.J. Evans (ed.), *The German Underworld: Deviants and Outcasts in German History*, London and New York: Routledge, 1988, pp. 108–40 notes that infanticide was the most frequent type of homicide in eighteenth-century Germany, and that its incidence began to drop in the second half of the nineteenth century as social conditions improved.

5 P.C. Hoffer and N.E.H. Hull, *Murdering Mothers: Infanticide in England and New England 1558–1803*, New York and London: New York University Press, 1984; K.L. Moseley, 'The history of infanticide in western society', *Issues in Law & Medicine*, 1986, vol. 1, 345–61; R. Leboutte, 'Offense against family order: infanticide in Belgium from the fifteenth through the early twentieth centuries', *Journal of the History of Sexuality*, 1991, vol. 2, 159–85; D. Tinková, 'Protéger ou punir? Les voies de la décriminalisation de l'infanticide en France et dans le domaine des Habsbourg (XVIIIe – XIXe siècles)', *Crime, History & Societies*, 2005, vol. 9, 43–72; D.J.R. Grey, 'Discourses of infanticide in England, 1880–1922', PhD thesis, Roehampton University, 2008, Ch. 3.

6 H. Oosterhuis, *Stepchildren of Nature: Krafft-Ebing, Psychiatry, and the Making of Sexual Identity*, Chicago and London: University of Chicago Press, 2000, pp. 275–85.

7 R.D. Goldney, J.A. Schioldann and K.I. Dunn, 'Suicide research before Durkheim', *Health and History*, 2008, vol. 10, 73–93.

8 G. Minois, *History of Suicide: Voluntary Death in Western Culture*, trans. L.G. Cochrane, Baltimore, MD and London: Johns Hopkins University Press, 1999, pp. 2–3, 42–54.

9 D. Lederer, 'Honfibú: nationhood, manhood, and the culture of self-sacrifice in Hungary', in J.R. Watt (ed.), *From Sin to Insanity: Suicide in Early Modern Europe*, Ithaca, NY: Cornell University Press, 2004, pp. 125–32.

10 Minois, *History of Suicide*, pp. 3, 54–55.

11 Ibid., pp. 3, 181–83; A. Murray, *Suicide in the Middle Ages, Vol. 1, The Violent against Themselves*, Oxford: Oxford University Press, 1998, pp. 38–40; D.M. Shepherd and B.M. Barraclough, 'Suicide – a traveller's tale: a study of the adoption of the word "suicide" into the main romance languages', *History of Psychiatry*, 1997, vol. 8, 395–406. The importance of this word lies in its more neutral tone in relation to the pejorative and condemnatory term 'self-murder', which it replaced. In German the term *Selbstmord* still implies negative associations with homicide, the more positive act being *Freitod* (voluntary death).

12 M. MacDonald and T.R. Murphy, *Sleepless Souls: Suicide in Early Modern England* (1990), Oxford: Clarendon Press, 1993, pp. 132–36; J.R. Watt, 'Introduction: toward a history of suicide in early modern Europe', in Watt (ed.), *From Sin to Insanity*, pp. 1–8; J.R. Watt, *Choosing Death: Suicide and Calvinism in Early Modern Geneva*, Kirksville, MO: Truman State University Press, 2001, pp. 265–76; H.I. Kushner, *Self-destruction in the Promised Land: A Psychocultural Biology of American Suicide* (1989), New Brunswick, NJ and London: Rutgers University Press, 1991, pp. 13–34; R. Healy, 'Suicide in early modern and modern Europe', *Historical Journal*, 2006, vol. 49, 903–19.

13 Minois, *History of Suicide*, pp. 3, 24–41.

14 L. Vandekerckhove, *On Punishment: The Confrontation of Suicide in Old-Europe*, Leuven: Leuven University Press, 2000, pp. 43–71; MacDonald and Murphy, *Sleepless Souls*, pp. 15–41, 138–39; A. Murray, *Suicide in the Middle Ages, Vol. 2, The Curse on Self-Murder*, Oxford: Oxford University Press, 2000, pp. 10–53. On the Continent the bodies of suicides could be dragged through the streets on hurdles then publicly hanged and left to rot, or burned, but were most commonly buried

without the usual religious ceremonies outside churchyards, in fields, under gallows or in rubbish pits. Superstitious fears that suicides might rise from the dead and haunt the living meant that their bodies were sometimes buried at crossroads with a stake through the heart, as in England and occasionally America, or removed by any route except over the threshold from the building they were found in, as in Germany.

15 Minois, *History of Suicide*, pp. 135–42; Watt, *Choosing Death*, pp. 80–98; M. Bosman, 'The judicial treatment of suicide in Amsterdam', in Watt (ed.), *From Sin to Insanity*, pp. 15–21. A typical example of suicide committed from despair or a bad conscience, which attracted the harshest sanctions, was that of criminals awaiting trial or execution who killed themselves to avoid the consequences of their crime.

16 Minois, *History of Suicide*, pp. 74–76.

17 C. Koslofsky, 'Suicide and the secularization of the body in early modern Saxony', *Continuity and Change*, 2001, vol. 16, 45–70.

18 Minois, *History of Suicide*, pp. 40–41; MacDonald and Murphy, *Sleepless Souls*, pp. 57–58, 78–86; S.M. Butler, 'Degrees of culpability: suicide verdicts, mercy, and the jury in medieval England', *Journal of Medieval and Early Modern Studies*, 2006, vol. 36, 263–90. G. Seabourne and A. Seabourne, 'The law on suicide in medieval England', *Journal of Legal History*, 2000, vol. 21, 21–48 question the notion of community leniency even on the grounds of insanity.

19 V. Lind, 'The suicidal mind and body: examples from northern Germany', in Watt (ed.), *From Sin to Insanity*, pp. 67–77.

20 Minois, *History of Suicide*, pp. 138–42. For an example of how the defence process worked, and the factors tending to lead to acquittal (insufficient evidence, insanity, accident), see M. Lorcy, 'Les procès à cadavres d'après la jurisprudence criminelle bretonne au XVIIIe siècle', Mémoire pour le Diplôme d'Études Supérieures d'Histoire du Droit, Université de Rennes, 1971, pp. 102–9, 142–45. My thanks to Tijl Vanneste for finding and photographing this reference.

21 MacDonald and Murphy, *Sleepless Souls*, pp. 114–25.

22 Kushner, *Self-destruction in the Promised Land*, pp. 13–30, 209n62.

23 Vandekerckhove, *On Punishment*, pp. 125–37; Minois, *History of Suicide*, pp. 294–97; Watt, *Choosing Death*, pp. 121–25.

24 Healy, 'Suicide in early modern and modern Europe', p. 909.

25 Minois, *History of Suicide*, pp. 241–46.

26 Ibid., p. 318.

27 E. Esquirol, *Mental Maladies: A Treatise on Insanity*, trans. E.K. Hunt, Philadelphia: Lea and Blanchard, 1845, pp. 253–317 (quotes on pp. 275, 307).

28 F. Winslow, *The Anatomy of Suicide*, London: Henry Renshaw, 1840, pp. v, 227–29, 280–82.

29 For more on the uniquely American nineteenth-century phenomenon of will disputes and their medico-legal importance regarding mental competence, see J.C. Mohr, *Doctors and the Law: Medical Jurisprudence in Nineteenth-Century America*, Baltimore, MD and London: Johns Hopkins University Press, 1993, pp. 60–66.

30 I. Ray, *A Treatise on the Medical Jurisprudence of Insanity*, London: G. Henderson, 1839, pp. 335–44.

31 Goldney et al, 'Suicide research before Durkheim', pp. 79, 81–82, 84.

32 A.S. Taylor, *Medical Jurisprudence*, 5th American edn, Philadelphia: Blanchard and Lea, 1861, pp. 677–80.

33 O. Anderson, *Suicide in Victorian and Edwardian England*, Oxford: Clarendon Press, 1987, pp. 266–69.

34 Ibid., pp. 282–311, 376–417.

35 A. Lacassagne, *Précis de médecine judiciaire*, 2nd edn (1886), Chestnut Hill, MA: Elibron Classics, 2006, pp. 451–64.

36   C. Lombroso, *Criminal Man*, translated with a new introduction by M. Gibson and N.H. Rafter, Durham, NC and London: Duke University Press, 2006, pp. 101–4; C. Lombroso and G. Ferrero, *Criminal Woman, the Prostitute, and the Normal Woman*, translated and with a new introduction by N.H. Rafter and M. Gibson, Durham, NC and London: Duke University Press, 2004, pp. 209–12.

37   I. Paperno, *Suicide as a Cultural Institution in Dostoevsky's Russia*, Ithaca, NY and London: Cornell University Press, 1997, pp. 20–41.

38   S. Timmermans, *Postmortem: How Medical Examiners Explain Suspicious Deaths*, Chicago and London: University of Chicago Press, 2006, pp. 74–112.

39   R.C. Trexler, 'Infanticide in Florence: new sources and first results', *History of Childhood Quarterly*, 1973, vol. 1, 98–116; K. Wrightson, 'Infanticide in European history', *Criminal Justice History*, 1982, vol. 3, pp. 1–5.

40   Wrightson, 'Infanticide in European history', pp. 5–11; C.B. Backhouse, 'Desperate women and compassionate courts: infanticide in nineteenth-century Canada', *University of Toronto Law Journal*, 1984, vol. 34, 447–78; J.K. Burton, 'Human rights issues affecting women in Napoleonic legal medicine textbooks', *History of European Ideas*, 1987, vol. 8, 427–34; C. Damme, 'Infanticide: the worth of an infant under law', *Medical History*, 1978, vol. 22, 1–24; G.S. Rowe, 'Infanticide, its judicial resolution, and criminal code revision in early Pennsylvania', *Proceedings of the American Philosophical Society*, 1991, vol. 135, 200–232; A. Rowlands, '"In great secrecy": the crime of infanticide in Rothenburg ob der Tauber, 1501–1618', *German History*, 1997, vol. 15, 179–99.

41   Trexler, 'Infanticide in Florence', pp. 105, 114n42.

42   Rowlands, '"In great secrecy"', pp. 185–92; Mark Jackson, 'Suspicious infant deaths: the statute of 1624 and medical evidence at coroners' inquests', in M. Clark and C. Crawford (eds), *Legal Medicine in History*, Cambridge: Cambridge University Press, 1994, pp. 67–69; N.H. Steenburg, *Children and the Criminal Law in Connecticut, 1635–1855: Changing Perceptions of Childhood*, New York: Routledge, 2005, pp. 151–53; H. Brock and C. Crawford, 'Forensic medicine in early colonial Maryland, 1633–83', in Clark and Crawford (eds), *Legal Medicine in History*, pp. 38–40.

43   Jackson, 'Suspicious infant deaths', pp. 75–76; R.P. Brittain, 'The hydrostatic and similar tests of live birth: a historical review', *Medico-Legal Journal*, 1963, vol. 31, pp. 189–90.

44   E. Fischer-Homberger, *Medizin vor Gericht: Gerichtsmedizin von der Renaissance bis zur Aufklärung*, Bern: Verlag Hans Huber, pp. 280–82.

45   Brittain, 'The hydrostatic and similar tests of live birth', pp. 190–92. For examples of Victorian medico-legal views see the textbooks of A.S. Taylor, A. Lacassagne, and J.L. Casper, *A Handbook of the Practice of Forensic Medicine*, Vol. 3, 3rd edn, trans. W. Balfour, London: The New Sydenham Society, 1864.

46   Backhouse, 'Desperate women and compassionate courts'; G.K. Behlmer, 'Deadly motherhood: infanticide and medical opinion in mid-Victorian England', *Journal of the History of Medicine and Allied Sciences*, 1979, vol. 34, 403–27; J.M. Donovan, 'Infanticide and the juries in France, 1825–1913', *Journal of Family History*, 1991, vol. 16, 157–76; J.S. Richter, 'Infanticide, child abandonment, and abortion in Imperial Germany', *Journal of Interdisciplinary History*, 1998, vol. 28, p. 511; Rowe, 'Infanticide, its judicial resolution, and criminal code revision in early Pennsylvania'.

47   Tinková, 'Protéger ou punir?', pp. 55–59; H. Marland, *Dangerous Motherhood: Insanity and Childbirth in Victorian Britain*, Basingstoke: Palgrave Macmillan, 2004, pp. 28–35.

48   Marland, *Dangerous Motherhood*, Ch. 6.

49   Ibid., pp. 201–9.

50   Donovan, 'Infanticide and the juries in France', p. 169.

51 Backhouse, 'Desperate women and compassionate courts'; M. Oberman, 'Understanding infanticide in context: mothers who kill, 1870–1930 and today', *Journal of Criminal Law and Criminology*, 2003, vol. 92, pp. 726–28.

52 Damme, 'Infanticide', pp. 13–15; T. Ward, 'Legislating for human nature: legal responses to infanticide, 1860–1938', in M. Jackson (ed.), *Infanticide: Historical Perspectives on Child Murder and Concealment, 1550–2000*, Aldershot: Ashgate, 2002, pp. 253–61.

53 I. Lambie, 'Mothers who kill: the crime of infanticide', *International Journal of Law and Psychiatry*, 2001, vol. 24, 71–80.

54 K. O'Donovan, 'The medicalisation of infanticide', *Criminal Law Review*, 1984, 259–64; T. Ward, 'The sad subject of infanticide: law, medicine and child murder, 1860–1938', *Social & Legal Studies*, 1999, vol. 8, 163–80.

55 The Canadian law of 1948 was modelled on the English Act of 1922, and then revised in 1955 along the lines of the 1938 Act. See K.J. Kramar and W.D. Watson, 'Canadian infanticide legislation, 1948 and 1955: reflections on the medicalization/autopoiesis debate', *Canadian Journal of Sociology*, 2008, vol. 33, 237–63.

56 R. Ogle and D. Maier-Katkin, 'A rationale for infanticide laws', *Criminal Law Review*, Dec. 1993, 903–14.

57 Lambie, 'Mothers who kill', p. 75.

58 K. Park, 'The rediscovery of the clitoris: French medicine and the tribade, 1570–1620', in D. Hillman and C. Mazzio (eds), *The Body in Parts: Fantasies of Corporeality in Early Modern Europe*, New York and London: Routledge, 1997, p. 174.

59 W. Naphy, *Sex Crimes from Renaissance to Enlightenment*, Stroud: Tempus, 2002, p. 129; P. Darmon, *Trial by Impotence: Virility and Marriage in Pre-Revolutionary France* (1979), trans. P. Keegan, London: Chatto & Windus, 1985, pp. 41–51; E. Behrend-Martínez, 'Manhood and the neutered body in early modern Spain', *Journal of Social History*, 2005, vol. 38, 1073–93.

60 See for example P. Cassar, 'A medico-legal report of the sixteenth century from Malta', *Medical History*, 1974, vol. 18, 354–59.

61 J. Murray, 'On the origins and role of "wise women" in causes for annulment on the grounds of male impotence', *Journal of Medieval History*, 1990, vol. 16, 235–49; Darmon, *Trial by Impotence*; A. Lefebvre-Teillard, 'A défaut d'expert expert', in A. Deperchin, N. Derasse and B. Dubois (eds), *Figures de Justice: Études en l'honneur de Jean-Pierre Royer*, Lille: Centre d'Histoire Judiciaire, 2005, pp. 665–78.

62 Murray, 'On the origins and role of "wise women" in causes for annulment on the grounds of male impotence', pp. 242–45.

63 Ibid., pp. 241, 243, 247; Lefebvre-Teillard, 'A défaut d'expert expert", pp. 670–72 seems to be unaware of Murray's article.

64 Darmon, *Trial by Impotence*, pp. 118–22.

65 E. Behrend-Martínez, 'Female sexual potency in a Spanish church court, 1673–1735', *Law and History Review*, 2006, vol. 24, pp. 308–9. This author makes no mention of trial by congress; rather, Spanish church courts ordered medical teams to examine the person accused of impotence, but not their spouse.

66 Darmon, *Trial by Impotence*, pp. 161–85.

67 Ibid., pp. 210–28.

68 Behrend-Martínez, 'Female sexual potency in a Spanish church court', p. 309.

69 A.N. Gilbert, 'Conceptions of homosexuality and sodomy in Western history', in S.J. Licata and R.P. Petersen (eds), *Historical Perspectives on Homosexuality*, New York: The Haworth Press, 1981, pp. 61–64.

70 L. Crompton, 'The myth of lesbian impunity: capital laws from 1270 to 1791', in Licata and Petersen (eds), *Historical Perspectives*, pp. 11–25. The death penalty

for sodomy was abolished gradually: Pennsylvania (1786), Austria (1787), France (1791), Prussia (1794), Britain (1861), and Canada (1869).

71 B. Eriksson, 'A lesbian execution in Germany, 1721: the trial records', in Licata and Petersen (eds), *Historical Perspectives*, pp. 27–40

72 G. Ruggiero, *The Boundaries of Eros: Sex Crime and Sexuality in Renaissance Venice*, Oxford: Oxford University Press, 1985, pp. 114–15.

73 Ibid., pp. 117–18, 121–25. See also, briefly, A. Pastore, *Il medico in tribunale: La perizia medica nella procedura penale d'antico regime (secoli XVI–XVIII)*, Bellinzona: Edizioni Casagrande, 1998, pp. 149–50.

74 K. Borris, 'Introduction: the prehistory of homosexuality in the early modern sciences', in K. Borris and G. Rousseau (eds), *The Sciences of Homosexuality in Early Modern Europe*, London and New York: Routledge, 2008, pp. 11–12.

75 W. Naphy, 'Sodomy in early modern Geneva: various definitions, diverse verdicts', in T. Betteridge (ed.), *Sodomy in Early Modern Europe*, Manchester and New York: Manchester University Press, 2002, pp. 97, 106.

76 C. Berco, 'Syphilis and the silencing of sodomy in Juan Calvo's *Tratado del morbo gálico*', in Borris and Rousseau (eds), *The Sciences of Homosexuality*, pp. 104–5; F. Garza Carvajal, *Butterflies Will Burn: Prosecuting Sodomites in Early Modern Spain and Mexico*, Austin, TX: University of Texas Press, 2003.

77 G. Rousseau, 'Policing the anus: Stuprum and sodomy according to Paolo Zacchia's forensic medicine', in Borris and Rousseau (eds), *The Sciences of Homosexuality*, pp. 72–91.

78 R. Brooks, '"Vices once adopted": theorising male homoeroticism in German-language legal and forensic discourses, 1752–1869', *Reinvention: A Journal of Undergraduate Research*, 1 (2008), online at http://www2.warwick.ac.uk/go/reinventionjournal/issues/volume1issue2/Brooks (accessed 27 October 2008).

79 H. Oosterhuis, 'Medical science and the modernisation of sexuality', in F.X. Eder, L.A. Hall and G. Hekma (eds), *Sexual Cultures in Europe: National Histories*, Manchester and New York: Manchester University Press, 1999, p. 222.

80 G. Hekma, 'A history of sexology: social and historical aspects of sexuality', in J. Bremmer (ed.), *From Sappho to De Sade: Moments in the History of Sexuality*, London and New York: Routledge, 1989, pp. 174–76; I.D. Crozier, 'The medical construction of homosexuality and its relation to the law in nineteenth-century England', *Medical History*, 2001, vol. 45, p. 62; V.L. Bullough, 'Homosexuality and the medical model', *Journal of Homosexuality*, 1974, vol. 1, pp. 100–101.

81 Hekma, 'A history of sexology', pp. 176–81; Oosterhuis, 'Medical science and the modernisation of sexuality', pp. 224–26; Brooks, '"Vices once adopted"'.

82 Gilbert, 'Conceptions of homosexuality and sodomy in Western history', p. 61; Brooks, '"Vices once adopted"'; Hekma, 'A history of sexology', pp. 178–81; Oosterhuis, 'Medical science and the modernisation of sexuality', pp. 226–27; Bullough, 'Homosexuality and the medical model', pp. 105–7. Westphal's article is online at Born Eunuchs Library, http://www.well.com/user/aquarius/westphal.htm (accessed 4 October 2009).

83 Lombroso, *Criminal Woman, the Prostitute, and the Normal Woman*, pp. 21–22.

84 Oosterhuis, 'Medical science and the modernisation of sexuality', p. 230; Crozier, 'The medical construction of homosexuality and its relation to the law in nineteenth-century England', p. 67.

85 Hekma, 'A history of sexology', pp. 181–86; Bullough, 'Homosexuality and the medical model', p. 108; Oosterhuis, 'Medical science and the modernisation of sexuality', pp. 229–37; Oosterhuis, *Stepchildren of Nature*, pp. 69–72, 241–52; Crozier, 'The medical construction of homosexuality and its relation to the law in nineteenth-century England', pp. 76–81; T. Delessert, 'Entre justice et psychiatrie: l'homosexualité dans le project de Code pénal suisse (1918)', *Gesnerus*, 2005, vol. 62, pp. 246–50; J. Terry, *An American Obsession: Science, Medicine, and*

Homosexuality in Modern Society, Chicago: University of Chicago Press, 1999, pp. 40–55.

86 Crozier, 'The medical construction of homosexuality and its relation to the law in nineteenth-century England', pp. 66–73; J. Dixon Mann, *Forensic Medicine and Toxicology*, 6th edn, rev. W.A. Brend, London: Charles Griffin and Company, 1922, pp. 92–94; L. Thoinot, *Medicolegal Aspects of Moral Offenses*, trans. and enlarged by A.W. Weysse (1923), Whitefish, MT: Kessinger Publishing, 2005, pp. 29–30, 256.

87 Terry, *An American Obsession*, Ch. 3.

88 K.A. Martin, 'Gender and sexuality: medical opinion on homosexuality, 1900–950', *Gender and Society*, 1993, vol. 7, p. 248.

89 Hekma, 'A history of sexology', p. 186.

90 Martin, 'Gender and sexuality', pp. 248–55.

91 Terry, *An American Obsession*, pp. 275–96.

6 Twentieth-century developments in forensic medicine and science

1 See, for example, A. Lacassagne, *Précis de médecine judiciaire*, 2nd edn (1886), Chestnut Hill, MA: Elibron Classics, 2006, pp. 214–38, in which he noted (p. 238) the importance that stains had recently attained in legal medicine. The usefulness of hair and fibres as forms of evidence, and the chemical and microscopical examination of blood stains were discussed by A.S. Taylor in *The Principles and Practice of Medical Jurisprudence*, London: John Churchill & Sons, 1865, pp. 428–32, 443–62.

2 S. Smith, 'The history and development of forensic medicine', *British Medical Journal*, 24 March 1951, 599–607; S. Bell, *Crime and Circumstance: Investigating the History of Forensic Science*, Westport, CT and London: Praeger, 2008.

3 P.B. Ainsworth, *Offender Profiling and Crime Analysis*, Cullompton: Willan Publishing, 2001.

4 C-A. Hooper, 'Rethinking the politics of child abuse', *Social History of Medicine*, 1989, vol. 2, p. 356; L. Gordon, 'The politics of child sexual abuse: notes from American history', *Feminist Review*, 1988, vol. 28, 56–64; E. Olafson, D.L. Corwin and R.C. Summit, 'Modern history of child sexual abuse awareness: cycles of discovery and suppression', *Child Abuse & Neglect*, 1993, vol. 17, 7–24.

5 R. Davidson, '"This pernicious delusion": law, medicine, and child sexual abuse in early-twentieth-century Scotland', *Journal of the History of Sexuality*, 2001, vol. 10, pp. 68–70; L.A. Jackson, *Child Sexual Abuse in Victorian England*, London and New York: Routledge, 2000, Ch. 4; L. Sacco, *Unspeakable: Father–Daughter Incest in American History*, Baltimore, MD: Johns Hopkins University Press, 2009, Ch. 2.

6 R. von Krafft-Ebing, *Psychopathia Sexualis, with especial reference to the Antipathetic Sexual Instinct: A Medico-Forensic Study*, 12th edn, Stuttgart: Ferdinand Enke, 1903, trans. F.S. Klaf, London: Staples Press, 1965, pp. 333–34; L. Thoinot, *Medicolegal Aspects of Moral Offenses*, trans. and enlarged by A.W. Weysse (1923), Whitefish, MT: Kessinger Publishing, 2005, pp. 10–21.

7 J.M. Donovan, 'Combatting the sexual abuse of children in France, 1825–1913', *Criminal Justice History*, 1994, vol. 15, pp. 62–65; F. Giuliani, 'Monsters in the village? Incest in nineteenth century France', *Journal of Social History*, 2009, vol. 42, 919–32. Incest was subject to stronger societal disapproval in France from the 1880s, and could be prosecuted under laws against rape and sexual abuse in the Napoleonic penal code of 1810, but it was not criminalized until January 2010. See http://www.telegraph.co.uk/news/worldnews/europe/france/7085759/France-makes-incest-a-crime.html (accessed on 27 May 2010).

8 S.J. Pfohl, 'The "discovery" of child abuse', *Social Problems*, 1977, vol. 24, 310–23; Hooper, 'Rethinking the politics of child abuse'.

9   M. Lynch, 'Child abuse before Kempe: an historical literature review', *Child Abuse & Neglect*, 1985, vol. 9, pp. 7–8.

10   Ibid., pp. 8–9.

11   J. Devaux, *L'art de faire les raports en chirurgie*, Paris: Laurent D'Houry, 1703, pp. 297–99.

12   Lynch, 'Child abuse before Kempe', p. 9.

13   The first was Professor A. Toulmouche of Rennes, in an article published in the *Annales d'hygiène publique et de médecine légale* in 1856.

14   A. Tardieu, *Étude médico-légale sur les attentats aux moeurs*, 3rd edn, Paris: J-B. Baillière et Fils, 1859, pp. 8–9, 45–46. The first edition appeared in 1857.

15   A. Tardieu, 'Étude médico-légale sur les sévices et mauvais traitements exercés sur des enfants', *Annales d'hygiène publique et de médecine légale*, 1860, vol. 13, 361–98; A.J. Roche, G. Fortin, J. Labbé, J. Brown and D. Chadwick, 'The work of Ambroise Tardieu: the first definitive description of child abuse', *Child Abuse & Neglect*, 2005, vol. 29, 325–34. The article's title in English is 'Medico-legal study on cruelty and the ill treatment of children'.

16   R.G. Fuchs, 'Crimes against children in nineteenth-century France: child abuse', *Law and Human Behavior*, 1982, vol. 6, 237–59.

17   J. Labbé, 'Ambroise Tardieu: the man and his work on child maltreatment a century before Kempe', *Child Abuse & Neglect*, 2005, vol. 29, p. 321; Olafson et al, 'Modern history of child sexual abuse awareness', pp. 9–10.

18   Donovan, 'Combatting the sexual abuse of children in France'.

19   Giuliani, 'Monsters in the village?', p. 938.

20   Krafft-Ebing, *Psychopathia Sexualis*, p. 371.

21   Pfohl, 'The "discovery of child abuse"', pp. 312–13; Sacco, *Unspeakable*, pp. 44–50. The argument can be summarized as one of immorality versus abnormality.

22   Sacco, *Unspeakable*, Ch. 2; Davidson, '"This pernicious delusion"'; J.B. Lyons, 'Sir William Wilde's medico-legal observations', *Medical History*, 1997, vol. 41, 437–54; S. Robertson, 'Signs, marks and private parts: doctors, legal discourses, and evidence of rape in the United States, 1823–1930', *Journal of the History of Sexuality*, 1998, vol. 8, 345–88; L. Sacco, 'Sanitized for your protection: medical discourse and the denial of incest in the United States, 1890–1940', *Journal of Women's History*, 2002, vol. 14, 80–104.

23   Sacco, *Unspeakable*, Ch. 5; Davidson, '"This pernicious delusion"', pp. 68–75; Robertson, 'Signs, marks and private parts', pp. 382–85.

24   S. West, 'Acute periosteal swellings in several young infants of the same family, probably rickety in nature', *British Medical Journal*, 1888, vol. 1, 856–57; Lynch, 'Child abuse before Kempe', pp. 9–10.

25   Labbé, 'Ambroise Tardieu', p. 322; P. Parisot and L. Caussade, 'Les sévices envers les enfants', *Annales de médecine légale*, 1929, vol. 9, 398–426.

26   Lynch, 'Child abuse before Kempe', pp. 10–12; Labbé, 'Ambroise Tardieu', p. 322; S.X. Radbill, 'Children in a world of violence: a history of child abuse', in C.H. Kempe and R.E. Helfer (eds), *The Battered Child*, 3rd edn, Chicago and London: University of Chicago Press, 1980, p. 17. The French often refer to child physical abuse as the 'syndrome of Silverman', while Silverman himself suggested calling it the 'syndrome of Tardieu' (Labbé, p. 322).

27   P. Conrad and J.W. Schneider, *Deviance and Medicalization: From Badness to Sickness* (1980), revised edn, Philadelphia: Temple University Press, 1992, pp. 161–69.

28   R.W. ten Bensel, M.M. Rheinberger and S.X. Radbill, 'Children in a world of violence: the roots of child maltreatment', in M.E. Helfer, R.S. Kempe and R.D. Krugman (eds), *The Battered Child*, 5th edn, Chicago and London: University of Chicago Press, 1997, p. 26.

29   Pfohl, 'Discovery of child abuse', pp. 315–32.

30 Sacco, *Unspeakable*, pp. 210–27; Olafson et al, 'Modern history of child sexual abuse awareness', pp. 16–18; Gordon, 'The politics of child sexual abuse', pp. 60–62.

31 In Britain the cases of Victoria Climbié (2000) and Baby P. (2009) have highlighted failures by the public services mandated to identify children at risk, while in Austria the case of Josef Fritzl (2008) brought incest back into the public eye.

32 Association of Clinical Pathologists, online, http://www.pathologists.org.uk/sub-spec-page/forensic/forensic.htm (accessed 5 March 2010).

33 Home Office Register of Forensic Pathologists, 1 February 2010, online at http://www.npia.police.uk/en/docs/Current_Home_Office_Register.pdf (accessed 5 March 2010).

34 E.A. Cawthon, *Medicine on Trial: A Sourcebook with Cases, Laws, and Documents*, Indianapolis, IN: Hackett Publishing Company, 2004, p. 22.

35 W.J. Tilstone, K.A. Savage and L.A. Clark, *Forensic Science: An Encyclopedia of History, Methods, and Techniques*, Santa Barbara, CA and Oxford: ABC-CLIO, 2006, p. 14; Brian Lane, *The Encyclopedia of Forensic Science*, London: Headline, 1992, pp. 417–18.

36 Institut National de Police Scientifique, online at http://www.inps.interieur.gouv.fr/ (accessed 5 March 2010).

37 Tilstone et al, *Forensic Science*, p. 15.

38 Lane, *The Encyclopedia of Forensic Science*, p. 418; J. David Rogers, Forensic Geology Case Histories, online at http://web.mst.edu/~rogersda/forensic_geology/Geoforensics%20Case%20Histories.htm (accessed 5 March 2010).

39 Tilstone et al, *Forensic Science*, p. 60.

40 Ibid., p. 15; N. Ambage and M. Clark, 'Unbuilt Bloomsbury: medico-legal institutes and forensic science laboratories in England between the wars', in M. Clark and C. Crawford (eds), *Legal Medicine in History*, Cambridge: Cambridge University Press, 1994, p. 293.

41 E. Malkoc and W. Neuteboom, 'The current status of forensic science laboratory accreditation in Europe', *Forensic Science International*, 2007, vol. 167, 121–26. ENFSI includes all European countries: members of the EU, EU candidate countries, and non-members.

42 Tilstone et al, *Forensic Science*, pp. 16–19, 27–28.

43 Bell, *Crime and Circumstance*, pp. 195–96; D.M. Lucas, 'North of 49 – the development of forensic science in Canada', *Science & Justice*, 1997, vol. 37, pp. 50–51.

44 M. Benecke, 'A brief history of forensic entomology', *Forensic Science International*, 2001, vol. 120, p. 3; Lane, *The Encyclopedia of Forensic Science*, p. 415.

45 *The Trial of Professor John White Webster*, with an introduction by George Dilnot, London: Geoffrey Bles, 1928; J.W. Stone (ed.), *Report of the Trial of Prof. John W. Webster*, Boston: Phillips, Sampson & Company, 1850; J. Ward, *Crimebusting: Breakthroughs in Forensic Science*, London: Blandford Press, 1998, pp. 40–46; W.R. Maples and M. Browning, *Dead Men Do Tell Tales: The Strange and Fascinating Cases of a Forensic Anthropologist*, New York and London: Doubleday, 1994, pp. 91–92.

46 Bell, *Crime and Circumstance*, pp. 158–59; D. Patzelt, 'History of forensic serology and molecular genetics in the sphere of activity of the German Society for Forensic Medicine', *Forensic Science International*, 2004, vol. 144, p. 185. Polish-born Ludwig Karl Teichmann was an anatomy professor at the University of Göttingen.

47 M.A. Crowther and B. White, *On Soul and Conscience. The Medical Expert and Crime: 150 Years of Forensic Medicine in Glasgow*, Aberdeen: Aberdeen University Press, 1988, pp. 20–21; C. Henssge and B. Madea, 'Estimation of the time since death in the early post-mortem period', *Forensic Science International*, 2004, vol. 144, p. 167.

48 Lane, *The Encyclopedia of Forensic Science*, pp. 526–27.
49 A. Lacassagne, *Vacher l'éventreur et les crimes sadiques* (1899), Chestnut Hill, MA: Elibron Classics, 2006.
50 F. Young (ed.), *The Trial of Hawley Harvey Crippen*, Edinburgh: William Hodge, 1920; K.D. Watson, *Crime Archive: Dr Crippen*, Kew: The National Archives, 2007, Ch. 2.
51 Tilstone et al, *Forensic Science*, pp. 80, 118–20, 132–33, 154–60, 226–28, 258–59; Ainsworth, *Offender Profiling and Crime Analysis*, pp. 7–9.
52 G.S.W. de Saram, G. Webster and N. Kathirgamatamby, 'Post-mortem temperature and the time of death', *Journal of Criminal Law, Criminology, and Police Science*, 1955, vol. 46, 562–77. For an obituary of de Saram, see the *Journal of Pathology and Bacteriology*, 1965, vol. 89, 411–14.
53 Bell, *Crime and Circumstance*, pp. 73–74; Henssge and Madea, 'Estimation of the time since death in the early post-mortem period'; S.A. Koehler and C.H. Wecht, *Postmortem: Establishing the Cause of Death*, Buffalo, NY: Firefly Books, 2006, pp. 29–30; C. Henssge, B. Knight, T. Krompecher, B. Madea and L. Nokes, *The Estimation of the Time Since Death in the Early Postmortem Period*, 2nd edn, London: Arnold, 2002, pp. 4–9, 40–41.
54 Bell, *Crime and Circumstance*, pp. 72–73; Henssge and Madea, 'Estimation of the time since death in the early post-mortem period', p. 172; Koehler and Wecht, *Postmortem*, p. 31; Tilstone et al, *Forensic Science*, pp. 114–15; Henssge et al, *The Estimation of the Time Since Death in the Early Postmortem Period*, pp. 144–60; Robin Peress, 'What causes rigor mortis?', online at http://www.howstuffworks.com/rigor-mortis-cause.htm/printable (accessed 5 March 2010).
55 Koehler and Wecht, *Postmortem*, p. 32; Tilstone et al, *Forensic Science*, p. 115; Henssge and Madea, 'Estimation of the time since death in the early post-mortem period', p. 172; Henssge et al, *The Estimation of the Time Since Death in the Early Postmortem Period*, pp. 206–8.
56 Tilstone et al, *Forensic Science*, p. 115 (quote); Lane, *The Encyclopedia of Forensic Science*, pp. 24, 533–37; Watson, *Crime Archive*, pp. 44–45.
57 B. Bass and J. Jefferson, *Death's Acre: Inside the Legendary 'Body Farm'*, London: Time Warner, 2003, Ch. 5 (quote on p. 79).
58 Ibid., pp. 275–76.
59 Ibid., Ch. 8; Koehler and Wecht, *Postmortem*, pp. 118–19; Tilstone et al, *Forensic Science*, pp. 132–33; Bell, *Crime and Circumstance*, pp. 215–17; C.P. Campobasso and F. Introna, 'The forensic entomologist in the context of the forensic pathologist's role', *Forensic Science International*, 2001, vol. 120, p. 136.
60 Benecke, 'Forensic entomology', pp. 3–4.
61 Ibid., pp. 4–8; Bass and Jefferson, *Death's Acre*, pp. 115–16.
62 Benecke, 'Forensic entomology', pp. 6–7; H. Klotzbach, R. Krettek, H. Bratzke, K. Püschel, R. Zehner and J. Amendt, 'The history of forensic entomology in German-speaking countries', *Forensic Science International*, 2004, vol. 144, pp. 259–61.
63 Benecke, 'Forensic entomology', pp. 10–11; Klotzbach et al, 'The history of forensic entomology in German-speaking countries', pp. 260–61; Bass and Jefferson, *Death's Acre*, Ch. 8; J. Leclercq, 'Marcel Leclercq (1924–2008), médecin, diptériste, parasitologue et pionnier de l'entomologie forensique (Part 1)', *Faunistic Entomology*, 2008, vol. 61, 129–50, online at http://popups.ulg.ac.be/NFG/document.php?id=983 (accessed on 27 May 2010).
64 Klotzbach et al, 'The history of forensic entomology in German-speaking countries', pp. 261–62; Campobasso and Introna, 'The forensic entomologist in the context of the forensic pathologist's role', p. 137; E. Gaudry, J-B. Myskowiak, B. Chauvet, T. Pasquerault, F. Lefebvre and Y. Malgorn, 'Activity of the forensic entomology department of the French Gendarmerie', *Forensic Science International*, 2001, vol. 120, 68–71.

65 Tilstone et al, *Forensic Science*, p. 11; Bell, *Crime and Circumstance*, pp. 157–60; Patzelt, 'History of forensic serology and molecular genetics in the sphere of activity of the German Society for Forensic Medicine', pp. 185–86. Takayama published in the *Japanese Journal of Toxicology*.
66 Tilstone et al, *Forensic Science*, pp. 11–12; Bell, *Crime and Circumstance*, p. 159.
67 Tilstone et al, *Forensic Science*, p. 11; Lane, *The Encyclopedia of Forensic Science*, pp. 571–72.
68 Tilstone et al, *Forensic Science*, pp. 10–11, 255–56; Lane, *The Encyclopedia of Forensic Science*, pp. 570–71, 573–75; Bell, *Crime and Circumstance*, pp. 160–66.
69 Bell, *Crime and Circumstance*, pp. 166–71; Lane, *The Encyclopedia of Forensic Science*, p. 575.
70 Tilstone et al, *Forensic Science*, pp. 47–58; Bell, *Crime and Circumstance*, Ch. 17 (quote on p. 178); Ward, *Crimebusting*, Chs 19 and 20.
71 Ainsworth, *Offender Profiling and Crime Analysis*, Ch. 1; Lane, *The Encyclopedia of Forensic Science*, pp. 526–27; D. Owen, *Criminal Minds: The Science and Psychology of Profiling*, New York: Barnes & Noble Books, 2004, pp. 24–31.
72 Owen, *Criminal Minds*, pp. 12–14.
73 Ibid., pp. 19–22; Lane, *The Encyclopedia of Forensic Science*, pp. 527–28; J.A. Brussel, *Casebook of a Crime Psychiatrist*, London: New English Library, 1969, Ch. 1.
74 B.E. Turvey, *Criminal Profiling: An Introduction to Behavioral Evidence Analysis*, 3rd edn, San Diego: Academic Press, 2008, pp. 35–38.
75 Lane, *The Encyclopedia of Forensic Science*, pp. 372–75, 528–30.
76 Ainsworth, *Offender Profiling and Crime Analysis*, Ch. 6.
77 Ibid., Ch. 7.
78 Ibid., Ch. 8.
79 A.K. Mant (ed.), *Taylor's Principles and Practice of Medical Jurisprudence*, 13th edn, London: Churchill Livingstone, 1984, pp. 1–10.

Bibliography

Primary Sources

Bass, Bill and Jon Jefferson, *Death's Acre: Inside the Legendary 'Body Farm'*, London: Time Warner, 2003.

Beccaria, Cesare, *On Crimes and Punishments* (1764), trans. David Young, Indianapolis, IN: Hackett Publishing, 1986.

Browne, G. Lathom and C.G. Stewart, *Reports of Trials for Murder by Poisoning*, London: Stevens and Sons, 1883.

Brussel, James A., *Casebook of a Crime Psychiatrist*, London: New English Library, 1969.

Casper, Johann Ludwig, *A Handbook of the Practice of Forensic Medicine*, Vol. 3, 3rd edn, trans. William Balfour, London: The New Sydenham Society, 1864.

Christison, Robert, *A Treatise on Poisons, in Relation to Medical Jurisprudence, Physiology, and the Practice of Physic*, Edinburgh: Adam Black, 1829.

Devaux, Jean, *L'art de faire les raports en chirurgie*, Paris: Laurent D'Houry, 1703.

The Digest of Justinian, Vol.1, trans. Charles Henry Monro, Cambridge: Cambridge University Press, 1904.

Dixon Mann, J., *Forensic Medicine and Toxicology*, 6th edn, revised by William A. Brend, London: Charles Griffin and Company, 1922.

Edbury, Peter W. (ed.), *John of Ibelin: Le Livre des Assises*, Leiden and Boston, MA: Brill, 2003.

Esquirol, Jean-Etienne, 'Note sur la monomanie-homicide', in Johann-Christoph Hoffbauer, *Médecine légale relative aux aliénés et aux sourds-muets*, trans. A-M. Chambeyron, Paris: J-B. Baillière, 1827, 309–59.

——*Mental Maladies: A Treatise on Insanity*, trans. E.K. Hunt, Philadelphia: Lea and Blanchard, 1845.

Gilbert, Sir Geoffrey, *The Law of Evidence, considerably enlarged by Capel Lofft*, 4 vols, London: A. Strahan and W. Woodfall, 1791.

Glaister, John and James Couper Brash, *Medico-Legal Aspects of the Ruxton Case*, Edinburgh: E. & S. Livingstone, 1937.

Guy, William A., *Principles of Forensic Medicine*, 2nd edn, London: Henry Renshaw, 1861.

Hale, Sir Mathew, *The History of the Pleas of the Crown*, Vol. 1, 1st American edn, Philadelphia: Robert H. Small, 1847.

Hall, Sir John (ed.), *Trial of Abraham Thornton*, Glasgow: William Hodge, 1926.

Henderson, Ernest F. (trans. and ed.), *Select Historical Documents of the Middle Ages*, London: G. Bell and Sons, 1910.

Henssge, Claus, Bernard Knight, Thomas Krompecher, Burkhard Madea and Leonard Nokes, *The Estimation of the Time Since Death in the Early Postmortem Period*, 2nd edn, London: Arnold, 2002.

Hunnisett, R.F. (ed.), *Calendar of Nottinghamshire Coroners' Inquests 1485–1558*, Nottingham: Thoroton Society, 1969.

——(ed.), *Wiltshire Coroners' Bills 1752–1796*, Devizes: Wiltshire Record Society, 1981.

——(ed.), *East Sussex Coroners' Records 1688–1838*, Lewes: Sussex Record Society, 2005.

Krafft-Ebing, Richard von, *Psychopathia Sexualis, with especial reference to the Antipathetic Sexual Instinct: A Medico-Forensic Study*, 12th edn, Stuttgart: Ferdinand Enke, 1903, trans. Franklin S. Klaf, London: Staples Press, 1965.

Lacassagne, Alexandre, *Précis de médecine judiciaire*, 2nd edn (1886), Chestnut Hill, MA: Elibron Classics, 2006.

——*Vacher l'éventreur et les crimes sadiques* (1899), Chestnut Hill, MA: Elibron Classics, 2006.

Lombroso, Cesare, *Criminal Man*, translated with a new introduction by Mary Gibson and Nicole Hahn Rafter, Durham, NC and London: Duke University Press, 2006.

Lombroso, Cesare and Guglielmo Ferrero, *Criminal Woman, the Prostitute, and the Normal Woman*, translated and with a new introduction by Nicole Hahn Rafter and Mary Gibson, Durham, NC and London: Duke University Press, 2004.

Mant, A. Keith (ed.), *Taylor's Principles and Practice of Medical Jurisprudence*, 13th edn, London: Churchill Livingstone, 1984.

Maples, William R. and Michael Browning, *Dead Men Do Tell Tales: The Strange and Fascinating Cases of a Forensic Anthropologist*, New York and London: Doubleday, 1994.

Mora, George (ed.), *Witches, Devils, and Doctors in the Renaissance: Johann Weyer, De praestigiis daemonum*, Binghamton, NY: Center for Medieval and Early Renaissance Studies, State University of New York at Binghamton, 1991.

Orfila, Mathieu J.B., *Traité des poisons tirés des règnes minéral, végétal et animal, ou toxicologie générale, considérée sous les rapports de la physiologie, de la pathologie et de la médecine légale*, 2 vols, Paris: Crochard, 1814–15.

Parisot, P. and L. Caussade, 'Les sévices envers les enfants', *Annales de médecine légale*, 1929, vol. 9: 398–426.

Ray, Isaac, *A Treatise on the Medical Jurisprudence of Insanity*, London: G. Henderson, 1839.

Roughead, William (ed.), *Trial of Mary Blandy* (1914), Charleston, SC: BiblioBazaar, 2006.

Saram, G.S.W. de, G. Webster and N. Kathirgamatamby, 'Post-mortem temperature and the time of death', *Journal of Criminal Law, Criminology, and Police Science*, 1955, vol. 46: 562–77.

Scott, Samuel Parsons (trans.), *The Visigothic Code: Forum Judicum*, Boston, MA: Boston Book Company, 1910.

Stone, James W. (ed.), *Report of the Trial of Prof. John W. Webster*, Boston, MA: Phillips, Sampson & Company, 1850.

Sung Tz'u, *The Washing Away of Wrongs: Forensic Medicine in Thirteenth-Century China*, trans. Brian E. McKnight, Ann Arbor, MI: Center for Chinese Studies, University of Michigan, 1981.

Tardieu, Ambroise, *Étude médico-légale sur les attentats aux moeurs*, 3rd edn, Paris: J-B. Baillière et Fils, 1859.

Tardieu, Ambroise, 'Étude médico-légale sur les sévices et mauvais traitements exercés sur des enfants', *Annales d'hygiène publique et de médecine légale*, 1860, vol. 13: 361–98.

——*Étude médico-légal sur l'infanticide*, Paris: J-B. Baillière et Fils, 1868.

Taylor, Alfred S., *Medical Jurisprudence*, 5th American edn, Philadelphia: Blanchard and Lea, 1861.

——*The Principles and Practice of Medical Jurisprudence*, London: John Churchill & Sons, 1865.

The Trial of Professor John White Webster, with an introduction by George Dilnot, London: Geoffrey Bles, 1928.

Thoinot, Leon, *Medicolegal Aspects of Moral Offenses*, trans. and enlarged by Arthur W. Weysse (1923), Whitefish, MT: Kessinger Publishing, 2005.

Tourdes, Gabriel and Edmond Metzquer, *Traité de médecine légale: théorique et pratique*, Paris: Asselin et Houzeau, 1896.

Virchow, Rudolf, *Post-Mortem Examinations: With Especial Reference to Medico-Legal Practice*, trans. T.P. Smith, 3rd American edn, Philadelphia: P. Blakiston, 1896.

West, Samuel, 'Acute periosteal swellings in several young infants of the same family, probably rickety in nature', *British Medical Journal*, 1888, vol. 1: 856–57.

Winslow, Forbes, *The Anatomy of Suicide*, London: Henry Renshaw, 1840.

Young, Filson (ed.), *The Trial of Hawley Harvey Crippen*, Edinburgh: William Hodge, 1920.

Secondary sources

Ackerknecht, Erwin H., 'Midwives as experts in court', *Bulletin of the New York Academy of Medicine*, 1976, vol. 52: 1224–28.

——'Early history of legal medicine', in Chester R. Burns (ed.), *Legacies in Law and Medicine*, New York: Science History Publications, 1977, 249–71.

Ainsworth, Peter B., *Offender Profiling and Crime Analysis*, Cullompton: Willan Publishing, 2001.

Ambage, Norman and Michael Clark, 'Unbuilt Bloomsbury: medico-legal institutes and forensic science laboratories in England between the wars', in Michael Clark and Catherine Crawford (eds), *Legal Medicine in History*, Cambridge: Cambridge University Press, 1994, 293 313.

Amundsen, Darrel W., 'Visigothic medical legislation', *Bulletin of the History of Medicine*, 1971, vol. 45: 553–69.

Amundsen, Darrel W. and Gary B. Ferngren, 'The physician as an expert witness in Athenian law', *Bulletin of the History of Medicine*, 1977, vol. 51: 202–13.

——'The forensic role of physicians in Ptolemaic and Roman Egypt', *Bulletin of the History of Medicine*, 1978, vol. 52: 336–53.

——'The forensic role of physicians in Roman law', *Bulletin of the History of Medicine*, 1979, vol. 53: 39–56.

Anderson, Olive, *Suicide in Victorian and Edwardian England*, Oxford: Clarendon Press, 1987.

Andrews, Richard Mowery, *Law, Magistracy, and Crime in Old Regime Paris, 1735–1789, Vol. 1, The System of Criminal Justice*, Cambridge: Cambridge University Press, 1994.

Asen, Daniel, 'Vital spots, mortal wounds, and forensic practice: finding cause of death in nineteenth-century China', *East Asian Science, Technology and Society*, 2009, vol. 3: 453–74.

Ash, Eric H., *Power, Knowledge and Expertise in Elizabethan England*, Baltimore, MD and London: Johns Hopkins University Press, 2004.

Baccino, E., A. Dorandeu, E. Margueritte, P. Fornes and A. Soussy, 'Medicolegal activity in France: who really are the médecins légistes', *Journal of Clinical Forensic Medicine*, 1999, vol. 6: 208.

Backhouse, Constance B., 'Desperate women and compassionate courts: infanticide in nineteenth-century Canada', *University of Toronto Law Journal*, 1984, vol. 34: 447–78.

Baker, J.H., *An Introduction to English Legal History*, 4th edn, London: Butterworths, 2002.

Barbero, Alessandro, *Charlemagne: Father of a Continent*, trans. Allan Cameron, Berkeley, CA: University of California Press, 2004.

Barnwell, P.S., 'Emperors, jurists and kings: law and custom in the late Roman and early medieval west', *Past and Present*, 2000, vol. 168: 6–29.

Barras, Vincent and Jacques Bernheim, 'The history of law and psychiatry in Europe', in Robert Bluglass and Paul Bowden (eds), *Principles and Practice of Forensic Psychiatry*, Edinburgh: Churchill Livingstone, 1990, 103–9.

Bartlett, Robert, *Trial by Fire and Water: the Medieval Judicial Ordeal*, Oxford: Oxford University Press, 1986.

Basten, John, 'The court expert in civil trials – a comparative appraisal', *Modern Law Review*, 1977, vol. 40: 174–91.

Bauer, G., 'Austrian forensic medicine', *Forensic Science International*, 2004, vol. 144: 143–49.

Behlmer, George K., 'Deadly motherhood: infanticide and medical opinion in mid-Victorian England', *Journal of the History of Medicine and Allied Sciences*, 1979, vol. 34: 403–27.

Behrend-Martínez, Edward, 'Manhood and the neutered body in early modern Spain', *Journal of Social History*, 2005, vol. 38: 1073–93.

——'Female sexual potency in a Spanish church court, 1673–1735', *Law and History Review*, 2006, vol. 24: 297–330.

Bell, Suzanne, *Crime and Circumstance: Investigating the History of Forensic Science*, Westport, CT and London: Praeger, 2008.

Benecke, Mark, 'A brief history of forensic entomology', *Forensic Science International*, 2001, vol. 120: 2–14.

Benedek, Thomas G., 'The changing relationship between midwives and physicians during the Renaissance', *Bulletin of the History of Medicine*, 1977, vol. 51: 550–64.

Bensel, Robert W. ten, Marguerite M. Rheinberger and Samuel X. Radbill, 'Children in a world of violence: the roots of child maltreatment', in Mary Edna Helfer, Ruth S. Kempe and Richard D. Krugman (eds), *The Battered Child*, 5th edn, Chicago and London: University of Chicago Press, 1997, 3–28.

Berco, Christian, 'Syphilis and the silencing of sodomy in Juan Calvo's *Tratado del morbo gálico*', in Kenneth Borris and George Rousseau (eds), *The Sciences of Homosexuality in Early Modern Europe*, London and New York: Routledge, 2008, 92–113.

Berman, Harold J., *Law and Revolution I: The Formation of the Western Legal Tradition*, Cambridge, MA and London: Harvard University Press, 1983.

——*Law and Revolution II: The Impact of the Protestant Reformations on the Western Legal Tradition*, Cambridge, MA and London: Belknap Press, 2003.

Bertomeu-Sánchez, José Ramón, 'Sense and sensitivity: Mateu Orfila, the Marsh test and the Lafarge Affair', in J.R. Bertomeu-Sánchez and A. Nieto-Galan (eds), *Chemistry, Medicine and Crime: Mateu J.B. Orfila (1787–1853) and His Times*, Sagamore Beach, MA: Science History Publications, 2006, 207–42.

Bertomeu-Sánchez, José Ramón and Agustí Nieto-Galan (eds), *Chemistry, Medicine and Crime: Mateu J.B. Orfila (1787–1853) and His Times*, Sagamore Beach, MA: Science History Publications, 2006.

Bodde, Derk, 'Forensic medicine in pre-Imperial China', *Journal of the American Oriental Society*, 1982, vol. 102: 1–15.

Bonner, Thomas Neville, *Becoming a Physician: Medical Education in Britain, France, Germany, and the United States, 1750–1945* (1995), Baltimore, MD and London: Johns Hopkins University Press, 2000.

Borris, Kenneth, 'Introduction: the prehistory of homosexuality in the early modern sciences', in Kenneth Borris and George Rousseau (eds), *The Sciences of Homosexuality in Early Modern Europe*, London and New York: Routledge, 2008, 1–40.

Borris, Kenneth and George Rousseau (eds), *The Sciences of Homosexuality in Early Modern Europe*, London and New York: Routledge, 2008.

Bosman, Machiel, 'The judicial treatment of suicide in Amsterdam', in Jeffrey R. Watt (ed.), *From Sin to Insanity: Suicide in Early Modern Europe*, Ithaca, NY: Cornell University Press, 2004, 9–24.

Brittain, Robert P., 'The hydrostatic and similar tests of live birth: a historical review', *Medico-Legal Journal*, 1963, vol. 31: 189–94.

——'Cruentation in legal medicine and in literature', *Medical History*, 1965, vol. 9: 82–88.

——'Origins of legal medicine: Constitutio Criminalis Carolina', *Medico-Legal Journal*, 1965, vol. 33: 124–27.

——'Origins of legal medicine: the origin of legal medicine in Italy', *Medico-Legal Journal*, 1965, vol. 33: 168–73.

——'Origins of legal medicine: Leges Barbarorum', *Medico-Legal Journal*, 1966, vol. 34: 21–23.

——'The history of legal medicine: Charlemagne', *Medico-Legal Journal*, 1966, vol. 34: 122–23.

——'The history of legal medicine: the Assizes of Jerusalem', *Medico-Legal Journal*, 1966, vol. 34: 72–73.

——'Origins of legal medicine: the origin of legal medicine in France', *Medico-Legal Journal*, 1966, vol. 34: 168–74.

——'Origins of legal medicine: Roman law: Lex Duodecim Tabularum', *Medico-Legal Journal*, 1967, vol. 35: 71–72.

——'Origins of legal medicine: the origin of legal medicine in France: Henri IV and Louis XIV', *Medico-Legal Journal*, 1967, vol. 35: 25–28.

Brock, Helen and Catherine Crawford, 'Forensic medicine in early colonial Maryland, 1633–83', in Michael Clark and Catherine Crawford (eds), *Legal Medicine in History*, Cambridge: Cambridge University Press, 1994, 25–44.

Brockliss, Laurence and Colin Jones, *The Medical World of Early Modern France*, Oxford: Oxford University Press, 1997.

Brooks, Ross, '"Vices once adopted": theorising male homoeroticism in German-language legal and forensic discourses, 1752–1869', *Reinvention: A Journal of Undergraduate Research*, 2008, vol. 1, http://www2.warwick.ac.uk/go/reinventionjournal/issues/volume1issue2/Brooks (accessed on 27 May 2010).

Bud, Robert F. and Gerrylynn K. Roberts, *Science Versus Practice: Chemistry in Victorian Britain*, Manchester: Manchester University Press, 1984.

Bullough, Vern L., 'Homosexuality and the medical model', *Journal of Homosexuality*, 1974, vol. 1: 99–110.

Burg, Thomas N., 'Forensic medicine in the nineteenth-century Habsburg monarchy', University of Minnesota, Center for Austrian Studies, June 1996, http://cas.umn.edu/assets/pdf/wp962.pdf (accessed on 25 May 2010).

Burney, Ian A., 'A poisoning of no substance: the trials of medico-legal proof in mid-Victorian England', *Journal of British Studies*, 1999, vol. 38: 59–92.

——*Bodies of Evidence: Medicine and the Politics of the English Inquest, 1830–1926*, Baltimore, MD and London: Johns Hopkins University Press, 2000.

——*Poison, Detection, and the Victorian Imagination*, Manchester and New York: Manchester University Press, 2006.

Burns, Chester R. (ed.), *Legacies in Law and Medicine*, New York: Science History Publications, 1977.

Burton, June K., 'Human rights issues affecting women in Napoleonic legal medicine textbooks', *History of European Ideas*, 1987, vol. 8: 427–34.

Butler, Sara M., 'Degrees of culpability: suicide verdicts, mercy, and the jury in medieval England', *Journal of Medieval and Early Modern Studies*, 2006, vol. 36: 263–90.

Bynum, W.F., E.J. Browne and Roy Porter (eds), *Macmillan Dictionary of the History of Science*, London: The Macmillan Press, 1983.

Caenegem, R.C. van, 'Reflexions on rational and irrational modes of proof in medieval Europe', *Legal History Review*, 1990, vol. 58: 263–79.

——*Legal History: A European Perspective*, London and Rio Grande: The Hambledon Press, 1991.

Campobasso, Carlo Pietro and Francesco Introna, 'The forensic entomologist in the context of the forensic pathologist's role', *Forensic Science International*, 2001, vol. 120: 132–39.

Cassar, Paul, 'A medico-legal report of the sixteenth century from Malta', *Medical History*, 1974, vol. 18: 354–59.

——*Landmarks in the Development of Forensic Medicine in the Maltese Islands*, Valetta: International Academy of Legal Medicine and Social Medicine, 1974.

Cavallar, Osvaldo, 'Agli albori della medicina legale: I trattati *"De percussionibus"* e *"De vulneribus"'*, *Ius Commune: Zeitschrift für Europäische Rechtsgeschichte*, 1999, vol. 26: 27–89.

——'La "benefundata sapientia" dei periti: Feritori, feriti e medici nei commentari e consulti di Baldo degli Ubaldi', *Ius Commune: Zeitschrift für Europäische Rechtsgeschichte*, 2000, vol. 27: 215–81.

Cawthon, Elisabeth A., *Medicine on Trial: A Sourcebook with Cases, Law, and Documents*, Indianapolis, IN: Hackett Publishing, 2004.

Chaillé, Stanford Emerson, 'Origins and progress of medical jurisprudence, 1776–1876' (1876), *Journal of Criminal Law and Criminology*, 1949, vol. 40: 397–444.

Chauvaud, Frédéric, *Les experts du crime: la médecine légale en France au XIXe siècle*, Paris: Aubier, 2000.

Chauvaud, Frédéric and Laurence Dumoulin, *Experts et expertise judiciaire: France, XIXe et XXe siècles*, Rennes: Presses Universitaires de Rennes, 2003.

Clark, Michael and Catherine Crawford (eds), *Legal Medicine in History*, Cambridge: Cambridge University Press, 1994.

——'Introduction', in Michael Clark and Catherine Crawford (eds), *Legal Medicine in History*, Cambridge: Cambridge University Press, 1994, 1–21.

Cody, Lisa Forman, *Birthing the Nation: Sex, Science, and the Conception of Eighteenth-Century Britons*, Oxford: Oxford University Press, 2005.

Cohen, Esther, *The Crossroads of Justice: Law and Culture in Late Medieval France*, Leiden: E.J. Brill, 1993.

Colaizzi, Janet, *Homicidal Insanity, 1800–1985*, Tuscaloosa, AL and London: University of Alabama Press, 1989.

Cole, Simon A., *Suspect Identities: A History of Fingerprinting and Criminal Identification*, Cambridge, MA and London: Harvard University Press, 2001.

Coley, Noel G., 'Alfred Swaine Taylor, MD, FRS (1806–80): forensic toxicologist', *Medical History*, 1991, vol. 35: 409–27.

Collard, Franck, *Pouvoir et Poison: histoire d'un crime politique de l'Antiquité à nos jours*, Paris: Éditions du Seuil, 2007.

Conrad, Peter and Joseph W. Schneider, *Deviance and Medicalization: From Badness to Sickness* (1980), revised edn, Philadelphia: Temple University Press, 1992.

Crawford, Catherine, 'A scientific profession: forensic medicine and professional reform in British periodicals of the early nineteenth century', in Roger French and Andrew Wear (eds), *British Medicine in an Age of Reform*, London and New York: Routledge, 1991, 203–30.

——'Legalizing medicine: early modern legal systems and the growth of medico-legal knowledge', in Michael Clark and Catherine Crawford (eds), *Legal Medicine in History*, Cambridge: Cambridge University Press, 1994, 89–116.

Crompton, Louis, 'The myth of lesbian impunity: capital laws from 1270 to 1791', in Salvatore J. Licata and Robert P. Petersen (eds), *Historical Perspectives on Homosexuality*, New York: The Haworth Press, 1981, 11–25.

Crowther, M.A. and B.M. White, 'Medicine, property and the law in Britain 1800–1914', *Historical Journal*, 1988, vol. 31: 853–70.

Crowther, M. Anne and Brenda White, *On Soul and Conscience. The Medical Expert and Crime: 150 Years of Forensic Medicine in Glasgow*, Aberdeen: Aberdeen University Press, 1988.

Crozier, Ivan Dalley, 'The medical construction of homosexuality and its relation to the law in nineteenth-century England', *Medical History*, 2001, vol. 45: 61–82.

Curran, William J., 'Titles in the medicolegal field: a proposal for reform', *American Journal of Law and Medicine*, 1975, vol. 1: 1–11.

Damaška, Mirjan, 'The death of legal torture', *Yale Law Journal*, 1978, vol. 87: 860–84.

Damme, Catherine, 'Infanticide: the worth of an infant under law', *Medical History*, 1978, vol. 22: 1–24.

Darmon, Pierre, *Trial by Impotence: Virility and Marriage in Pre-Revolutionary France* (1979), trans. Paul Keegan, London: Chatto & Windus, 1985.

Daston, Lorraine and Katharine Park, 'The hermaphrodite and the orders of nature: sexual ambiguity in early modern France', in Louise Fradenburg and Carla Freccero (eds), *Premodern Sexualities*, New York and London: Routledge, 1996.

Davidson, Roger, '"This pernicious delusion": law, medicine, and child sexual abuse in early-twentieth-century Scotland', *Journal of the History of Sexuality*, 2001, vol. 10: 62–77.

Delessert, Thierry, 'Entre justice et psychiatrie: l'homosexualité dans le project de Code pénal suisse (1918)', *Gesnerus*, 2005, vol. 62: 237–56.

De Renzi, Silvia, 'Witnesses of the body: medico-legal cases in seventeenth-century Rome', *Studies in History and Philosophy of Science*, 2002, vol. 33: 219–42.

——'Medical expertise, bodies, and the law in early modern courts', *Isis*, 2007, vol. 98: 315–22.

Desmaze, Charles, *Histoire de la médecine légale en France*, Paris: G. Charpentier, 1880.

Digby, Anne, *Making a Medical Living: Doctors and Patients in the English Market for Medicine, 1720–1911*, Cambridge: Cambridge University Press, 1994.

Donovan, James M., 'Infanticide and the juries in France, 1825–1913', *Journal of Family History*, 1991, vol. 16: 157–76.

——'Combatting the sexual abuse of children in France, 1825–1913', *Criminal Justice History*, 1994, vol. 15: 59–93.

Duffin, Jacalyn, *History of Medicine: A Scandalously Short Introduction*, Basingstoke: Macmillan, 2000.

Dülmen, Richard van, *Theatre of Horror: Crime and Punishment in Early Modern Germany*, trans. Elisabeth Neu, Cambridge: Polity Press, 1990.

Dwyer, Déirdre M., 'Expert evidence in the English civil courts, 1550–1800', *Journal of Legal History*, 2007, vol. 28: 93–118.

Eigen, Joel Peter, *Witnessing Insanity: Madness and Mad-doctors in the English Court*, New Haven, CT and London: Yale University Press, 1995.

Elsakkers, Marianne, 'Inflicting serious bodily harm: the Visigothic *Antiquae* on violence and abortion', *Legal History Review*, 2003, vol. 71: 55–63.

Emsley, Clive, *Crime and Society in England 1750–1900*, 3rd edn, Harlow: Pearson Education, 2005.

Engstrom, Eric J., Volker Hess and Ulrike Thoms (eds), *Figurationen des Experten: Ambivalenzen der Wissenschaftlichen Expertise im ausgehenden 18. und fruhen 19. Jahrhundert*, Frankfurt: Peter Lang, 2005.

Eriksson, Brigitte, 'A lesbian execution in Germany, 1721: the trial records', in Salvatore J. Licata and Robert P. Petersen (eds), *Historical Perspectives on Homosexuality*, New York: The Haworth Press, 1981, 27–40.

Esmein, Adhémar, *A History of Continental Criminal Procedure with special reference to France*, trans. J. Simpson (1913), Union, NJ: Lawbook Exchange, 2000.

Essig, Mark, 'Poison murder and expert testimony: doubting the physician in late nineteenth-century America', *Yale Journal of Law and the Humanities*, 2002, vol. 14: 177–210.

Ewing, Charles Patrick, *Insanity: Murder, Madness, and the Law*, Oxford: Oxford University Press, 2008.

Fischer, F., M. Graw and W. Eisenmenger, 'Legal medicine in the Federal Republic of Germany and after reunification', *Forensic Science International*, 2004, vol. 144: 137–41.

Fischer-Homberger, Esther, *Medizin vor Gericht: Gerichtsmedizin von der Renaissance bis zur Aufklärung*, Bern: Verlag Hans Huber, 1983.

Forbes, Thomas R., 'London coroner's inquests for 1590', *Journal of the History of Medicine and Allied Sciences*, 1973, vol. 28: 376–86.

——'Crowner's quest', *Transactions of the American Philosophical Society*, 1978, vol. 68: 5–52.

——*Surgeons at the Bailey: English Forensic Medicine to 1878*, New Haven, CT and London: Yale University Press, 1985.

Forshaw, David and Henry Rollin, 'The history of forensic psychiatry in England', in Robert Bluglass and Paul Bowden (eds), *Principles and Practice of Forensic Psychiatry*, Edinburgh: Churchill Livingstone, 1990, 61–101.

Foucault, Michel, 'About the concept of the dangerous individual in nineteenth-century legal psychiatry', *International Journal of Law and Psychiatry*, 1987, vol. 1: 1–18.

Fraher, Richard M., 'Conviction according to conscience: the medieval jurists' debate concerning judicial discretion and the law of proof', *Law and History Review*, 1989, vol. 7: 23–88.

Freckelton, Ian R., *The Trial of the Expert: A Study of Expert Evidence and Forensic Experts*, Melbourne and Oxford: Oxford University Press, 1987.

Fuchs, Rachel Ginnis, 'Crimes against children in nineteenth-century France: child abuse', *Law and Human Behavior*, 1982, vol. 6: 237–59.

Fullmer, June Z., 'Technology, chemistry, and the law in early 19th-century England', *Technology and Culture*, 1980, vol. 21: 1–28.

Garza Carvajal, Federico, *Butterflies Will Burn: Prosecuting Sodomites in Early Modern Spain and Mexico*, Austin, TX: University of Texas Press, 2003.

Gaudry, Emmanuel, Jean-Bernard Myskowiak, Bernard Chauvet, Thierry Pasquerault, Fabrice Lefebvre and Yvan Malgorn, 'Activity of the forensic entomology department of the French Gendarmerie', *Forensic Science International*, 2001, vol. 120: 68–71.

Gee, D.J. and J.K. Mason, *The Courts and the Doctor*, Oxford: Oxford University Press, 1990.

Geis, Gilbert and Ivan Bunn, *A Trial of Witches: A Seventeenth-century Witchcraft Prosecution*, London: Routledge, 1997.

Gilbert, Arthur N., 'Conceptions of homosexuality and sodomy in Western history', in Salvatore J. Licata and Robert P. Petersen (eds), *Historical Perspectives on Homosexuality*, New York: The Haworth Press, 1981, 57–68.

Giuliani, Fabienne, 'Monsters in the village? Incest in nineteenth century France', *Journal of Social History*, 2009, vol. 42: 919–32.

Golan, Tal, 'The history of scientific expert testimony in the English court-room', *Science in Context*, 1999, vol. 12: 7–32.

——*Laws of Men and Laws of Nature: The History of Scientific Expert Testimony in England and America*, Cambridge, MA and London: Harvard University Press, 2004.

Goldney, Robert D., Johan A. Schioldann and Kirsten I. Dunn, 'Suicide research before Durkheim', *Health and History*, 2008, vol. 10: 73–93.

Goldstein, Jan, *Console and Classify: The French Psychiatric Profession in the Nineteenth Century*, Cambridge: Cambridge University Press, 1987, rev ed. 2001.

——'Professional knowledge and professional self-interest: the rise and fall of monomania in 19th-century France', *International Journal of Law and Psychiatry*, 1998, vol. 21: 385–96.

Goold, Imogen and Catherine Kelly (eds), *Lawyers' Medicine: The Legislature, the Courts and Medical Practice, 1760–2000*, Oxford and Portland, OR: Hart Publishing, 2009.

Gordon, Linda, 'The politics of child sexual abuse: notes from American history', *Feminist Review*, 1988, vol. 28: 56–64.

Green, Monica H., 'Gendering the history of women's healthcare', *Gender & History*, 2008, vol. 20: 487–518.

——*Making Women's Medicine Masculine: The Rise of Male Authority in Pre-Modern Gynaecology*, Oxford: Oxford University Press, 2008.

Guarnieri, Patrizia, 'Alienists on trial: conflict and convergence between psychiatry and law (1876–1913)', *History of Science*, 1991, vol. 29: 393–410.

Guignard, Laurence, 'Aliénation mentale, irresponsabilité pénale et dangerosité sociale face à la justice du XIXe siècle: étude d'un cas de fureur', *Crime, History & Societies*, 2006, vol. 10: 83–100.

Gwei-Djen, Lu and Joseph Needham, 'A history of forensic medicine in China', *Medical History*, 1988, vol. 32: 357–400.

Halsall, Guy, 'Violence and society in the early medieval west: an introductory survey', in Guy Halsall (ed.), *Violence and Society in the Early Medieval West*, Woodbridge: The Boydell Press, 1998.

Halttunen, Karen, *Murder Most Foul: The Killer and the American Gothic Imagination*, Cambridge, MA and London: Harvard University Press, 2000.

Hamlin, Christopher, 'Scientific method and expert witnessing: Victorian perspectives on a modern problem', *Social Studies of Science*, 1986, vol. 16: 485–513.

Harding, Timothy, 'A comparative survey of medico-legal systems', in John Gunn and Pamela J. Taylor (eds), *Forensic Psychiatry: Clinical, Legal and Ethical Issues*, Oxford: Butterworth-Heinemann, 1993, 118–66.

Harley, David, 'Historians as demonologists: the myth of the midwife-witch', *Social History of Medicine*, 1990, vol. 3: 1–26.

——'Political post-mortems and morbid anatomy in seventeenth-century England', *Social History of Medicine*, 1994, vol. 7: 1–28.

Harris, Ruth, *Murders and Madness: Medicine, Law, and Society in the Fin de Siècle*, Oxford: Clarendon Press, 1989.

Hasson, Ezra, 'Capability to marry: law, medicine and conceptions of insanity', *Social History of Medicine*, 2010, vol. 23: 1–20.

Havard, J.D.J., *The Detection of Secret Homicide: A Study of the Medico-legal System of Investigation of Sudden and Unexplained Deaths*, London: Macmillan, 1960.

Healy, Róisín, 'Suicide in early modern and modern Europe', *Historical Journal*, 2006, vol. 49: 903–19.

Hekma, Gert, 'A history of sexology: social and historical aspects of sexuality', in Jan Bremmer (ed.), *From Sappho to De Sade: Moments in the History of Sexuality*, London and New York: Routledge, 1989, 173–93.

Helmholtz, R.H., 'Crime, compurgation and the courts of the medieval church', *Law and History Review*, 1983, vol. 1: 1–26.

Henssge, C. and B. Madea, 'Estimation of the time since death in the early post-mortem period', *Forensic Science International*, 2004, vol. 144: 167–75.

Hoffer, Peter C. and N.E.H. Hull, *Murdering Mothers: Infanticide in England and New England 1558–1803*, New York and London: New York University Press, 1984.

Holmes, Frederic Lawrence, *Eighteenth-Century Chemistry as an Investigative Enterprise*, Berkeley, CA: Office for History of Science and Technology, University of California, 1989.

Hooper, Carol-Ann, 'Rethinking the politics of child abuse', *Social History of Medicine*, 1989, vol. 2: 356–64.

Hunnisett, R.F. 'The origins of the office of coroner', *Transactions of the Royal Historical Society*, 5th series, 1958, vol. 8: 85–104.

Hurnard, Naomi D., *The King's Pardon for Homicide before AD 1307*, Oxford: Clarendon Press, 1969.

Jackson, Louise A., *Child Sexual Abuse in Victorian England*, London and New York: Routledge, 2000.

Jackson, Mark, 'Suspicious infant deaths: the statute of 1624 and medical evidence at coroners' inquests', in Michael Clark and Catherine Crawford (eds), *Legal Medicine in History*, Cambridge: Cambridge University Press, 1994, 64–86.

——'"It begins with the goose and ends with the goose": medical, legal and lay understandings of imbecility in Ingram v Wyatt, 1824–32', *Social History of Medicine*, 1998, vol. 11: 361–80.

——(ed.), *Infanticide: Historical Perspectives on Child Murder and Concealment, 1550–2000*, Aldershot: Ashgate, 2002.

Jager, Eric, *The Last Duel: A True Story of Crime, Scandal, and Trial by Combat in Medieval France*, New York: Broadway Books, 2004.

Janin, Hunt, *Medieval Justice: Cases and Laws in France, England, and Germany, 500–1500*, Jefferson, NC and London: McFarland, 2004.

Johnson, Julie, 'William Scott Wadsworth: an appreciation of an anomalous career', *Transactions and Studies of the College of Physicians of Philadelphia*, 1990, vol. 12: 335–46.

——'Coroners, corruption and the politics of death: forensic pathology in the United States', in Michael Clark and Catherine Crawford (eds), *Legal Medicine in History*, Cambridge: Cambridge University Press, 1994, 268–89.

Johnson-McGrath, Julie, 'Speaking for the dead: forensic pathologists and criminal justice in the United States', *Science, Technology & Human Values*, 1995, vol. 20: 438–59.

Jones, Carol A.G., *Expert Witnesses: Science, Medicine, and the Practice of Law*, Oxford: Clarendon Press, 1994.

Jones, Kingsley, 'The Windham Case: the enquiry held in London in 1861 into the state of mind of William Frederick Windham, heir to the Felbrigg Estate', *British Journal of Psychiatry*, 1971, vol. 119: 425–33.

Kaufman, Matthew H., 'Origin and history of the Regius Chair of Medical Jurisprudence and Medical Police established in the University of Edinburgh in 1807', *Journal of Forensic and Legal Medicine*, 2007, vol. 14: 121–30.

Kaufmann, Doris, 'Boundary disputes: criminal justice and psychiatry in Germany, 1760–1850', *Journal of Historical Sociology*, 1993, vol. 6: 276–87.

Keil, W., A. Berzlanovich and B. Madea, 'Textbooks on legal medicine in the German-speaking countries', *Forensic Science International*, 2004, vol. 144: 289–302.

Kelly, Howard A. and Walter L. Burrage, *American Medical Biographies*, Baltimore, MD: The Norman, Remington Company, 1920.

Kerr, Margaret H., Richard D. Forsyth and Michael J. Plyley, 'Cold water and hot iron: trial by ordeal in England', *Journal of Interdisciplinary History*, 1992, vol. 22: 573–95.

King, Lester S. and Marjorie C. Meehan, 'A history of the autopsy', *American Journal of Pathology*, 1973, vol. 73: 514–44.

Klotzbach, H., R. Krettek, H. Bratzke, K. Püschel, R. Zehner and J. Amendt, 'The history of forensic entomology in German-speaking countries', *Forensic Science International*, 2004, vol. 144: 259–63.

Koehler, Steven A. and Cyril H. Wecht, *Postmortem: Establishing the Cause of Death*, Buffalo, NY: Firefly Books, 2006.

Koslofsky, Craig, 'Suicide and the secularization of the body in early modern Saxony', *Continuity and Change*, 2001, vol. 16: 45–70.

Kramar, Kirsten Johnson and William D. Watson, 'Canadian infanticide legislation, 1948 and 1955: reflections on the medicalization/autopoiesis debate', *Canadian Journal of Sociology*, 2008, vol. 33: 237–63.

Krauland, W., 'The history of the German Society of Forensic Medicine', *Forensic Science International*, 2004, vol. 144: 95–108.

Kushner, Howard I., *Self-destruction in the Promised Land: A Psychocultural Biology of American Suicide* (1989), New Brunswick, NJ and London: Rutgers University Press, 1991.

Labbé, Jean, 'Ambroise Tardieu: the man and his work on child maltreatment a century before Kempe', *Child Abuse & Neglect*, 2005, vol. 29: 311–24.

Lambie, Ian, 'Mothers who kill: the crime of infanticide', *International Journal of Law and Psychiatry*, 2001, vol. 24: 71–80.

Landsman, Stephan, 'Of witches, madmen, and products liability: a historical survey of the use of expert testimony', *Behavioral Sciences and the Law*, 1995, vol. 13: 131–57.

——'One hundred years of rectitude: medical witnesses at the Old Bailey, 1717–1817', *Law and History Review*, 1998, vol. 16: 445–94.

Lane, Brian, *The Encyclopedia of Forensic Science*, London: Headline, 1992.

Langbein, John H., *Prosecuting Crime in the Renaissance: England, Germany, France* (1974), Clark, NJ: Lawbook Exchange, 2005.

——*Torture and the Law of Proof: Europe and England in the Ancien Régime* (1976), Chicago: University of Chicago Press, 2006.

——*The Origins of Adversary Criminal Trial*, Oxford: Oxford University Press, 2003.

Leboutte, René, 'Offense against family order: infanticide in Belgium from the fifteenth through the early twentieth centuries', *Journal of the History of Sexuality*, 1991, vol. 2: 159–85.

Leclercq, Jean, 'Marcel Leclercq (1924–2008), médecin, diptériste, parasitologue et pionnier de l'entomologie forensique (Part 1)', *Faunistic Entomology*, 2008, vol. 61: 129–50.

Lederer, David, 'Honfibú: nationhood, manhood, and the culture of self-sacrifice in Hungary', in Jeffrey R. Watt (ed.), *From Sin to Insanity: Suicide in Early Modern Europe*, Ithaca, NY: Cornell University Press, 2004, 116–37.

Lefebvre-Teillard, Anne, 'A défaut d'expert expert', in Annie Deperchin, Nicolas Derasse and Bruno Dubois (eds), *Figures de Justice: Études en l'honneur de Jean-Pierre Royer*, Lille: Centre d'Histoire Judiciaire, 2005, 665–78.

Levack, Brian P., *The Witch-hunt in Early Modern Europe*, 3rd edn, Harlow: Pearson Education Limited, 2006.

Licata, Salvatore J. and Robert P. Petersen (eds), *Historical Perspectives on Homosexuality*, New York: The Haworth Press, 1981.

Lind, Vera, 'The suicidal mind and body: examples from northern Germany', in Jeffrey R. Watt (ed.), *From Sin to Insanity: Suicide in Early Modern Europe*, Ithaca, NY: Cornell University Press, 2004, 64–80.

Lucas, D.M., 'North of 49 – the development of forensic science in Canada', *Science & Justice*, 1997, vol. 37: 47–54.

Lynch, Margaret, 'Child abuse before Kempe: an historical literature review', *Child Abuse & Neglect*, 1985, vol. 9: 7–17.

Lyons, J. B., 'Sir William Wilde's medico-legal observations', *Medical History*, 1997, vol. 41: 437–54.

MacDonald, Michael and Terence R. Murphy, *Sleepless Souls: Suicide in Early Modern England* (1990), Oxford: Clarendon Press, 1993.

Magherini, Graziella and Vittorio Biotti, 'Madness in Florence in the 14th–18th centuries: judicial inquiry and medical diagnosis, care, and custody', *International Journal of Law and Psychiatry*, 1998, vol. 21: 355–68.

Malkoc, Ekrem and Wim Neuteboom, 'The current status of forensic science laboratory accreditation in Europe', *Forensic Science International*, 2007, vol. 167: 121–26.

Mant, A. Keith, 'Milestones in the development of the British medicolegal system', *Medicine, Science and the Law*, 1977, vol. 17: 155–63.

Marland, Hilary (ed.), *The Art of Midwifery: Early Modern Midwives in Europe*, London and New York: Routledge, 1993.

——*Dangerous Motherhood: Insanity and Childbirth in Victorian Britain*, Basingstoke: Palgrave Macmillan, 2004.

Martin, Benjamin F., *Crime and Criminal Justice Under the Third Republic: The Shame of Marianne*, Baton Rouge, LA and London: Louisiana State University Press, 1990.

Martin, Karin A., 'Gender and sexuality: medical opinion on homosexuality, 1900–1950', *Gender and Society*, 1993, vol. 7: 246–60.

Mausen, Yves, 'Ex scientia et arte sua testificatur: A propos de la spécificité du statut de l'expert dans la procédure judiciaire médiévale', *Rechtsgeschichte*, 2007, vol. 10: 127–35.

McClive, Cathy, 'Blood and expertise: the trials of the female medical expert in the ancien-régime courtroom', *Bulletin of the History of Medicine*, 2008, vol. 82: 86–108.

McEwan, Jenny, *The Verdict of the Court: Passing Judgment in Law and Psychology*, Oxford: Hart Publishing, 2003.

McMahon, Vanessa, 'Reading the body: dissection and the "murder" of Sarah Stout, Hertfordshire, 1699', *Social History of Medicine*, 2006, vol. 19: 19–35.

Mendelson, Danuta, 'The expert deposes, but the court disposes: the concept of malingering and the function of a medical expert witness in the forensic process', *International Journal of Law and Psychiatry*, 1995, vol. 18: 425–36.

——'English medical experts and the claims for shock occasioned by railway collisions in the 1860s: issues of law, ethics, and medicine', *International Journal of Law and Psychiatry*, 2002, vol. 25: 303–29.

Merrick, Jeffrey, 'Patterns and prosecutions of suicide in eighteenth-century Paris', *Historical Reflections*, 1989, vol. 16: 1–53.

Midelfort, H.C. Erik, *A History of Madness in Sixteenth-Century Germany*, Stanford, CA: Stanford University Press, 1999.

Minois, Georges, *History of Suicide: Voluntary Death in Western Culture*, trans. Lydia G. Cochrane, Baltimore, MD and London: Johns Hopkins University Press, 1999.

Mitchell, Piers D., *Medicine in the Crusades: Warfare, Wounds and the Medieval Surgeon*, Cambridge: Cambridge University Press, 2004.

Mohr, James C., 'The trial of John Hendrickson, Jr: medical jurisprudence at mid-century', *New York History*, 1989, vol. 70: 23–53.

——*Doctors and the Law: Medical Jurisprudence in Nineteenth-Century America*, Baltimore, MD and London: Johns Hopkins University Press, 1993.

——'The origins of forensic psychiatry in the United States and the great nineteenth-century crisis over the adjudication of wills', *Journal of the American Academy of Psychiatry and the Law*, 1997, vol. 25: 273–84.

Moran, Richard, *Knowing Right from Wrong: The Insanity Defense of Daniel McNaughtan*, New York and London: The Free Press, 1981.

——'The origin of insanity as a special verdict: the trial for treason of James Hadfield (1800)', *Law and Society Review*, 1985, vol. 19: 487–519.

Moseley, Kathryn L., 'The history of infanticide in western society', *Issues in Law & Medicine*, 1986, vol. 1: 345–61.

Murray, Alexander, *Suicide in the Middle Ages, Vol. 1, The Violent against Themselves*, Oxford: Oxford University Press, 1998.

——*Suicide in the Middle Ages, Vol. 2, The Curse on Self-Murder*, Oxford: Oxford University Press, 2000.

Murray, Jacqueline, 'On the origins and role of "wise women" in causes for annulment on the grounds of male impotence', *Journal of Medieval History*, 1990, vol. 16: 235–49.

Naphy, William, *Sex Crimes: From Renaissance to Enlightenment*, Stroud: Tempus, 2002.

——'Sodomy in early modern Geneva: various definitions, diverse verdicts', in Tom Betteridge (ed.), *Sodomy in Early Modern Europe*, Manchester and New York: Manchester University Press, 2002, 94–111.

Nemec, Jaroslav, *Highlights in Medicolegal Relations*, Bethesda: National Library of Medicine, 1968, http://www.nlm.nih.gov/hmd/pdf/highlights.pdf (accessed on 25 May 2010).

Nutton, Vivian, 'Continuity or rediscovery? The city physician in classical antiquity and mediaeval Italy', in Andrew W. Russell (ed.), *The Town and State Physician in Europe from the Middle Ages to the Enlightenment*, Wolfenbüttel: Herzog August Bibliothek, 1981, 9–46.

Oberman, Michelle, 'Understanding infanticide in context: mothers who kill, 1870–1930 and today', *Journal of Criminal Law and Criminology*, 2003, vol. 92: 707–37.

O'Donovan, Katherine, 'The medicalisation of infanticide', *Criminal Law Review*, 1984, 259–64.

Ogle, Robin and Daniel Maier-Katkin, 'A rationale for infanticide laws', *Criminal Law Review*, Dec 1993, 903–14.

Olafson, Erna, David L. Corwin and Roland C. Summit, 'Modern history of child sexual abuse awareness: cycles of discovery and suppression', *Child Abuse & Neglect*, 1993, vol. 17: 7–24.

Oldham, James C., 'The origins of the special jury', *University of Chicago Law Review*, 1983, vol. 50: 137–221.

——'On pleading the belly: a history of the jury of matrons', *Criminal Justice History*, 1985, vol. 6: 1–64.

O'Neill, Ynes Violé, 'Innocent III and the evolution of anatomy', *Medical History*, 1976, vol. 20: 429–33.

O'Neill, Ynez Violé and Gerald L. Chan, 'A Chinese coroner's manual and the evolution of anatomy', *Journal of the History of Medicine and Allied Sciences*, 1976, vol. 31: 3–16.

Oosterhuis, Harry, 'Medical science and the modernisation of sexuality', in Franz X. Eder, Lesley A. Hall and Gert Hekma (eds), *Sexual Cultures in Europe: National Histories*, Manchester and New York: Manchester University Press, 1999, 221–41.

——*Stepchildren of Nature: Krafft-Ebing, Psychiatry, and the Making of Sexual Identity*, Chicago and London: University of Chicago Press, 2000.

Oppenheimer, Heinrich, *The Criminal Responsibility of Lunatics: A Study in Comparative Law*, London: Sweet and Maxwell, 1909.

Ortolani, Marc, 'L'empoisonnement à Nice sous la Restauration: enquête judiciaire et expertise toxicologique', *Legal History Review*, 2008, vol. 76: 95–131.

Owen, David, *Criminal Minds: The Science and Psychology of Profiling*, New York: Barnes & Noble Books, 2004.

Paperno, Irina, *Suicide as a Cultural Institution in Dostoevsky's Russia*, Ithaca, NY and London: Cornell University Press, 1997.

Pardo-Tomás, José and Àlvar Martínez-Vidal, 'Victims and experts: medical practitioners and the Spanish Inquisition', in John Woodward and Robert Jütte (eds), *Coping with Sickness: Medicine, Law and Human Rights – Historical Perspectives*, Sheffield: European Association for the History of Medicine and Health Publications, 2000, 11–27.

Park, Katharine, 'The criminal and the saintly body: autopsy and dissection in Renaissance Italy', *Renaissance Quarterly*, 1994, vol. 47: 1–33.

——'The life of the corpse: division and dissection in late medieval Europe', *Journal of the History of Medicine and Allied Sciences*, 1995, vol. 50: 111–32.

——'The rediscovery of the clitoris: French medicine and the tribade, 1570–1620', in David Hillman and Carla Mazzio (eds), *The Body in Parts: Fantasies of Corporeality in Early Modern Europe*, New York and London: Routledge, 1997, 170–93.

——*Secrets of Women: Gender, Generation, and the Origins of Human Dissection*, New York: Zone Books, 2006.

Partridge, Ralph, *Broadmoor: A History of Criminal Lunacy and its Problems*, London: Chato and Windus, 1953.

Pastore, Alessandro, *Il medico in tribunale: La perizia medica nella procedura penale d'antico regime (secoli XVI–XVIII)*, Bellinzona: Edizioni Casagrande, 1998.

Pastore, Alessandro and Giovanni Rossi (eds), *Paolo Zacchia: alle origini della medicina legale 1584–1659*, Milan: FrancoAngeli, 2008.

Patzelt, D., 'History of forensic serology and molecular genetics in the sphere of activity of the German Society for Forensic Medicine', *Forensic Science International*, 2004, vol. 144: 185–91.

Pfohl, Stephen J., 'The "discovery" of child abuse', *Social Problems*, 1977, vol. 24: 310–23.

Porter, Roy, *The Greatest Benefit to Mankind: A Medical History of Humanity from Antiquity to the Present*, London: Harper Collins, 1997.

Prior, Pauline, *Madness and Murder: Gender, Crime and Mental Disorder in Nineteenth-Century Ireland*, Dublin: Irish Academic Press, 2008.

Quen, Jacques M., 'The history of law and psychiatry in America', in Robert Bluglass and Paul Bowden (eds), *Principles and Practice of Forensic Psychiatry*, Edinburgh: Churchill Livingstone, 1990, 111–16.

Rabier, Christelle, 'Introduction: expertise in historical perspectives', in Christelle Rabier (ed.), *Fields of Expertise: A Comparative History of Expert Procedures in Paris and London, 1600 to Present*, Newcastle: Cambridge Scholars Publishing, 2007, 1–33.

Rabin, Dana, *Identity, Crime and Legal Responsibility in Eighteenth-Century England*, Basingstoke: Palgrave Macmillan, 2004.

Radbill, Samuel X., 'Children in a world of violence: a history of child abuse', in C. Henry Kempe and Ray E. Helfer (eds), *The Battered Child*, 3rd edn, Chicago and London: University of Chicago Press, 1980, 3–20.

Rafter, Nicole, 'The unrepentant horse-slasher: moral insanity and the origins of criminological thought', *Criminology*, 2004, vol. 42: 979–1008.

——'The murderous Dutch fiddler: criminology, history and the problem of phrenology', *Theoretical Criminology*, 2005, vol. 9: 65–96.

Redmayne, Mike, *Expert Evidence and Criminal Justice*, Oxford: Oxford University Press, 2001.

Renneville, Marc, *Crime et folie: deux siècles d'enquêtes médicales et judiciaires*, Paris: Fayard, 2003.

Restier-Melleray, Christiane, 'Experts et expertise scientifique: le cas de la France', *Revue française de science politique*, 1990, vol. 40: 546–85.

Richardson, Ruth, *Death, Dissection and the Destitute*, 2nd edn with a new afterword, London: Phoenix Press, 2001.

Richter, Jeffrey S., 'Infanticide, child abandonment, and abortion in Imperial Germany', *Journal of Interdisciplinary History*, 1998, vol. 28: 511–51.

Robertson, Stephen, 'Signs, marks and private parts: doctors, legal discourses, and evidence of rape in the United States, 1823–1930', *Journal of the History of Sexuality*, 1998, vol. 8: 345–88.

Robinson, Daniel N., *Wild Beasts and Idle Humours: The Insanity Defense from Antiquity to the Present*, Cambridge, MA and London: Harvard University Press, 1996.

Robisheaux, Thomas, 'Witchcraft and forensic medicine in seventeenth-century Germany', in Stuart Clark (ed.), *Languages of Witchcraft: Narrative, Ideology and Meaning in Early Modern Culture*, Basingstoke: Macmillan, 2001, 197–215.

Roche, Albert John, Gilles Fortin, Jean Labbé, Jocelyn Brown and David Chadwick, 'The work of Ambroise Tardieu: the first definitive description of child abuse', *Child Abuse & Neglect*, 2005, vol. 29: 325–34.

Roemer, Milton I., 'Government's role in American medicine – a brief historical survey', in Chester R. Burns (ed.), *Legacies in Law and Medicine*, New York: Science History Publications, 1977, 183–205.

Rose, Lionel, *Massacre of the Innocents: Infanticide in Great Britain 1800–1939*, London: Routledge & Kegan Paul, 1986.

Rosenberg, Charles E., *The Trial of the Assassin Guiteau: Psychiatry and Law in the Gilded Age*, Chicago: University of Chicago Press, 1968.

Rousseau, George, 'Policing the anus: Stuprum and sodomy according to Paolo Zacchia's forensic medicine', in Kenneth Borris and George Rousseau (eds), *The Sciences of Homosexuality in Early Modern Europe*, London and New York: Routledge, 2008, 72–91.

Rowe, G.S., 'Infanticide, its judicial resolution, and criminal code revision in early Pennsylvania', *Proceedings of the American Philosophical Society*, 1991, vol. 135: 200–232.

Rowlands, Alison, '"In great secrecy": the crime of infanticide in Rothenburg ob der Tauber, 1501–1618', *German History*, 1997, vol. 15: 179–99.

Rubin, Stanley, 'The bot, or composition in Anglo-Saxon law: a reassessment', *Journal of Legal History*, 1996, vol. 17: 144–54.

Ruggiero, Guido, 'The cooperation of physicians and the state in the control of violence in Renaissance Venice', *Journal of the History of Medicine and Allied Sciences*, 1978, vol. 33: 156–66.

——'Excusable murder: insanity and reason in early Renaissance Venice', *Journal of Social History*, 1982, vol. 16: 109–19.

——*The Boundaries of Eros: Sex Crime and Sexuality in Renaissance Venice*, Oxford: Oxford University Press, 1985.

Russell, A.W. (ed.), *The Town and State Physician in Europe from the Middle Ages to the Enlightenment*, Wolfenbüttel: Herzog August Bibliothek, 1981.

Russell, M.J., 'Trial by battle and the appeals of felony', *Journal of Legal History*, 1980, vol. 1: 135–64.

——'Trial by battle and the writ of right', *Journal of Legal History*, 1980, vol. 1: 111–34.

——'Trial by battle procedure in writs of right and criminal appeals', *Legal History Review*, 1983, vol. 51: 123–34.

Sacco, Lynn, 'Sanitized for your protection: medical discourse and the denial of incest in the United States, 1890–1940', *Journal of Women's History*, 2002, vol. 14: 80–104.

——*Unspeakable: Father–Daughter Incest in American History*, Baltimore, MD: Johns Hopkins University Press, 2009.

Savoja, Valeria, Pierre François Godet and Jacques Dubuis, 'Compulsory treatments in France', *International Journal of Mental Health*, 2008–9, vol. 37: 17–32.

Schulte, Regina, *The Village in Court: Arson, Infanticide, and Poaching in the Court Records of Upper Bavaria, 1848–1910*, Cambridge: Cambridge University Press, 1994.

Schwartz, Vanessa R., *Spectacular Realities: Early Mass Culture in Fin-de-Siècle Paris*, Berkeley, CA and London: University of California Press, 1998.

Seabourne, Gwen and Alice Seabourne, 'The law on suicide in medieval England', *Journal of Legal History*, 2000, vol. 21: 21–48.

Sharpe, J.A., *Judicial Punishment in England*, London: Faber & Faber, 1990.

Shatzmiller, Joseph, *Médecine et Justice en Provence Médiévale: Documents de Manosque, 1262–1348*, Aix-en-Provence: Université de Provence, 1989.

——'The jurisprudence of the dead body: medical practition (sic) at the service of civic and legal authorities', *Micrologus*, 1999, vol. 7: 223–30.

Shepherd, D.M. and B.M. Barraclough, 'Suicide – a traveller's tale: a study of the adoption of the word "suicide" into the main romance languages', *History of Psychiatry*, 1997, vol. 8: 395–406.

Sim, Joe, *Medical Power in Prisons: The Prison Medical Service in England 1774–1989*, Milton Keynes: Open University Press, 1990.

Simili, Allessandro, 'The beginnings of forensic medicine in Bologna', in Heinrich Karplus (ed.), *International Symposium on Society, Medicine and Law: Jerusalem, March 1972*, Amsterdam: Elsevier, 1973, 91–100.

Skoda, Hannah, 'Violent discipline or disciplining violence? Experience and reception of domestic violence in late thirteenth- and early fourteenth-century Paris and Picardy', *Cultural and Social History*, 2009, vol. 6: 9–27.

Smith, Roger, *Trial by Medicine: Insanity and Responsibility in Victorian Trials*, Edinburgh: Edinburgh University Press, 1981.

Smith, Roger and Brian Wynne (eds), *Expert Evidence: Interpreting Science in the Law*, London and New York: Routledge, 1989.

Smith, Sydney, 'The history and development of forensic medicine', *British Medical Journal*, 24 March 1951: 599–607.

Spierenburg, Pieter, 'Faces of violence: homicide trends and cultural meanings: Amsterdam, 1431–1816', *Journal of Social History*, 1994, vol. 27: 701–16.

Steenburg, Nancy Hathaway, *Children and the Criminal Law in Connecticut, 1635–1855: Changing Perceptions of Childhood*, New York: Routledge, 2005.

Steinberg, Holger, Adrian Schmidt-Recla and Sebastian Schmideler, 'Forensic psychiatry in nineteenth-century Saxony: the case of Woyzeck', *Harvard Review of Psychiatry*, 2007, vol. 15: 169–80.

Stürzbecher, Manfred, 'The physici in German-speaking countries from the Middle Ages to the Enlightenment', in Andrew W. Russell (ed.), *The Town and State Physician in Europe from the Middle Ages to the Enlightenment*, Wolfenbüttel: Herzog August Bibliothek, 1981, 123–29.

Summers, Ralph D., 'History of the police surgeon', *The Practitioner*, 1978, vol. 221: 383–87.

Terry, Jennifer, *An American Obsession: Science, Medicine, and Homosexuality in Modern Society*, Chicago: University of Chicago Press, 1999.

Thorwald, Jürgen, *Proof of Poison*, trans. Richard and Clara Winston, London: Thames and Hudson, 1966.

Tighe, Janet A., 'The New York Medico-Legal Society: legitimating the union of law and psychiatry (1867–1918)', *International Journal of Law and Psychiatry*, 1986, vol. 9: 231–43.

Tilstone, William J., Kathleen A. Savage and Leigh A. Clark, *Forensic Science: An Encyclopedia of History, Methods, and Techniques*, Santa Barbara, CA and Oxford: ABC-CLIO, 2006.

Timmermans, Stefan, *Postmortem: How Medical Examiners Explain Suspicious Deaths*, Chicago and London: University of Chicago Press, 2006.

Tinková, Daniela, 'Protéger ou punir? Les voies de la décriminalisation de l'infanticide en France et dans le domaine des Habsbourg (XVIIIe – XIXe siècles)', *Crime, History & Societies*, 2005, vol. 9: 43–72.

Trexler, Richard C., 'Infanticide in Florence: new sources and first results', *History of Childhood Quarterly*, 1973, vol. 1: 98–116.

Turvey, Brent E., *Criminal Profiling: An Introduction to Behavioral Evidence Analysis*, 3rd edn, San Diego: Academic Press, 2008.

Ulbricht, Otto, 'Infanticide in eighteenth-century Germany', in Richard J. Evans (ed.), *The German Underworld: Deviants and Outcasts in German History*, London and New York: Routledge, 1988, 108–40.

Vandekerckhove, Lieven, *On Punishment: The Confrontation of Suicide in Old-Europe*, Leuven: Leuven University Press, 2000.

Volk, Peter and Hans Jurgen Warlo, 'The role of medical experts in court proceedings in the medieval town', in Heinrich Karplus (ed.), *International Symposium on Society, Medicine and Law: Jerusalem, March 1972*, Amsterdam: Elsevier, 1973, 101–16.

Waelkens, Laurent, 'Traces Romano-canoniques dans les preuves "Germaniques"', *Legal History Review*, 2007, vol. 75: 321–31.

Wagner, Hans-Joachim, 'On the prehistory of the German Society of Legal Medicine', *Forensic Science International*, 2004, vol. 144: 89–93.

Walker, Nigel, *Crime and Insanity in England, Vol. 1: The Historical Perspective*, Edinburgh: Edinburgh University Press, 1968.

——'McNaughtan's innings: a century and a half not out', *Journal of Forensic Psychiatry and Psychology*, 1993, vol. 4: 207–13.

Wambaugh, Joseph, *The Blooding*, London: Bantam Books, 1989.

Ward, Jenny, *Crimebusting: Breakthroughs in Forensic Science*, London: Blandford Press, 1998.

Ward, Tony, 'Law, common sense and the authority of science: expert witnesses and criminal insanity in England, ca. 1840–1940', *Social and Legal Studies*, 1997, vol. 6: 343–62.

——'The sad subject of infanticide: law, medicine and child murder, 1860–1938', *Social & Legal Studies*, 1999, vol. 8: 163–80.

——'Legislating for human nature: legal responses to infanticide, 1860–1938', in Mark Jackson (ed.), *Infanticide: Historical Perspectives on Child Murder and Concealment, 1550–2000*, Aldershot: Ashgate, 2002, 249–69.

——'A mania for suspicion: poisoning, science, and the law', in Judith Rowbotham and Kim Stevenson (eds), *Criminal Conversations: Victorian*

Crimes, Social Panic, and Moral Outrage, Columbus, OH: Ohio State University Press, 2005, 140–56.

——'English law's epistemology of expert testimony', *Journal of Law and Society*, 2006, vol. 33: 572–95.

Watson, Katherine D., 'The chemist as expert: the consulting career of Sir William Ramsay', *Ambix*, 1995, vol. 42: 143–59.

——*Poisoned Lives: English Poisoners and their Victims*, London: Hambledon and London, 2004.

——'Medical and chemical expertise in English trials for criminal poisoning, 1750–1914', *Medical History*, 2006, vol. 50: 373–90.

——*Crime Archive: Dr Crippen*, Kew: The National Archives, 2007.

Watson, Katherine D. and Philip Wexler, 'History of toxicology', in Philip Wexler (ed.), *Information Resources in Toxicology*, 4th edn, San Diego and Oxford: Academic Press, 2009, 11–29.

Watt, Jeffrey R., *Choosing Death: Suicide and Calvinism in Early Modern Geneva*, Kirksville, MO: Truman State University Press, 2001.

——(ed.), *From Sin to Insanity: Suicide in Early Modern Europe*, Ithaca, NY: Cornell University Press, 2004.

——'Introduction: toward a history of suicide in early modern Europe', in Jeffrey R. Watt (ed.), *From Sin to Insanity: Suicide in Early Modern Europe*, Ithaca, NY: Cornell University Press, 2004, 1–8.

Wecht, Cyril H., 'The history of legal medicine', *Journal of the American Academy of Psychiatry and the Law*, 2005, vol. 33: 245–51.

Wetzell, Richard F., 'The medicalization of criminal law reform in Imperial Germany', in Norbert Finzsch and Robert Jütte (eds), *Institutions of Confinement: Hospitals, Asylums, and Prisons in Western Europe and North America, 1500–1950*, Cambridge: Cambridge University Press, 1996, 275–83.

White, Brenda, 'Training medical policemen: forensic medicine and public health in nineteenth-century Scotland', in Michael Clark and Catherine Crawford (eds), *Legal Medicine in History*, Cambridge: Cambridge University Press, 1994, 145–63.

Wiener, Martin J., *Reconstructing the Criminal: Culture, Law, and Policy in England, 1830–1914*, Cambridge: Cambridge University Press, 1990.

——*Men of Blood: Violence, Manliness, and Criminal Justice in Victorian England*, Cambridge: Cambridge University Press, 2004.

Williams, Mark, *Suicide and Attempted Suicide* (1997), London: Penguin, 2001.

Williams, Owen, 'Exorcising madness in late Elizabethan England: *The Seduction of Arthington* and the criminal culpability of demoniacs', *Journal of British Studies*, 2008, vol. 47: 30–52.

Winkler, John Frederick, 'Roman law in Anglo-Saxon England', *Journal of Legal History*, 1992, vol. 13: 101–27.

Wright, Gordon, *Between the Guillotine and Liberty: Two Centuries of the Crime Problem in France*, Oxford: Oxford University Press, 1983.

Wrightson, Keith, 'Infanticide in European history', *Criminal Justice History*, 1982, vol. 3: 1–20.

Unpublished theses

Crawford, Catherine J., 'The emergence of English forensic medicine: medical evidence in common-law courts, 1730–1830', DPhil thesis, Oxford University, 1987.

Fisher, Pamela Jane, 'The politics of sudden death: the office and role of the coroner in England and Wales, 1726–1888', PhD thesis, University of Leicester, 2007.

Grey, Daniel John Ross, 'Discourses of infanticide in England, 1880–1922', PhD thesis, Roehampton University, 2008.

Lorcy, Maryvonne, 'Les procès à cadavres d'après la jurisprudence criminelle bretonne au XVIIIe siècle', Mémoire pour le Diplôme d'Études Supérieures d'Histoire du Droit, Université de Rennes, 1971.

Septon, Monique I., 'Les femmes et le poison: l'empoisonnement devant les jurisdictions criminelles en Belgique au XIXe siècle, 1795–1914', PhD thesis, Marquette University, 1996.

Websites

Association of Clinical Pathologists: Forensic Pathology, http://www.pathologists.org.uk/sub-spec-page/forensic/forensic.htm.

The Avalon Project: Documents in Law, History and Diplomacy, http://avalon.law.yale.edu/default.asp.

Home Office Register of Forensic Pathologists, http://www.npia.police.uk/en/docs/Current_Home_Office_Register.pdf.

Institut National de Police Scientifique, http://www.inps.interieur.gouv.fr/.

Internet Medieval Sourcebook, http://www.fordham.edu/halsall/sbook.html.

Museo Criminologico, Rome, http://www.museocriminologico.it/index_uk.htm.

National Library of Wales, Crime and Punishment Database, http://www.llgc.org.uk/sesiwn_fawr/index_s.htm.

The Newgate Calendar, http://exclassics.com/newgate/ngintro.htm.

Peress, Robin, 'What causes rigor mortis?', http://www.howstuffworks.com/rigor-mortis-cause.htm/printable.

The Proceedings of the Old Bailey, 1674–1913, http://www.oldbaileyonline.org.

Rogers, J. David, Forensic Geology Case Histories, http://web.mst.edu/~rogersda/forensic_geology/Geoforensics%20Case%20Histories.htm.

Index

16, 34, 35, 42, 43, 73, 80, 112,
113, 114, 115; customary 10, 11,
16, 18, 37, 153n8; *see also*
common law; Roman law
laws 1, 8, 9, 24, 29, 42, 43, 76, 78, 98;
against child abuse 128, 130, 175n7;
barbarian 30, 73; civil 9; criminal
9; ecclesiastical 15; feudal 32, 43;
in German states 37, 38; against
homosexuality 118, 121, 122;
against infanticide 23, 43, 105,
106, 108, 111; Norman 33; Salic
Law Code 30; Visigothic Code 30
lawyers 13, 34, 47, 49, 61, 76, 83,
86, 91, 94, 95; American 62, 63,
94, 129; Austrian 56; canon 73,
74, 77; English 57, 58, 61, 94;
French 49, 54, 92; German 90;
Italian 73; Scottish 58, 61
Le Gris, Jacques (trial by battle) 14
Leclercq, Marcel 141
legal systems 1, 8, 9, 10, 12, 14, 15,
16, 18, 20, 23, 24, 27, 29, 32, 43,
48, 78, 95, 114, 153n5, 157n27
leprosy 35
Lewis, Meriwether (case study) 102–4
Littlejohn, Henry H. 60
Locard, Edmond 59, 132–33, 134
Lombroso, Cesare 91, 93, 104, 118,
132, 135
London 56, 57, 58, 60, 74, 78, 80–81,
133, 165n101; Medico-Legal
Society 58; Society of
Apothecaries 56, 57
Low Countries 19

magistrates 19, 20, 23, 24, 28, 29,
36, 55, 58, 65, 72, 104;
investigating 3, 28, 51, 52, 59, 142
Magrath, George Burgess 60
Malevoda, Master Albertus 33
mania 77, 78, 82, 83, 88, 100, 102, 108
manslaughter 3, 11, 34, 40, 89, 105,
106, 108, 110
Marcis, Marie le (case study) 112–13

marriage 35, 104, 112, 113, 115;
dissolution of 42, 99, 104, 114,
115; *see also* divorce
Marsh, James 52
Matthews, Rose (case study) 109–10
McAfee, Melba (case study) 129
McNaughtan, Daniel (case study)
80, 88–89
McNaughtan Rules 88–89, 90, 95,
111, 169n87
Mearns, Dr Alexander 139
medical education 5–7, 29, 46, 50,
51, 56–57, 61, 70, 152n18
medical examiners 60, 62–63, 132,
143, 149
medical licensing 5, 6, 7, 35, 41, 50,
54, 56, 57
medical police 3, 58; *see also* state
medicine
medical practitioners 5, 9, 46, 50;
see also apothecaries; midwives;
physicians; surgeons
medical professionalization 5–7, 41,
50–51, 54–57
medical schools: *see* universities
medicine 1, 4, 6, 8, 26, 27, 29, 30,
34, 36, 37, 38, 40, 41, 43, 46, 47,
48, 50, 51, 54, 55, 56, 57, 61, 62,
70, 99, 134, 145, 149; and
infanticide 106–11; and insanity
72, 75–78, 95; and sexuality
111–22; and suicide 100–102
medico-legal practice 4, 8, 24,
26–44, 52, 60, 108, 117, 134, 149;
in ancient Egypt 27, 29; in
ancient Greece 27–28; in ancient
Rome 27, 28, 41; early medieval
29–32, 41; early modern 35–37,
38–40, 42–43; and infanticide
106–11; and insanity 72–97;
medieval 31–35, 37–38, 41–42;
and sexuality 111–22; and suicide
100–102, 104–5; and torture 35;
twentieth-century 134–49; by
women 40–43

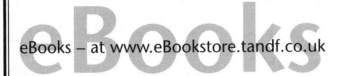

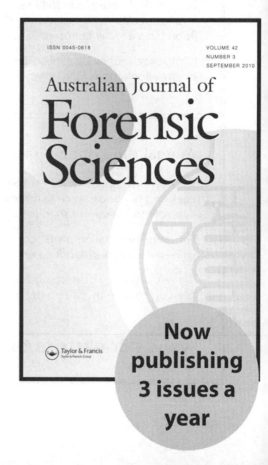
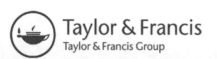

Forensic Science in Healthcare
Caring for Patients, Preserving the Evidence
Connie Darnell

This book contains basic forensic information necessary for healthcare professionals to assess and manage victims of trauma and criminal behavior. Chapters cover information on types of wounds and how to describe them; various types of evidence which may be encountered in the healthcare setting; and general principles of evidence collection. Common evidentiary items such as clothing, foreign objects, trace evidence, biological evidence, and bite marks are discussed and collection procedures are identified. A glossary of terms is included and a downloadable CD-ROM with information and printable templates such as human body diagrams supplements the text.

Pb: 978-1-4398-4490-8

For ordering and further information please visit:
www.routledge.com